EMERGENCY MEDICINE

PreTest® Self-Assessment and Review

NOTICE

EMERGENCY MEDICINE

PreTest® *Self-Assessment and Review*

SECOND EDITION

Kristi L. Koenig, MD, FACEP
Director, Emergency Management Strategic Healthcare Group
Veterans Health Administration
Washington, DC

MᴄGʀᴀᴡ-Hɪʟʟ

Health Professions Division

PreTest® Series

New York   St. Louis   San Francisco   Auckland   Bogotá   Caracas   Lisbon   London
Madrid   Mexico City   Milan   Montreal   New Delhi   San Juan   Singapore   Sydney   Tokyo   Toronto

McGraw-Hill

A Division of The McGraw·Hill Companies

Emergency Medicine:
PreTest® Self-Assessment and Review, Second Edition

1 2 3 4 5 6 7 8 9 0   PBTPBT   0 9 8 7 6 5 4 3 2 1 0

ISBN 0-07-135144-2

This book was set in Times Roman by V&M Graphics, Inc.
The editors were John Dolan and Jeanmarie Roche.
The production supervisor was Richard C. Ruzycka.
Phoenix Book Technologies was printer and binder.
This book is printed on acid-free paper.

Library of Congress Cataloging-in-Publication Data

Emergency medicine pretest / edited by Kristi L. Koenig. — 2 ed.
      p. ; cm.
    Rev. ed. of: Clinical emergency medicine. c1996.
    Review of: Emergency medicine / Judith E. Tintinalli. 5th ed. 1999.
    Includes bibliographical references.
    ISBN 0-07-135144-2
      1. Emergency medicine—Examinations, questions, etc.   I. Koenig, Kristi L. II.
Tintinalli, Judith E. Emergency medicine.
    [DNLM: 1. Emergencies—United States—Examination Questions.   2. Emergency
Medical Services—United States—Examination Questions.   WB 18.2 E527 2000]
RC86.9 .C57 2000
616.02′5′076—dc21
                                                                                    99-059151

To my mother, the wisest and most supportive person I know.

CONTENTS

CONTRIBUTORS

Kristi L. Koenig, MD, FACEP
Director, Emergency Management
  Strategic Healthcare Group
Veterans Health Administration
Washington, DC

R. Carter Clements, MD, FACEP
Department of Emergency Medicine
Alameda County Medical Center, Highland Campus
Oakland, California
Toxicologic Emergencies

Elizabeth Dorn, MD
Department of Emergency Medicine
Alameda County Medical Center, Highland Campus
Oakland, California
Cardiologic Emergencies

Rochelle Eggleston, MD
Department of Emergency Medicine
Alameda County Medical Center, Highland Campus
Oakland, California
Gastroenterologic Emergencies

David K. English, MD, FACEP
Director of Informatics
Department of Emergency Medicine
Alameda County Medical Center, Highland Campus
Oakland, California
Assistant Clinical Professor of Medicine
University of California, San Francisco
San Francisco, California
Administration, Ethics, and Legal Aspects
Cardiologic Emergencies
Geriatric Emergencies

Cherie A. Hargis, MD
Attending Physician
Department of Emergency Medicine
Alameda County Medical Center, Highland Campus
Oakland, California
Hematologic and Oncologic Emergencies
Pediatric Emergencies

H. Gene Hern, Jr., MD, MS
Department of Emergency Medicine
Alameda County Medical Center, Highland Campus
Oakland, California
Eye, Ear, Nose, Throat, and Maxillofacial Emergencies

Amy M. Hutson, MD
Department of Emergency Medicine
Alameda County Medical Center, Highland Campus
Oakland, California
Metabolic, Endocrinologic, and Rheumatologic
  Emergenices

Loretta Jackson-Williams, MD PhD
Assistant Professor
Emergency Medicine Department
University of Mississippi
Jackson, Mississippi
Neurologic and Psychiatric Emergencies

Amin Antoine Kazzi, MD, FAAEM, FACEP
Associate Division Chief
Associate Clinical Professor
Division of Emergency Medicine
University of California, Irvine
Dermatologic Emergencies
Pulmonary Emergencies

Linda E. Keyes, MD
Department of Emergency Medicine
Alameda County Medical Center, Highland Campus
Oakland, California
Environmental Emergencies
Renal and Urologic Emergencies

Susan Lambe, MD
Robert Wood Johnson Clinical Scholars Program
University of California, Los Angeles
Los Angeles, California
Anesthesia and Analgesia
Orthopedic Emergencies

Daniel McDermott, MD
Assistant Clinical Professor of Medicine
Division of Emergency Medicine
University of California, San Francisco
San Francisco, California
Pulmonary Emergencies

Flavia Nobay, MD
Department of Emergency Medicine
Alameda County Medical Center, Highland Campus
Oakland, California
Trauma

Susan B. Promes, MD, FACEP
Associate Residency Director
Department of Emergency Medicine
Alameda County Medical Center, Highland Campus
Oakland, California
Assistant Professor of Clinical Medicine
University of California, San Francisco
San Francisco, California
Metabolic, Endocrinologic, and Rheumatologic Emergencies
Obstetric and Gynecologic Emergencies

Augusta J. Saulys, MD, FAAP, FACEP
Associate Director, Emergency Department
Children's Hospital Oakland
Fellowship Director, Pediatric Emergency Medicine
Children's Hospital Oakland
Oakland, California
Pediatric Emergencies

Angelo Salvucci, Jr., MD, FACEP
Assistant Clincial Professor of Emergency Medicine
University of Southern California School of Medicine
Los Angeles, California
Medical Director, Emergency Medical Services
Santa Barbara and Ventura Counties, California
Trauma

Eric Snoey, MD
Residency Director
Department of Emergency Medicine
Alameda County Medical Center, Highland Campus
Oakland, California
Assistant Clinical Professor
Department of Internal Medicine
University of California, San Francisco
San Francisco, California
Eye, Ear, Nose, Throat, and Maxillofacial Emergencies

Susan Stroud, MD
Department of Emergency Medicine
Alameda County Medical Center, Highland Campus
Oakland, California
Infectious Disease Emergencies

Gary W. Tamkin, MD
Assistant Medical Director
Emergency Services
NorthBay Medical Center
Fairfield, California
Assistant Clinical Professor
University of California San Francisco
San Francisco, California
Emergency Medical Services and Disaster Medicine
Gastroenterologic Emergencies

William D. Whetstone, MD
Assistant Clinical Professor of Medicine
School of Medicine
Division of Emergency Medicine
University of California, San Francisco
San Francisco, California
Cardiologic Emergencies

PREFACE

This text is intended to help emergency physicians preparing for the written board certification examination. It was developed by reviewing the core content areas on the residency in-service exam, then creating questions with a proportionately equal emphasis on each section. I wish the users of this book great success in their careers in emergency medicine. I hope this book contributes to expanding their knowledge base, not only in order to pass the boards, but also to help them care for patients in the day-to-day practice of emergency medicine.

I am deeply grateful to the 20 contributors who spent countless hours developing questions and answers for this text. The contributors show a true commitment to teaching emergency medicine.

I also wish to thank my friends, family, and co-workers for their patience and guidance. Finally, I am gravely indebted to my administrative assistant, Liz McCarty, without whom this book would not have been possible.

EMERGENCY MEDICINE

PreTest® Self-Assessment and Review/2e

ADMINISTRATION, ETHICS, AND LEGAL ASPECTS

QUESTIONS

DIRECTIONS: Each question below contains five suggested responses. Select the **one best** response to each question.

1. All of the following are elements of a hospital's disaster plan EXCEPT

   (A) activation mechanism
   (B) capacity assessment
   (C) communication
   (D) discharge of predisaster patients
   (E) training and drills

2. All of the following are helpful strategies to cope with shift work EXCEPT

   (A) counterclockwise shift rotation
   (B) isolated night shifts
   (C) bright light (>10,000 lux) for 2 h after rising
   (D) regular exercise
   (E) anchor sleep and naps

3. All of the following statements are true of sexual assault EXCEPT

   (A) The physician's first responsibility is to the patient, not to the legal system
   (B) All patients should be offered follow-up
   (C) Lack of genital injuries makes involuntary intercourse unlikely
   (D) Facial or extremity injuries are common
   (E) Every female patient should have a pregnancy test

4. Each of the following is an ethical justification to terminate or withhold cardiopulmonary resuscitation EXCEPT

   (A) preexisting poor quality of life
   (B) a valid do-not-resuscitate order
   (C) known irreversible and untreatable terminal illness
   (D) nonsurviveable trauma, such as decapitation
   (E) failure to respond to standard protocols according to advanced cardiac life support

5. Each of the following is an expected physician response to a malpractice suit EXCEPT

   (A) disbelief
   (B) anger
   (C) depression
   (D) threats against the suing patient
   (E) self-doubt and difficulty making decisions

6. In a case of suspected child abuse, which of the following statements is TRUE?

   (A) A physician must report evidence of abuse but is not required to report mere suspicions
   (B) Physicians are required to report any clear evidence of abuse but can be successfully sued for incorrect reports
   (C) Physicians are at great legal risk when they report suspected abuse cases that turn out to be unfounded
   (D) Physicians in all states are required by law to report any suspected abuse, and complete legal immunity is provided in every state
   (E) The physician should take custody of the child

7. A 14-month-old male infant is brought to the ED for evaluation of diarrhea. The child has an area of alopecia over the occiput. Ribs are prominent and the skin is loose, but muscle tone is increased. The child weighs only 11 pounds. What is the BEST course of action?

   (A) Urgent outpatient referral to an endocrinologist
   (B) Admission, skeletal survey, and social service evaluation
   (C) Elimination diet for evaluation of food allergies
   (D) Stool culture and test for fecal leukocytes
   (E) Evaluation by a pediatric neurologist for muscular dystrophy

8. A 28-year-old woman presents at 2:00 A.M. with a leg laceration that she sustained the previous afternoon. She states she struck a coffee table. Examination shows a healing periorbital contusion and several other ecchymoses of various ages. When questioned, she relates these to falls sustained while pursuing her active 2-year-old son. A nurse recalls this patient as a "frequent flyer" who often receives opiates to treat pain. Review of the records shows a series of visits for various injuries, including a facial laceration, a wrist fracture, and back strains and contusions. What is the MOST appropriate course of action?

(A) Repair the laceration and provide nonopioid analgesics
(B) Confront the patient about her excessive use of prescription drugs and offer a referral to substance abuse counseling
(C) Question the patient about her use of alcohol and administer a standardized diagnostic questionnaire
(D) Question the patient about domestic violence and offer referral to a shelter and support services
(E) Report the case to child protective services

9. With regard to the patient discussed in question 8, goals of the ED encounter include all of the following EXCEPT

(A) providing the patient with information about risks and options
(B) having the spouse arrested
(C) assessing risk of suicide or homicide
(D) assessing safety of the patient and children
(E) offering referral to battered women's shelters and services

10. Each of the following is an appropriate question to ask in a case of suspected domestic violence EXCEPT

(A) Are you in a relationship in which you have been physically hurt or threatened by your partner?
(B) What do you do that makes your partner hit you?
(C) Has your partner ever threatened or abused your children?
(D) Has your partner ever forced you to have sex when you did not want to?
(E) What happens when you and your partner fight or disagree?

11. Each of the following is a risk factor for violent behavior in the ED EXCEPT

(A) male sex
(B) previous violent behavior
(C) depression
(D) alcohol abuse
(E) paranoid schizophrenia

12. The Emergency Medical Treatment and Active Labor Act (EMTALA) has many provisions that affect emergency care in U.S. EDs. All of the following provisions are true of EMTALA EXCEPT

(A) A patient in active labor is not considered "stabilized" until the baby and placenta are delivered
(B) If capacity exists, a hospital with a "special service" (such as a burn center) is required to accept transfers, regardless of the patient's financial status
(C) A patient may never be transferred for purely financial reasons
(D) A hospital must provide a medical screening examination to anyone who presents requesting care
(E) Fines under EMTALA are not covered by traditional malpractice insurance

13. All of the following are appropriate actions to preserve evidence in cases of penetrating trauma EXCEPT

(A) picking up bullet and metal fragments with a metal instrument to avoid contaminating the surface with glove residue or skin oils
(B) not incising through skin wounds whenever possible
(C) when cutting clothing, cut around rather than through bullet holes and knife holes
(D) not scrubbing wounds
(E) collecting and preserving clothing and belongings and storing them in a secure area

14. Each of the following is a true statement about the use of restraints in the ED EXCEPT

(A) The law requires that the minimal force necessary be used when restraining a patient

(B) As few people as possible should participate in restraining the patient

(C) From a legal standpoint, restraining patients against their will is generally better than allowing patients to harm themselves or others

(D) The medical chart must reflect the reason for placing the patient in restraints

(E) Patients who require restraints should not be allowed to sign out against medical advice

15. All of the following are ethical duties of a physician EXCEPT

(A) protect and preserve life

(B) prevent disability

(C) relieve suffering

(D) respect patient autonomy

(E) provide treatment that is in society's best interest

ADMINISTRATION, ETHICS, AND LEGAL ASPECTS

ANSWERS

1. **The answer is D.** *(Chapter 5)* A good hospital disaster plan includes a mechanism of activation, assessment of the hospital's capacity, establishment of disaster command, communication, supplies, administrative and treatment areas, and training and drills. Although immediate discharge of predisaster patients may augment capacity, it is not contemplated in the regulations of the Joint Commission of the Accreditation of Healthcare Organizations. Good disaster planning also includes assessment of likely hazards and cooperation between the hospital and the community.

2. **The answer is A.** *(Chapter 288)* When shifts must be rotated, they should be rotated in a clockwise manner (each change to a later, not earlier, shift), ideally with 1 month or more per rotation. Sporadic night shifts are less disruptive than longer stretches of nights to circadian rhythms. Anchor sleep involves sleeping for the same 4-h period each night, regardless of the shift worked.

3. **The answer is C.** *(Chapter 290)* Lack of genital injuries does not imply consensual intercourse, although their presence may suggest force. Toluene dye staining with colposcopy may identify lesions in the posterior fourchette suggestive of rape that are not visible on routine examination. Because rape is a violent crime, nongenital injuries are common, particularly of the face and extremities. Preexisting pregnancy must be ruled out before offering pregnancy prophylaxis. Follow-up is necessary to assess the effectiveness of pregnancy and sexually transmitted disease prophylaxis, and patients frequently require additional counseling.

4. **The answer is A.** *(Chapter 13)* Judgments about quality of life are highly subjective and individual, and physicians should refrain from making such judgments about their patients. When a patient is known to have an untreatable terminal illness, it is appropriate to withhold resuscitation, but this level of knowledge is rarely available in the emergency setting. Often, only the failure to respond to resuscitation efforts will determine that the patient has "irreversible cessation of circulatory and respiratory functions."

5. **The answer is D.** *(Chapter 288)* Malpractice stress syndrome is a pattern of response characterized by disbelief, anger, and depression, followed by isolation, embarrassment, and self-doubt. The greatest predictor of dysfunction is isolation. Peer support groups composed of other physicians who have experienced litigation are very helpful in preventing or relieving the sense of isolation.

6. **The answer is D.** *(Chapter 289)* Physicians and other licensed health care professionals are required to report any suspicion of child abuse. Every state provides complete legal immunity for any good-faith report of suspected abuse. Although parents are frequently angry and upset and may threaten lawsuits, a physician cannot be successfully sued for reporting child abuse unless the report is intentionally false.

7. **The answer is B.** *(Chapter 289)* Failure-to-thrive syndrome results from severe neglect starting in early infancy. Physical examination shows evidence of longstanding malnutrition, and the child often exhibits wide-eyed, wary behavior. Muscle tone is

usually increased, but is occasionally decreased. Admission to the hospital generally results in prompt weight gain, which is diagnostic. A skeletal survey is needed to evaluate for physical abuse, and an extensive social service assessment is mandatory.

8. **The answer is D.** *(Chapter 291)* Battered women seek care for a wide variety of complaints. The most significant reason for failing to make the diagnosis is simple failure to ask. However, only about one-third of battered women will speak to a physician or nurse about the violence in their lives if direct inquiry is made. Therefore, the diagnosis is not ruled out by a negative answer. Although battered women may resort to substance abuse, there is no established link between substance use and the cause of violence. Multiple injuries in various stages of healing, substantial delay between injury and presentation, and frequent visits for vague complaints are factors suggestive of a diagnosis of domestic violence.

9. **The answer is B.** *(Chapter 291)* When physicians have "getting her to a shelter" or "having him arrested" as the goal of the patient encounter in cases of domestic violence, they are rarely successful. Women stay in violent relationships for a variety of reasons, including the very real fear of escalating violence. The highest number of fatalities from domestic violence occur when the woman leaves or tries to leave the relationship. Leaving the relationship may not be the immediate goal of the patient, and she may be loath to have her husband and the father of her children arrested.

10. **The answer is B.** *(Chapter 291)* The presentations of battered women are so different that the diagnosis may be missed if the physician fails to ask directly about the presence of violence in the patient's life. Many battered women respond truthfully if questioned directly in a sensitive, nonjudgmental way. However, the woman needs to know that she does not deserve to be beaten. Questions that suggest or imply that the battering is the patient's fault must be avoided.

11. **The answer is C.** *(Chapter 293)* Most perpetrators of violence are males with a history of substance abuse. The best predictor of potential violence is the patient's history; any patient with a history of violence must be taken seriously and handled cautiously. The most common functional disorder related to violence is schizophrenia, especially the paranoid subtypes. Although the most dangerous functional disorder is mania, depression is not a strong predictor of violence.

12. **The answer is C.** *(Chapter 3)* Under EMTALA (also known as COBRA), every patient who presents with a request for medical care must receive a "medical screening examination" to rule out a medical emergency. If a medical emergency is present, the patient must be stabilized without regard for the financial status of the patient. A patient in active labor is defined as having an emergency under EMTALA and can only be stabilized by delivery of the infant and the placenta. Fines under EMTALA are not covered by malpractice insurance. Once a patient is "stable," EMTALA no longer applies, and the patient may be transferred for purely financial reasons. However, the burden of proving stability is with the transferring physician and hospital.

13. **The answer is A.** *(Chapter 256)* Bullets should not be handled with metal instruments because the instrument may leave marks that can confuse interpretation. Cutting through holes in clothing or through skin wounds can destroy valuable indications of the force, direction, and nature of the wounding instrument. Scrubbing wounds can destroy powder marks from gunshots and obscure abrasions. Clothing and belongings must be secured to prevent the possibility of tampering.

14. **The answer is B.** *(Chapter 293)* Each person who requires restraint should be approached by a team of four or five trained individuals with a single leader. Ideally, one person can control each extremity and another can control the head. Inadequate numbers

of personnel lead to increased injuries to both the staff and the patient. The minimum necessary force should be used, and not every patient requires four-point leather restraint. Patients who require restraint should not leave the ED without complete evaluation. The chart must reflect the reason for the restraints and a specific physician order for the type and duration of restraint. The patient must be reevaluated frequently.

15. **The answer is E.** *(Chapter 13)* Although there has been increasing attention to physicians' role in promoting greater social good and preserving resources, the physician is expected to be an advocate for the patient first and provide treatment that is in that patient's best interest. It is in resuscitation that the duties to protect and preserve life most often conflict with the duties to relieve suffering and respect autonomy. Patient autonomy is a highly prized ideal in U.S. society.

ANESTHESIA AND ANALGESIA

QUESTIONS

DIRECTIONS: Each question below contains five suggested responses. Select the **one best** response to each question.

16. Which of the following agents is LEAST likely to cause hypotension at standard doses?

    (A) Morphine
    (B) Meperidine
    (C) Fentanyl
    (D) Midazolam
    (E) Propofol

17. Which of the following agents may cause truncal and jaw muscle rigidity?

    (A) Morphine
    (B) Meperidine
    (C) Ketamine
    (D) Fentanyl
    (E) Etomidate

18. Which of the following agents may precipitate bronchospasm in patients with reactive airway disease?

    (A) Midazolam
    (B) Etomidate
    (C) Ketamine
    (D) Propofol
    (E) Methohexital

19. Which of the following statements regarding local anesthetics is FALSE?

    (A) Lidocaine and bupivicaine are both amide anesthetics
    (B) Warming and buffering has been shown to reduce the pain of injection
    (C) The duration of anesthesia is twice as long with bupivicaine as with lidocaine
    (D) Duration of anesthesia is prolonged with epinephrine
    (E) Epinephrine can damage local tissue defenses

20. EMLA is appropriate for all of the following procedures EXCEPT

    (A) venipuncture
    (B) laceration repair
    (C) lumbar puncture
    (D) myringotomy
    (E) cautery of genital warts

21. Which of the following statements regarding toxicity of local anesthetics is FALSE?

    (A) The first signs of toxicity are dizziness, tinnitus, periorbital tingling, and nystagmus
    (B) Systemic convulsions are rare and usually self-limited
    (C) Most allergic reactions are to aminoamide compounds
    (D) For patients allergic to local anesthetics, diphenhydramine hydrochloride 1 percent can be injected into the wound
    (E) To prevent toxicity, avoid rapid injections of local anesthetic into the wound

22. Which of the following statements about digital nerve blocks is FALSE?

    (A) Digital nerve blocks are more efficacious than metacarpal blocks
    (B) A 27-gauge needle is inserted through the skin into each side of the extensor tendon, just proximal to the web
    (C) The needle is advanced toward the palm until its tip is palpable beneath the volar surface of the finger
    (D) It is not necessary to anesthetize the dorsum of the involved digit
    (E) The total volume of anesthetic agent should not exceed 4 mL

23. A 32-year-old male presents with a laceration he sustained after stepping on broken glass at the beach. The examination reveals an 8-cm cut on the medial plantar aspect of the left foot. Which peripheral nerve block is appropriate?

(A) Saphenous nerve
(B) Sural nerve
(C) Posterior tibial nerve
(D) Superficial peroneal nerve
(E) Deep peroneal nerve

24. A 20-year-old male kick boxer sustains a lower lip laceration during a practice match. The wound is complex and crosses the vermilion border. Which is the best way to achieve anesthesia?

(A) Local infiltration with 1 percent lidocaine
(B) Local infiltration with 1 percent lidocaine with epinephrine
(C) Inferior alveolar nerve block
(D) Lingular nerve block
(E) Mental nerve block

ANESTHESIA AND ANALGESIA

ANSWERS

16. **The answer is C.** *(Chapter 33)* Fentanyl is a potent, synthetic opioid. Because it does not trigger histamine release like other opioid analgesics, it causes little hemodynamic compromise. All the other agents listed cause dose-dependent hypotension.

17. **The answer is D.** *(Chapter 33)* Truncal and jaw muscle rigidity are rare side effects of fentanyl that can lead to impaired ventilation. This rigidity most often occurs at high doses (>10–15 µg/kg) and may be reversed by parenteral naloxone. If naloxone is unsuccessful, paralysis and endotracheal intubation may be necessary.

18. **The answer is E.** *(Chapter 15)* Methohexital is an ultra-short-acting barbiturate that provides sedation and amnesia for short, invasive procedures. Barbiturate administration may precipitate bronchospasm in patients with moderate to severe reactive airway disease, thus limiting its use in those patients. There is some evidence that ketamine may have a mild, transient bronchodilatory effect. Midazolam, etomidate, and propofol have no clinically significant effect on bronchial smooth muscle tone. Of the listed agents, only ketamine provides analgesia in addition to sedation.

19. **The answer is C.** *(Chapter 32)* The duration of anesthesia after bupivicaine is nearly four times longer than that for lidocaine. With either agent, the duration of action is prolonged when combined with epinephrine. However, the local vasoconstrictive action of epinephrine may result in local hypoxia that impairs white blood cell function, thereby damaging local tissue defenses. Both lidocaine and bupivicaine are amide anesthetics.

20. **The answer is B.** *(Chapter 32)* EMLA (eutectic mixture of local anesthetics) is a eutectic mixture of 5 percent lidocaine and prilocaine that is used to produce anesthesia over intact skin. In the ED, its primary use is to produce anesthesia before venipuncture and lumbar puncture. In other settings, this cream has been used for anesthesia of split-thickness graft donor sites, curettage of molluscum contagiosum, cautery of genital warts, and myringotomy. EMLA is not recommended for topical anesthesia of lacerations because it induces an exaggerated inflammatory response, thereby damaging host defenses and inviting the development of infection.

21. **The answer is C.** *(Chapter 32)* Slow injections limit the chance for local anesthetic toxicity. When history of allergy is uncertain, an antihistamine such as diphenhydramine injected directly into the wound can be used as an alternative and achieves anesthesia in approximately 30 min. True allergic reactions to local anesthetics are rare, especially to aminoamide compounds such as lidocaine and bupivicaine. The ester derivatives of para-aminobenzoic acid, such as procaine, are responsible for most local anesthetic allergic reactions. Toxicity should be suspected in patients who complain of dizziness, tinnitus, and periorbital tingling. Rarely, systemic convulsions follow. These are usually self-limited because of rapid redistribution of the drug, with resultant lower serum levels.

22. **The answer is D.** *(Chapter 32)* The dorsal branch of the digital nerve supplies the dorsal aspect of each digit and should be included in the digital block. Digital nerve blocks are less time consuming and more efficacious than metacarpal blocks.

23. **The answer is C.** *(Chapter 32)* The posterior tibial nerve innervates the sole of the foot. To perform a peroneal nerve block, 1 percent lidocaine is injected into the subcutaneous tissue lateral to the posterior tibial artery at the upper border of the medial malleolus. None of the other nerves listed supply the plantar surface of the foot. The saphenous nerve provides sensation to the skin over the medial malleolus. The sural nerve supplies the lateral foot and fifth toe. The superficial peroneal nerve innervates the dorsum of the foot and the other toes, except the adjacent sides of the first and second toes, which derive sensation from the deep peroneal nerve.

24. **The answer is E.** *(Chapter 32)* A regional block is preferred for a complex lower lip laceration because it preserves tissue planes and landmarks, facilitating anatomically correct repair. The mental nerve supplies the skin and mucus membranes of the lower lip. The mental foramen is located inside the lower lip at its junction with the lower gum, just posterior to the first premolar tooth. To avoid nerve injury, 1 percent lidocaine with epinephrine is injected close to, but not into, the mental foramen. The inferior alveolar and lingular nerves do not supply the lower lip and thus would not be effective in this patient.

CARDIOLOGIC EMERGENCIES

QUESTIONS

DIRECTIONS: Each question below contains five suggested responses. Select the **one best** response to each question.

25. Stable angina is characterized by all of the following EXCEPT

(A) episodic chest pain lasting 30 to 45 min
(B) may be accompanied by light-headedness, palpitations, diaphoresis, dyspnea, nausea, or vomiting
(C) auscultation may reveal transient S4 or apical systolic murmur indicative of mitral regurgitation
(D) provoked by exertion or stress
(E) an ECG taken during an acute attack may show ST-segment depression or T-wave inversion

26. Unstable (crescendo or preinfarction) angina is characterized by all of the following EXCEPT

(A) exertional angina of recent onset, usually defined as within 4 to 8 weeks
(B) elevated troponin and new Q waves
(C) angina of worsening character, characterized by increasing severity and duration
(D) angina at rest (angina decubitus)
(E) increased requirement for nitroglycerin to control angina

27. What percentage of AMI patients have diagnostic changes on their *initial* ECG?

(A) 20
(B) 35
(C) 50
(D) 65
(E) 80

28. An ECG with abnormal Q waves and ST-segment elevation in I, aVL, and V_4–V_6 would represent infarction in which area of the myocardium?

(A) Inferior
(B) Anteroseptal
(C) Lateral
(D) Anterolateral
(E) Posterior

29. What percentage of unstable angina patients can be identified by positive troponin assays?

(A) 10
(B) 25
(C) 33
(D) 50
(E) 75

30. How long after coronary artery occlusion can echocardiography detect wall-motion abnormalities?

(A) Within a few heartbeats
(B) 5 to 10 min
(C) 30 min
(D) 1 h
(E) 2 to 4 h

31. Rupture of a papillary muscle is usually associated with an infarction of which area of myocardium?

(A) Inferior
(B) Inferior–posterior
(C) Lateral
(D) Anterior
(E) Anteroseptal

32. Postmyocardial infarction (Dressler's) syndrome is characterized by all of the following EXCEPT

(A) chest pain
(B) fever
(C) pleuropericarditis
(D) mediastinitis
(E) pleural effusion

33. All of the following should be used in the initial management of AMI EXCEPT

(A) nifedipine
(B) nitroglycerin
(C) oxygen
(D) aspirin
(E) heparin or low-molecular-weight heparin (LMWH)

34. The Global Utilization of Streptokinase and Tissue Plasminogen Activator for Occluded Coronary Arteries (GUSTO) trial found a reduced mortality rate in groups taking heparin intravenously with tPA rather than streptokinase. For which of the following subgroups of patients were these relatively small benefits of tPA over streptokinase fewer or nonexistent?

(A) Patients younger than 75 years
(B) Patients with anterior MI
(C) Patients with inferior MI
(D) Patients with posterior MI
(E) Patients in whom thrombolysis was not initiated within 2 h of symptom onset

35. Of the following criteria, which is the BEST for thrombolytic therapy?

(A) ≥ 1-mm ST-segment depression in a single limb lead
(B) ≥ 2-mm ST-segment elevation in two or more contiguous limb leads in a patient with signs of cardiogenic shock
(C) ≥ 2-mm ST-segment elevation in two or more contiguous precordial leads
(D) New right bundle branch block
(E) New left bundle branch block with evidence of cardiogenic shock

36. Absolute contraindications to thrombolytic therapy include all of the following EXCEPT

(A) recent head trauma
(B) stroke within the past 6 months or any history of hemorrhagic stroke
(C) suspected aortic dissection
(D) initial BP > 240/140
(E) suspected pericarditis

37. By which percentage does aspirin (by itself) reduce cardiovascular mortality when given in the early stages of coronary occlusion?

(A) 5
(B) 10
(C) 20
(D) 30
(E) 40

38. Nitrates have all of the following effects EXCEPT

(A) reducing cardiac preload
(B) reducing cardiac afterload
(C) dilating major capacitance vessels of the coronary system thereby improving collateral flow
(D) inhibiting vasospasm
(E) improving clinical outcome when used orally during AMI

39. Contraindications to β blockade include all of the following EXCEPT

(A) heart rate < 60 beats per minute
(B) first-degree AV block
(C) severe left ventricular dysfunction
(D) severe chronic obstructive pulmonary disease
(E) systolic blood pressure < 100 with signs of hypoperfusion

40. Which of the following is the MOST appropriate intravenous heparin dose in the setting of AMI?

(A) loading dose: 75 U/kg, maintenance infusion: 13 U/kg per hour
(B) loading dose: 7.5 U/kg, maintenance infusion: 13 U/kg per hour
(C) no loading dose, maintenance infusion: 1100 U/h
(D) loading dose: 10,000 U, maintenance infusion: 1000 U/h
(E) loading dose: 1000 U, maintenance infusion: 1200 U/h

41. A 70-year-old man presents to the ED after a 1-min episode of loss of consciousness while eating dinner. Potential cardiac causes of this syncopal episode include all of the following EXCEPT

(A) bradycardia
(B) tachycardia
(C) aortic stenosis
(D) aortic regurgitation
(E) ischemia

42. All of the following drugs may contribute to syncope EXCEPT

(A) spironolactone
(B) digitalis
(C) metoprolol
(D) nitrates
(E) synthroid

43. Which artery is MOST likely to be diseased in a patient who suffers a syncopal episode secondary to cerebral ischemia?

(A) Carotid
(B) Vertebrobasilar
(C) Anterior communicating artery
(D) Anterior cerebral artery
(E) Posterior communicating artery

44. A 44-year-old man complains of recurrent syncope associated with upper extremity exercise. What is the MOST likely cause?

(A) Trigeminal neuralgia
(B) Hypoglycemia
(C) Carotid sinus hypersensitivity
(D) Subclavian steal syndrome
(E) Vasovagal syncope

45. What diagnosis should be suspected in an elderly patient who experiences a syncopal episode after head turning or shaving?

(A) vasovagal syncope
(B) carotid sinus hypersensitivity
(C) orthostatic syncope
(D) cardiomyopathy
(E) seizure disorder

46. Which of the following conditions is NOT associated with a risk of aortic dissection?

(A) Aortic regurgitation
(B) Aortic stenosis
(C) Bicuspid aortic valve
(D) Marfan's syndrome
(E) Coarctation of the aorta

47. All of the following findings support the diagnosis of pericarditis EXCEPT

(A) pain relieved by sitting up and leaning forward
(B) presence of a pericardial friction rub
(C) ECG with diffuse ST segment depression
(D) ECG with PR segment depression
(E) pericardial effusion

48. Which of the following statements regarding chest pain is FALSE?

(A) Burning or gnawing pain may be present with AMI
(B) An acid or foul taste in the mouth suggests dypepsia is more likely than angina
(C) Tenderness to palpation in the epigastric region may be elicited with AMI
(D) Relief of pain with antacids strongly suggests a gastrointestinal etiology
(E) Epigastric or lower chest discomfort may be described with both cardiac and noncardiac causes

49. Risk factors for coronary artery disease include all of the following EXCEPT

(A) male sex
(B) hypercholesterolemia
(C) estrogen replacement medications
(D) diabetes
(E) cigarette smoking

50. Physical examination and laboratory findings that may be present in AMI include all of the following EXCEPT

(A) chest wall tenderness
(B) sinus tachycardia or bradycardia
(C) hypertension or hypotension
(D) crackles on pulmonary examination
(E) non–anion-gap metabolic acidosis

51. A patient has a blood pressure of 210/140 accompanied by severe headache, nausea, and vomiting. Which category of hypertension BEST describes this presentation?

(A) Hypertensive emergency
(B) Hypertensive urgency
(C) Uncomplicated hypertension
(D) Transient hypertension
(E) Chronic hypertension

52. How quickly and to what level should the blood pressure be lowered in a patient with a hypertensive emergency?

(A) 120/80 as quickly as possible
(B) 180/90 within 12 h
(C) 120/80 within 30 to 60 min
(D) A level that is "normal" for that patient within 30 to 60 min
(E) A level that is "normal" for that patient within 4 h

53. A patient, 8 months' pregnant, with no medical history presents with a BP of 160/100 and seizures. Which of the following is the BEST drug for lowering BP in this setting?

(A) Sodium nitroprusside
(B) Hydralazine
(C) Intravenous nitroglycerin
(D) Nifedipine
(E) Furosemide

54. Sodium nitroprusside has all of the following actions EXCEPT

(A) arteriolar dilator
(B) venodilator
(C) decreasing preload and afterload
(D) near immediate onset of action
(E) duration of action of 1 to 2 h

55. Labetalol is an excellent drug for lowering blood pressure in all of the following conditions EXCEPT

(A) pheochromocytoma
(B) MAO inhibitor–induced hypertensive emergencies
(C) clonidine withdrawal
(D) dissecting aortic aneurysm
(E) in patients with congestive heart failure and hypertension after AMI

56. Each of the following is a risk factor for venous thrombosis EXCEPT

(A) hormone replacement therapy
(B) CHF
(C) central line placement
(D) blood type O
(E) extensive burns

57. A 50-year-old man presents with a painful, swollen leg that occurred over 2 days. He smokes two packs of cigarettes per day, and he is moderately overweight. He recalls striking his calf against a coffee table 3 days before and suffered an abrasion. His temperature is 100.5°F, and the leg is visibly swollen to the groin with moderate erythema. Pulses are normal. Which of the following statements is correct?

(A) Absence of palpable cords and a negative Homans' sign make DVT unlikely
(B) The fever and erythema make a diagnosis of DVT very unlikely
(C) The patient may be started on heparin anticoagulation immediately
(D) Because there is no evidence of pulmonary embolism, the patient may be started on coumadin alone
(E) A venogram must be performed within 24 h

58. An elderly man with a history of smoking complains of sudden, severe pain in the left leg beginning 2 h previously. The leg is cool, pale, and mottled from the mid-thigh distally, and sensation is decreased. All of the following are true EXCEPT

(A) the patient likely had an embolus that originated in the heart
(B) the patient should immediately receive thrombolytic therapy with streptokinase or recombinant tPA because there is only a 4-h window during which reperfusion must be achieved to preserve limb function
(C) a vascular surgeon should be consulted immediately
(D) the patient has an overall mortality rate of about 15 percent
(E) intravenous heparin is indicated

59. In a heart transplant recipient, each of the following statements is true EXCEPT

(A) Sinus tachycardia at rest can be normal
(B) The effect of atropine is exaggerated in the denervated heart
(C) The response to β-adrenergic drugs is normal or increased
(D) The ECG is often read as atrial fibrillation or flutter
(E) The patient will be immunosuppressed for life

60. A 55-year-old man is 2 years post–heart transplantation for dilated cardiomyopathy. He presents with 1 day of fatigue, nausea, vomiting, and diarrhea. He is currently taking cyclosporine, prednisone, and azathioprine. All of the following statements are true EXCEPT

(A) The patient may have a cytomegalovirus infection
(B) The patient must be evaluated for possible acute rejection
(C) The patient should immediately receive 1 g intravenous methylprednisolone
(D) This illness may cause an episode of rejection
(E) The patient must receive antibiotics before endoscopic procedures

61. Regarding abdominal aortic aneurysms, all of the following statements are true EXCEPT

(A) Aneurysms larger than 5 cm should be treated surgically
(B) Fusiform aneurysms smaller than 4 cm can be managed conservatively
(C) Tenderness of an aneurysm may be an indication for surgery
(D) Most patients complain of back pain
(E) The most common presentation of an aneurysm is as an incidental finding

62. A 67-year-old man is brought to the ED by ambulance after a syncopal episode. He was well before the event, except for mild chronic hypertension. He fell on pavement, striking his head, so paramedics placed him in a cervical collar and strapped him to a spine board. He complains of low back pain, which he attributes to the spine board. BP is 100/50, and heart rate (HR) is 80 beats per minute. Which of the following is the best course of action?

(A) Analgesia, ECG, and outpatient referral to cardiologist

(B) ECG, cardiac enzymes, admit for telemetry monitoring

(C) Lateral abdominal x-ray, with aortogram if inconclusive

(D) Intravenous fluids, morphine, computed tomography (CT) of the abdomen

(E) Immediate surgical consultation, multiple large-bore intravenous lines, type and cross-match blood

63. A 60-year-old man presents with 1 h of chest and upper back pain "like I'm being ripped apart!" BP is 170/110 in the right arm and 110/50 in the left arm. ECG shows sinus rhythm with left ventricular hypertrophy. Chest x-ray is unremarkable. Which of the following is the most appropriate intervention?

(A) Nitroglycerin sublingual $\times$ 3, cardiac enzymes, admit

(B) Intravenous r-tPA or streptokinase, admit to cardiac care unit

(C) Intravenous heparin 80 U/kg bolus and 18 U/kg per hour as continuous infusion, ventilation/perfusion lung scan, admit

(D) Intravenous nitroprusside to keep systolic BP < 110, intravenous propranolol to keep HR < 60, contrast-enhanced CT of the thorax

(E) Intravenous morphine sulfate, emergency gastrointestinal consultation for endoscopy

64. All of the following are acceptable strategies for diagnosis of DVT EXCEPT

(A) duplex ultrasonography

(B) IPG

(C) contrast venography

(D) elevated D-dimer fragments

(E) MRI

65. Each of the following may be a manifestation of rejection in a cardiac transplant patient EXCEPT

(A) dysrhythmias

(B) myocardial infarction

(C) ascites

(D) renal insufficiency

(E) hypotension

66. All of the following statements are true of geriatric trauma patients EXCEPT

(A) Symptoms of intracranial hemorrhage may be delayed compared with symptoms in younger patients

(B) A normal heart rate is a good prognostic sign

(C) Cervical spine fractures are less common with increasing age

(D) Elderly patients have decreased pulmonary reserve

(E) Orthopedic injuries alone may cause significant hypovolemia

67. All of the following statements are TRUE with regard to mitral valve stenosis (MVS) EXCEPT

(A) Rheumatic heart disease is the most common cause

(B) Symptoms may be precipitated by atrial fibrillation, pregnancy, and anemia

(C) Syncope is the most common presenting symptom

(D) Hemoptysis is the second most common presenting symptom

(E) If the defect is not corrected, atrial fibrillation almost always develops

68. All of the following statements are TRUE regarding mitral valve prolapse (MVP) EXCEPT

(A) There is an increased incidence of sudden death and dysrhythmias

(B) In patients younger than 45 years, there is an increased incidence of TIAs

(C) Approximately 1 percent of the population has MVP

(D) A mid-systolic snap is a classic auscultatory finding

(E) Most patients are asymptomatic

69. Which of the following statements is FALSE with respect to aortic stenosis (AS)?

(A) Congential heart disease is the most common cause

(B) Left ventricular hypertrophy (LVH) is the most common ECG finding

(C) Sudden death occurs in 25 percent of patients

(D) Endocarditis occurs in 15 percent of patients

(E) Exertional angina is a common presenting symptom

70. For which of the following procedures should patients with valvular heart disease receive prophylactic antibiotics?

(A) Incision and drainage of an abscess
(B) Anoscopy
(C) Endotracheal intubation
(D) A and B only
(E) All of the above

71. Which valvular disease is MOST commonly associated with sudden death in younger patients?

(A) Aortic stenosis
(B) Mitral stenosis
(C) IHSS
(D) Tetralogy of Fallot
(E) Mitral valve prolapse

72. Afterload reduction is an important therapeutic modality in all of the following patients with symptomatic valvular disease EXCEPT

(A) a patient with BP of 125/70, with acute mitral incontinence secondary to an inferior MI
(B) a patient with aortic insufficiency (AI) with BP of 135/55 with pulmonary edema
(C) a patient with AS with a BP of 135/70 and angina
(D) a patient with mitral stenosis (MS) with a BP of 135/65 and pink frothy sputum
(E) a patient with chronic mitral and aortic insufficiency, a BP of 130/80 and CHF

73. A 25-year-old runner is brought to the ED by ambulance after experiencing witnessed syncope on the track. Paramedics arrived within 3 min and found the patient in ventricular fibrillation. A 200-J shock converted the rhythm to sinus tachycardia, and the patient has remained stable. He complains of some chest discomfort and tells you he has a familial heart problem and was told he should not run. BP is 100/80, respiratory rate (RR) is 20 breaths per minute, and pulse oximetry is 93 percent. The ECG shows sinus tachycardia at 115 beats per minute with septal Q and upright T waves. In addition to oxygen administration, which of the following is the MOST important therapeutic intervention?

(A) Aspirin and nitroglycerin
(B) Intravenous fluids and 5 mg intravenous labetalol
(C) Nitroglycerin and a lidocaine drip
(D) CPAP, nitroglycerin, and furosemide
(E) Aspirin, nitroglycerin, and dopamine

74. All of the following statements are TRUE regarding emergent pericardiocentesis EXCEPT

(A) Complications include pneumothorax, dysrhythmias, laceration of coronary arteries, and liver lacerations
(B) Associated mortality with a blind approach is 6 percent
(C) The technique of choice is the left paraxyphoid approach aiming toward the right shoulder
(D) An ECG unipolar electrode attached to V_1 is the guidance technique of choice
(E) There is a 7 to 15 percent complication rate with a blind approach

75. A 62-year-old man is brought to the ED by ambulance with confusion and dyspnea. BP is 80/60. With inspiration, SBP decreases to 55. The monitor shows a HR of 121 beats per minute, with vacillating amplitude of the QRS complex. RR is 26 breaths per minute, and oximetry saturation is 91 percent. Physical examination shows jugular venous distention (JVD), distant heart sounds, cool extremities, and diaphoresis. Chest x-ray is grossly normal. Which of the following would be the MOST effective therapeutic intervention?

(A) Large-volume resuscitation with crystalloid, oxygen, and emergent diagnostic spiral CT
(B) Large-volume resuscitation with crystalloid, oxygen, and dopamine
(C) Immediate intubation, large-volume resuscitation, and dopamine
(D) Large-volume resuscitation, oxygen, and immediate involvement of cardiology consult for placement of an intraaortic balloon pump
(E) Large-volume resuscitation, oxygen, and pericardiocentesis

76. Which of the following statements is FALSE with regard to cardiomyopathy (CM)?

(A) Hypertrophic CM is a familial disease associated with decreased compliance, outflow obstruction, and septal Q waves
(B) The work-up of a newly diagnosed dilated CM patient should include a check of thyroid-stimulating hormone (TSH), phosphate, and iron, HIV status, and an endocardial biopsy
(C) Patients with restrictive CM secondary to amyloidosis should be started on a triple regimen of diuretics, afterload reduction agents, and digoxin
(D) Fever and myalgias are not part of the presenting symptoms of CM
(E) Most CM patients are best treated with diuretics, afterload reduction agents, and digoxin

77. Which of the following statements is FALSE with regard to myocarditis?

(A) Most patients with myocarditis return to their baseline cardiac function within several months of initial presentation

(B) Up to 60 percent of patients with chronic cardiomyopathy have histologic evidence of myocarditis

(C) On polymerase chain reaction analysis of endocardial biopsy, adenovirus is found to be the most frequent etiologic agent of acute myocarditis

(D) Forty percent of patients with acute cardiomyopathy have histologic evidence of myocarditis

(E) Cocksackie, influenza B, and Epstein-Barr (EBV) viruses have all been implicated in acute myocarditis

78. A previously healthy 25-year-old woman with no medical history presents to the ED complaining of 4 h of substernal chest pain, shortness of breath, dyspnea on exertion, and "not feeling well" during the past few days. She denies illicit drug use or alcoholism. Vital signs are remarkable for a BP of 92/60, HR of 135, RR of 30, and temperature of 101.5°F. ECG shows normal sinus rhythm with nonspecific T-wave changes. Chest x-ray is normal. In addition to oxygen, which one of the following represents the BEST initial treatment regimen?

(A) Aspirin, nitroglycerin, check troponin and myoglobin levels

(B) Aspirin, β blocker, check TSH

(C) Intravenous fluids, analgesia, emergent echocardiogram

(D) Aspirin, nitroglycerin, emergent ventilation perfusion (V̇/Q̇) scan

(E) Intravenous fluids, lorazepam, antacids

79. All of the following statements are TRUE with regard to acute pericarditis EXCEPT

(A) Acute pericarditis is associated with transient dysrhythmias that are usually clinically insignificant

(B) Aspirin, 650 mg every 4 h for 7 days, should be initiated if the diagnosis is suspected, so long as no contraindications are present

(C) Electrical alternans or low-voltage ECG suggests the presence of pericardial effusion

(D) Concomitant pericardial effusion is common

(E) Sixty percent of patients have complete recovery within a week

80. All of the following statements are TRUE about uremic pericarditis EXCEPT

(A) Uremic pericarditis is one of most common causes of cardiac tamponade

(B) Pericarditis is detected clinically in 20 percent of uremic patients

(C) ECG changes of pericarditis are more common in uremic patients

(D) Hemodialysis daily for 2 to 6 weeks is the treatment of choice for uremic pericarditis

(E) Hemodialysis-associated pericarditis requires a diligent work-up for infectious causes

81. A 32-year-old man presents with 1 week of flulike symptoms and 2 days of sharp intermittent substernal chest and left shoulder pain that wakes him at night. The pain is partly relieved by sitting up. BP is 130/65, HR is 100, RR is 16, and temperature is 100.6°F. On physical examination, you hear a triphasic whispering heart sound over the precordium. All of the following are TRUE with regard to ECG findings associated with this condition EXCEPT

(A) Diffuse concave ST elevation and PR depression may be present

(B) ST-segment elevation of less than one-fourth of the T-wave amplitude is more consistent with this patient's condition than with early repolarization

(C) ST-segment elevation is most prominent in the limb leads and lateral precordial leads

(D) ST-segment elevation in this condition can be distinguished from that seen in AMI because there are no associated T-wave inversions

(E) The PR depression seen with this condition does not occur with early repolarization

82. Which represents the BEST matches of valvular diseases from the left column with ECG findings in the right column?

1. MS
2. AS
3. mitral valve prolapse
4. mitral insufficiency
5. IHSS

6. acute inferior ischemia
7. LVH and bundle branch block
8. biphasic P waves and right axis
9. normal sinus rhythm
10. pseudoinfarction pattern

(A) 1 + 8; 3 + 10
(B) 5 + 7; 2 + 10
(C) 4 + 6; 2 + 7
(D) 3 + 9; 1 + 6
(E) 2 + 9; 5 + 8

---

83. All of the following statements are TRUE regarding the treatment of valvular emergencies EXCEPT

(A) An intraaortic counterpulsation balloon is contraindicated in AI
(B) Thrombolytic agents may be helpful in acute mitral insufficiency
(C) Emergent surgery is usually indicated in acute aortic and mitral insufficiency
(D) Patients with AS and syncope require urgent surgical intervention
(E) Patients with decompensated MS and atrial fibrillation should be considered for cardioversion

84. A 28-year-old intravenous drug user presents with dyspnea, agitation, diaphoresis, cool extremities, and cough productive of pink frothy sputum. He has had fevers and chills for 2 days but suddenly became short of breath 1 h before. Vital signs are BP of 105/40, HR of 126, RR of 38 with oximetry saturation of 88 percent, and temperature of 103.5°F. He has quick, upsweeping pulses and a diastolic murmur. In addition to emergent intubation and intravenous furosemide administration, what is the MOST important immediate action?

(A) Administer naloxone and nitrates
(B) Call for a cardiac surgeon
(C) Perform emergent echocardiography
(D) Draw blood cultures and give intravenous antibiotics
(E) Administer naloxone and intravenous antibiotics and place an intraaortic counterpulsation balloon

85. All of the following statements are TRUE about infectious endocarditis EXCEPT

(A) Cardiac valve leaflets are susceptible to infection because of their limited blood supply
(B) Fatality rates for right-sided disease are greater than those for left-sided disease
(C) *Streptococcus viridans* is the most common organism implicated in left-sided disease
(D) More than three-fourths of cases of right-sided endocarditis are caused by *Staphyloccus aureus*
(E) Murmurs are detected in fewer than 50 percent of patients with right-sided disease

86. All of the following statements are TRUE concerning subacute infectious endocarditis EXCEPT

(A) The diagnosis is frequently missed
(B) Ten percent of patients have evidence of peripheral vasculitic embolic lesions
(C) Splenomegaly is present in 25 percent of patients
(D) Subacute presentations are unusual in right-sided disease
(E) Neurologic signs from septic emboli are seen in up to 40 percent of patients

87. All of the following statements are TRUE about CHF EXCEPT

(A) Patients with CHF have a 50 percent mortality risk within 5 years
(B) Ventricular ejection fraction is the best predictor of mortality
(C) Sudden death occurs in 40 percent of CHF patients
(D) ACE inhibitors have decreased the incidence of sudden death
(E) β Blockers have been shown to be a useful treatment adjunct

88. A 59-year-old man presents to the ED by ambulance with a 1-h history of severe substernal chest pain and diaphoresis 12 h before presentation. Several hours after initial resolution of the pain, he developed increasing shortness of breath and chest heaviness. The patient is pale, cyanotic, and dyspneic, puffing out one to two words at a time. Vital signs are BP 102/60, HR 121 (sinus tachycardia), and RR 36 with pulse oximetry showing 87 percent saturation. ECG shows deep Q waves in leads V_1 through V_4 and no ST-segment changes. The chest x-ray shows normal heart size, Kerly B lines, and bilateral perihilar infiltrates. All of the following statements are CORRECT with regard to this patient EXCEPT

(A) He should be placed on positive pressure ventilation by face mask and given intravenous furosemide and nitroglycerin
(B) On insertion of a pulmonary artery catheter, wedge pressure would be at least 20 mm Hg
(C) The principal role of morphine is to calm the patient
(D) Dopamine should be started to keep the SBP between 90 and 100 mm Hg
(E) The patient should receive aspirin and metoprolol

89. All of the following statements are TRUE with regard to the treatment of pulmonary edema EXCEPT

(A) Higher doses of nitroglycerin are needed to alleviate the symptoms of APE than to relieve stable angina
(B) An appropriate estimate of intravenous furosemide dose is 1 mg/kg
(C) Dopamine produces a more favorable balance between myocardial oxygen supply and demand than does dobutamine
(D) Nitroprusside may induce ischemia in patients with coronary artery disease
(E) Digoxin has no role in the acute management of CHF

90. You respond to a "code blue" on the labor-and-delivery ward. The nurse tells you that the patient is a previously healthy 41-year-old African-American woman, 4 days status post normal spontaneous vaginal delivery. She complained of chest pain and dyspnea and then fell to the floor unconscious. No seizure activity was noted. Although initially pulseless, vital signs returned with assisted ventilations. You find the patient confused, grunting, and cyanotic. Vital signs are BP 68/50 mm Hg, HR 121 beats per minute (sinus tachycardia), and RR 28, with pulse oximetry of 78 percent on high-flow oxygen. Physical examination shows distended neck veins, normal heart sounds with a prominent S_2, a thready pulse with cool, cyanotic extremities, and adequate tidal volume with no rales or wheezes. Chest x-ray is normal. Bedside ultrasound of the heart shows a dilated right ventricle with parodoxical septal wall motion. In addition to immediate intubation and fluid resuscitation, what is the MOST appropriate therapeutic intervention?

(A) Emergent diagnostic spiral CT
(B) Heparin bolus of 80 U/kg intravenously followed by 18 U/kg infusion
(C) LMWH 1 U/kg every 12 h
(D) r-tPA at a dose of 100 mg over 2 h
(E) Emergent transfer to the angiography suite for pulmonary arteriography and local infusion of urokinase

91. All of the following statements are TRUE about diagnostic tests for PE EXCEPT

(A) The $\dot{V}/\dot{Q}$ scan is 98 percent sensitive and 35 percent specific for PE
(B) Duplex ultrasound is 95 percent sensitive and 95 percent specific for DVT
(C) The difficulty in using $\dot{V}/\dot{Q}$ scan findings for the diagnosis of PE is the lack of a standardized definition for "clinical suspicion"
(D) A D-dimer of less than 500 U/mL has a negative predictive value of 90 percent
(E) Spiral CT is up to 90 percent sensitive and 96 percent specific for PE

92. A 29-year-old man presents to the ED complaining of the acute onset of shortness of breath and chest discomfort. He was discharged from the ICU 2 weeks before, after surgical correction of a perforated viscus secondary to blunt trauma. Vital signs are BP of 120/60 mm Hg, HR of 100 beats per minute, and RR of 17, with a room air pulse oximetry of 97 percent. Chest x-ray is normal, as are initial electrolytes and hematocrit. A Doppler duplex scan of the lower extremities is normal. All of the following statements are TRUE with regard to this presentation EXCEPT

(A) PE is more common in men than in women before age 50 years

(B) If the patient has a low-probability $\dot{V}/\dot{Q}$ scan, no further work-up is warranted

(C) A normal chest x-ray in the setting of acute dyspnea and hypoxemia is suggestive of PE

(D) Intravenous heparin administration should be strongly considered if the $\dot{V}/\dot{Q}$ scan is "intermediate probability"

(E) Diffuse wheezing on examination would not reduce clinical suspicion for PE

93. All of the following statements are TRUE about PE EXCEPT

(A) The risk for embolism from proximal DVT is highest in the first week

(B) The majority of the patients with PE have at least one risk factor

(C) Tachypnea is defined as a RR of greater than 16 breaths per minute

(D) Syncope is the presenting complaint in up to 5 percent of cases

(E) The right lower lobe is the most common part of the lung involved

94. All of the following statements are TRUE about PE EXCEPT

(A) Seventy percent of the pulmonary vasculature must be occluded to produce hypoxia and hypotension

(B) Massive PE presenting with hypotension and hypoxemia accounts for 5 percent of all cases

(C) The most common ECG abnormality is non-specific ST and T-wave changes

(D) ECG changes are seen in about 40 percent of patients with PE

(E) New right bundle branch block should raise the clinical suspicion for PE

---

95. Match the items in the left column with their MOST appropriate counterparts in the right column.

1. ankle brachial index = 0.6
2. ankle brachial index = 1.0
3. apteriovenous fistula
4. ankle brachial index = 0.3
5. monophasic wave every 3 s

6. vascular emergency
7. triphasic wave over tibialis pedis
8. Doppler flow sound in diastole
9. monophasic wave over dorsalis pedis
10. venous flow

(A) 1 + 9; 2 + 10
(B) 2 + 7; 3 + 10
(C) 4 + 6; 5 + 8
(D) 1 + 9; 4 + 6
(E) 2 + 9; 3 + 8

96. All of the following statements are TRUE about the use of nuclear medicine in cardiac disease EXCEPT

(A) Thallium 201 is a potassium cation analog that is taken up by active well-perfused myocytes during exercise and redistributes to less well-perfused myocardium during rest

(B) Technetium-99m sestamibi accumulates in well-perfused myocytes and does not redistribute at rest

(C) Thallium 201 has a stronger signal and shows better contrast on positron emission tomography than does technetium-99m sestamibi

(D) Nuclear stress tests for coronary ischemia are more sensitive than ECG stress tests

(E) The role of nuclear cardiac stress tests in the ED is to evaluate for coronary ischemia

97. A 56-year-old man with a history of hypertension and tobacco use complains of intermittent substernal chest pain without radiation or associated shortness of breath, nausea, or diaphoresis. Chest pain occurs both with exertion and at rest and lasts 5 to 10 min at a time. He is currently pain free, but his ECG shows LVH and inverted T waves in leads V_4 to V_6. Two sets of cardiac enzymes are negative. Which of the following diagnostic tests would be MOST appropriate?

(A) An ECG exercise stress test

(B) A T99 exercise stress test

(C) Echocardiography for evaluation of wall motion abnormalities

(D) Coronary angiography

(E) A 24-h Holter monitor

98. All of the following statements are TRUE regarding the role of echocardiography in the ED EXCEPT

(A) Normal left ventricular wall motion during chest pain suggests noncardiac chest pain

(B) Among patients with nonspecific ECG abnormalities and chest pain, echocardiography changes the admission diagnosis in up to 40 percent of cases

(C) The presence of thin hyperechoic myocardium implies an area of infarct more than 2 weeks before presentation

(D) Cardiac ultrasound is superior to clinical assessment of Killip classification and superior to ECG in predicting death and major complications

(E) Localized or small wall motion abnormalities may be apparent on echocardiogram, even in the presence of nonspecific ECG changes

CARDIOLOGIC EMERGENCIES

ANSWERS

25. The answer is A. *(Chapter 47)* Stable angina is characterized by episodic chest pain that lasts minutes (usually 5 to 15), is provoked by exertion or stress, and is relieved by rest or sublingual nitroglycerin. Other symptoms may accompany angina. In addition, transient electrocardiogram (ECG) changes and heart auscultation changes may exist.

26. The answer is B. *(Chapter 47)* Unstable angina is defined as (1) exertional angina of recent onset; (2) angina of worsening character, including an increased nitroglycerin requirement; and (3) angina at rest. In unstable angina, ST-segment or T-wave changes may persist up to several hours after the pain episode but without ECG evidence of new transmural infarction (new Q waves). Troponin is elevated in as many as one-third of unstable angina episodes, indicating the presence of a microinfarct.

27. The answer is C. *(Chapter 47)* Although the ECG is the most important diagnostic test in patients with chest pain, only about half of all patients with acute myocardial infarction (AMI) have diagnostic changes on their initial ECG. A normal or nonspecific ECG does not exclude ischemia or negate the need for hospital admission. History and clinical assessment should guide treatment decisions. Additional ECGs increase diagnostic yield.

28. The answer is C. *(Chapter 47)* When one area of the myocardium dies, electrical conduction detected by the ECG is characteristically affected. ST-segment elevation in leads II, III, and aVF represents inferior infarction. Elevations in leads V_1–V_3 occur with anteroseptal infarctions. Elevations in leads I, aVL, and V_4–V_6 suggest lateral infarction, whereas elevations in leads V_1–V_6 suggest anterolateral infarction. ST depression in V_1 and V_2 represents true posterior infarction. A right-sided ECG should be performed when inferior ischemia or infarction is detected to assess for right ventricular involvement. If present, extension to the right heart portends a worse prognosis.

29. The answer is C. *(Chapter 47)* With a monoclonal antibody assay, troponin I can be measured down to levels as low as 1 ng/mL. Advantages to measuring troponin I include more specificity than CK-MB in the setting of skeletal muscle damage (e.g., postoperative patients), more sensitivity in detecting unstable angina patients, and the ability to detect myocardial damage up to 1 week after the event.

30. The answer is A. *(Chapter 57)* Soon after the onset of myocardial ischemia, muscle contraction is impaired. This may manifest on echocardiography as a wall-motion abnormality. Experimentally, hypokinesis, akinesis, or dyskinesis can be seen within a few heartbeats after coronary occlusion. In selected patients in the critical care unit, echocardiography has a sensitivity greater than 70 percent in AMI. In studies of ED patients, where prevalence of AMI is lower and prevalence of coronary artery disease is higher, echo has been shown to be sensitive but not specific. Echocardiography is most useful in patients with cardiogenic shock to diagnose anatomic complications that may be amenable to surgical correction (i.e., septal or mitral ruptures).

31. **The answer is B.** *(Chapter 47)* Papillary muscle rupture is usually associated with an inferior–posterior infarction and involves the posterior papillary muscle. Outcome depends on whether the entire muscle body or only the head is ruptured. Rupture of an entire muscle body is associated with a high mortality rate (up to 50 percent within 24 h). Diagnosis of papillary muscle dysfunction or rupture may be made on echocardiography or by measuring large V waves in the pulmonary artery wedge pressure with a Swan-Ganz catheter.

32. **The answer is D.** *(Chapter 47)* Dressler's syndrome is characterized by chest pain, fever, pleuropericarditis, and pleural effusion. An immunologic reaction that occurs 2 to 6 weeks after AMI is responsible for this syndrome. Aspirin or indomethacin is standard initial therapy. Refractory cases are treated with steroids, but it is difficult to wean patients from this class of drugs, and recurrences are common. In addition to Dressler's syndrome, an acute form of pericarditis, manifested by pain and a friction rub, can develop during the first 7 days after infarction.

33. **The answer is A.** *(Chapter 47)* Currently available calcium channel antagonists are not recommended for early management of AMI patients. Nifedipine increases mortality in unstable angina and AMI patients. Verapamil is not recommended in the peri-infarct period but can be beneficial in the postinfarct phase for patients without heart failure.

34. **The answer is C.** *(Chapter 48)* The GUSTO investigators studied 41,021 patients with AMI from 1081 centers in 15 countries. They reported that front-loaded tissue plasminogen activator (tPA) with intravenous heparin resulted in a reduced mortality rate at 30 days after treatment (6.3 percent) compared with streptokinase and subcutaneous heparin (7.2 percent) or streptokinase and intravenous heparin (7.4 percent). However, subgroup analysis showed that the relatively small benefits of tPA over streptokinase were fewer or nonexistent for patients with inferior myocardial infarction (MI), age older than 75 years, or in whom thrombolysis was not initiated until more than 4 h after symptom onset.

35. **The answer is C.** *(Chapter 48)* For patients who are not in cardiogenic shock, ECG criteria for thrombolytic therapy include one or more of the following: (1) ≥ 1-mm ST segment elevation in two or more contiguous limb leads, (2) ≥ 2-mm ST segment elevation in two or more contiguous precordial leads, and (3) new left bundle branch block. Patients in cardiogenic shock should undergo emergent angiography and mechanical reperfusion, if available. If angioplasty cannot be performed within 60 min, "front-loaded" tPA is indicated.

36. **The answer is D.** *(Chapter 48)* Absolute contraindications to thrombolytic therapy include active internal bleeding; altered consciousness; stroke in the past 6 months or any history of hemorrhagic stroke; intracranial surgery within the past 2 months; known arteriovenous malformation (AVM), aneurysm, or intracranial neoplasm; known bleeding disorder; persistent hypertension greater than 200/120; recent head trauma; suspected aortic dissection; suspected pericarditis; and trauma or surgery within the past 2 weeks that could result in bleeding into a closed space.

37. **The answer is C.** *(Chapter 48)* During the early stages of acute coronary occlusion, platelets form the bulk of the clot. Aspirin is a cyclooxygenase inhibitor that binds irreversibly and thereby inhibits platelet aggregation. The ISIS-2 study randomized 18,000 patients to receive a placebo, low-dose aspirin (160 mg), streptokinase, or a combination of both aspirin and streptokinase. Administration of aspirin alone led to a significant reduction in cardiovascular deaths (20 percent). This mortality benefit increased to 40 percent when aspirin was combined with streptokinase.

38. **The answer is E.** *(Chapter 48)* Nitrates are vasodilators that reduce cardiac preload and, to a lesser extent, afterload. The result is a lower cardiac volume, reduced wall

stress, and decreased myocardial oxygen consumption. Nitrates dilate the major capacitance vessels of the coronary system and improve collateral blood flow in the myocardium. In addition, they inhibit vasospasm. The largest trial evaluating oral nitrates to date (ISIS-4) showed no improved outcome with nitrates versus placebo in the setting of AMI. Although there is no proven outcomes benefit, nitrates are useful in providing pain relief, an important component of treating AMI.

39. **The answer is B.** *(Chapter 48)* β-Blocker administration reduces both the short- and long-term mortality in patients with AMI. More than 28 randomized studies involving more than 27,000 patients have demonstrated a 14 percent reduction in mortality when acute β blockade was used during AMI. Contraindications to β blockade include type I and II second-degree atrioventricular (AV) block, severe chronic obstructive pulmonary disease, heart rate slower than 60 beats per minute, and hypotension. Because of the impressive mortality reduction, β blockers are now being used in patients with mild heart failure. First-degree AV block is a relative contraindication.

40. **The answer is A.** *(Chapter 48)* The protective benefits of heparin are dependent on appropriate dosing. In one study, more than 25 percent of patients' partial thromboplastin times (PTTs) were not within the therapeutic range during the first 24 h of therapy. Adherence to weight-based dosing significantly reduced this number to 8.8 percent. Many practitioners are now switching to a LMWH such as enoxaparin (dose, 1 mg/kg) given its ease of administration and the lack of need to follow PTTs.

41. **The answer is D.** *(Chapter 46)* Cardiac causes of syncope fall into three groups: rhythm disturbances, ventricular outflow obstructive processes, and myocardial ischemia. To be considered the cause of syncope, the heart rate should be more than 150 or fewer than 40 beats per minute. Any process causing acute or chronic obstruction to ventricular inflow or outflow may cause syncope. For the left ventricle, obstructions include aortic stenosis, atrial myxoma, or mitral stenosis. Syncope associated with cardiac ischemia is usually secondary to dysrhythmia.

42. **The answer is E.** *(Chapter 46)* Drugs may cause or contribute to syncope by several mechanisms. They may precipitate dysrhythmias, aggravate orthostatic hypotension (antihypertensives), or cause volume depletion (diuretics). The drugs most commonly associated with syncope are nitrates, diuretics, and antidysrhythmics. Synthroid is not associated with syncope.

43. **The answer is B.** *(Chapter 46)* Syncope is caused by disease affecting either (1) the bilateral cerebral hemispheres or (2) the reticular activating system (RAS). A vertebrobasilar transient ischemic attack (TIA) may result in a "drop attack" by causing ischemia to the RAS. An anterior circulation TIA would be unlikely to result in syncope because it would have to involve both cerebral hemispheres.

44. **The answer is D.** *(Chapter 46)* An association between upper extremity exercise and syncope suggests the presence of subclavian steal syndrome. If blood pressure is measured on each arm, a difference of at least 20 mm Hg is often noted. Obstruction of the brachiocephalic or subclavian artery causes shunting of blood through the vertebrobasilar system from the normal side past the obstruction, resulting in brain stem ischemia.

45. **The answer is B.** *(Chapter 46)* Although rare, carotid sinus hypersensitivity should be suspected in an elderly patient whose immediate presyncopal state is suggestive of carotid sinus stimulation, e.g., wearing a tight collar, shaving, or head turning. If carotid sinus hypersensitivity is suspected, confirmatory carotid sinus massage may be performed at the bedside. A positive response is asystole of 3 s or greater or a drop in systolic blood pressure of at least 50 mm Hg.

46. The answer is A. *(Chapter 45)* Aortic dissection is an uncommon cause of chest pain. Although it may present in all age groups, the majority of cases are seen in hypertensive men in the fifth to seventh decades. Patients with Marfan's syndrome, coarctation of the aorta, bicuspid aortic valves, and aortic stenosis are all predisposed to aortic dissection.

47. The answer is C. *(Chapter 51)* The pain of pericarditis is generally pleuritic, retrosternal in location, and may radiate to the back, neck, or jaw. Classically, pain is relieved when the patient sits up and leans forward. Pericardial effusion is often present and can be detected by echocardiogram. The presence of a pericardial friction rub supports the diagnosis. The ECG may show diffuse ST-segment elevation or T-wave inversions. PR segment depression is a highly specific finding.

48. The answer is D. *(Chapter 45)* Although various gastrointestinal syndromes may present with epigastic burning or gnawing pain, this description of pain may also represent angina. Pain associated with an acid or foul taste in the mouth and eructation is more suggestive of dyspepsia. Tenderness to palpation in the epigastric or upper quadrants suggests a gastrointestinal etiology, but AMI patients may also complain of tenderness on chest palpation. Chest discomfort relieved by antacids may be both cardiac and noncardiac in origin. Nitroglycerin is a smooth muscle dilator that may afford relief in cases of lower esophageal spasm or biliary colic. Diagnostic decisions should not be influenced by response to a therapeutic trial.

49. The answer is C. *(Chapter 45)* Risk factors include being a male or a postmenopausal female, hypertension, tobacco use, hypercholesterolemia, diabetes, obesity, and family history. Cocaine use has also been associated with AMI, even in young people with minimal or no coronary artery disease. Estrogen replacement therapy may be protective against heart disease.

50. The answer is E. *(Chapter 47)* Although patients with myocardial ischemia can present with almost any vital sign abnormality, a normal physical examination does not preclude the diagnosis of AMI. Sinus tachycardia may be reflective of increased sympathetic stimulation resulting from ischemia or of decreased left ventricular stroke volume. Patients with acute ischemia have a slightly higher incidence of abnormal heart sounds, and crackles on pulmonary examination are twice as common in patients with AMI as in those with nonischemic chest pain. In one study, chest wall tenderness was present in 36 percent of chest pain patients without myocardial infarction and in 15 percent of those with acute infarction. Non–anion-gap metabolic acidosis should not be attributed to AMI.

51. The answer is A. *(Chapter 53)* Category of hypertension is based on clinical presentation and the level of aggression required for treatment, not on the absolute number of the blood pressure. A hypertensive emergency is defined as elevated blood pressure with evidence of end-organ damage or dysfunction. A hypertensive urgency is an elevation of blood pressure to a level that may be potentially harmful, usually sustained at greater than 115 mm Hg diastolic without signs, symptoms, or other evidence of end-organ dysfunction. Mild, uncomplicated hypertension is defined as a blood pressure less than 115 mm Hg diastolic without symptoms of end-organ damage. Transient hypertension can be seen in many conditions such as pain states, anxiety, pancreatitis, thrombotic stroke, early dehydration, alcohol-withdrawal syndromes, epistaxis, and some overdoses. Treatment of the underlying condition rather than administration of antihypertensive medications is the rule.

52. The answer is D. *(Chapter 53)* The goal of treatment during a hypertensive emergency is to lower the blood pressure within 30 to 60 min to a level that is "normal" for the patient. A 30 percent reduction within the first 30 min is a useful guideline.

Resolution of signs and symptoms is a helpful endpoint, but in elderly patients improvements may lag behind the pressure drop. Absolute numbers for blood pressure are less important than the patient's baseline. For example, a young woman with a normal blood pressure (BP) of 90/60 may be suffering from a hypertensive emergency with a BP of only 120/80 if she has ingested phenylpropanolamine and complains of severe headache suggestive of intracranial bleed.

53. **The answer is B.** *(Chapter 101)* During pregnancy-induced hypertension (PIH), uterine blood flow decreases, placing the fetus at risk. Blood pressure reduction is best accomplished with magnesium sulfate and hydralazine. Hydralazine should be administered in 10- to 20-mg intravenous boluses every 30 min until the desired effect is achieved. Sodium nitroprusside can be used, but the infusion should be brief and thiocyanate levels must be monitored. Labetalol is another second-line agent in this setting. Diuretics are contraindicated because the patient with PIH is already volume-contracted. Angiotensin-converting enzyme (ACE) inhibitors should not be used because they cross the placenta and may depress angiotensin II levels in the fetus. The definitive treatment of PIH is delivery of the baby.

54. **The answer is E.** *(Chapter 53)* Sodium nitroprusside, a rapidly acting arteriolar and venous dilator, is useful for treating hypertensive emergencies. It causes both arterial and venous smooth muscles to dilate, decreasing preload and afterload and resulting in decreased myocardial oxygen demand. Nitroprusside has a rapid onset and short duration of action (plasma half-life of 3 to 4 min). It is initially metabolized to cyanide by sulfhydryl groups in the blood and then converted to thiocyanate in the liver by rhodanase.

55. **The answer is E.** *(Chapter 53)* In the setting of a hypertensive emergency, intravenous labetalol provides a steady, consistent drop in BP. Labetalol does not change cerebral blood flow and, therefore, is safe for use in patients with cerebral vascular disease. It is an ideal choice for conditions characterized by excessive catecholamine stimulation such as pheochromocytoma, monoamine oxidase (MAO) inhibitor–induced emergencies, and abrupt clonidine withdrawal. After an intravenous bolus, blood pressure falls in 5 min, with a maximum response in 10 min. BP control is maintained for up to 6 h after a single injection. Labetalol is the agent of choice in thoracic aortic dissection. Because labetalol is a nonselective β blocker, it can exacerbate heart failure and induce bronchospasm.

56. **The answer is D.** *(Chapter 55)* There are many risk factors for deep venous thrombosis. Blood group A is associated with an increased risk; type O is not. Common risks include trauma, hormonal and hypercoagulable states, injected drugs, being older than 40 years, obesity, pregnancy, surgery, smoking, immobilization, and a variety of medical illnesses including congestive heart failure (CHF), CVA, stroke, and nephrotic syndrome.

57. **The answer is C.** *(Chapter 55)* A patient with four or more risk factors has a high probability for deep venous thrombosis (DVT). It is reasonable to start anticoagulation with heparin or LMWH pending confirmation with diagnostic studies. Coumadin should never be started alone because it can cause a transient hypercoagulable state that promotes thrombus propagation and embolization. Homans' sign has no clinical predictive value. A mild fever is consistent with DVT, as is redness. Although venography was once the gold standard test, duplex ultrasonography is currently favored.

58. **The answer is B.** *(Chapter 55)* Systemic thrombolytics produce inferior results compared with either catheter embolectomy or intraarterial thrombolysis. If there are no contraindications, heparin should be administered immediately pending additional treatment. The heart is by far the most common source of peripheral arterial emboli, and mortality is usually related to underlying heart disease.

59. **The answer is B.** *(Chapter 56)* Atropine has no effect on the denervated heart because it acts by blocking actions of the vagus nerve. The response to catecholamines may be increased by upregulation of receptors in the denervated heart. The resting heart rate is usually between 90 and 100 beats per minute. The ECG often displays multiple P waves, from both the new heart and a residual portion of the original atria. Lifelong immunosuppression is mandatory to prevent rejection.

60. **The answer is C.** *(Chapter 56)* Although intravenous methylprednisolone is standard treatment for acute rejection, it should not be started without consulting the patient's transplant center. Every effort must be made to confirm rejection by endomyocardial biopsy because the severe immunosuppression of antirejection therapy may worsen infectious illnesses, including cytomegalovirus (CMV). Gastroenteritis and other illnesses may precipitate an episode of rejection by decreasing absorption of medications against rejection. The patient should receive antibiotic prophylaxis for any invasive procedure.

61. **The answer is D.** *(Chapter 54)* Most patients with intact aneurysms are asymptomatic. Even grossly obvious aneurysms are usually painless and nontender unless they are acutely or chronically ruptured. Tenderness is an indication for urgent surgical evaluation. Aneurysms larger than 5 cm are at risk for rupture, whereas aneurysms smaller than 4 cm rarely rupture unless they are saccular.

62. **The answer is E.** *(Chapter 54)* Unheralded syncope in an elderly patient, with new back or abdominal pain, is suspicious for acute rupture of an abdominal aortic aneurysm. Because the patient may suddenly become hypotensive, immediate surgical consultation and preparation for surgery is indicated. Aortography may be falsely negative, and the associated delay may be fatal. Likewise, delay for CT scanning may also result in death.

63. **The answer is D.** *(Chapter 54)* Tearing pain, pulse disparity, and hypertension make aortic dissection the most likely diagnosis. Emergency management includes reducing BP (with vasodilators such as nitroprusside), reducing shear forces of the aorta with β blockers, and testing to determine the extent of dissection. CT, aortography, magnetic resonance imaging (MRI), and transesophageal echocardiography have all been used successfully. Although testing protocols differ by institution and test availability, the goal is to determine the need for surgery. Dissections that involve the ascending aorta (Stanford type A) are usually best treated surgically, whereas dissections that involve only the descending aorta (type B) are managed medically unless major vessels or organs are seriously compromised.

64. **The answer is D.** *(Chapter 55)* Low levels of D-dimer can exclude DVT, but many other disorders can lead to elevation, including surgery, trauma, infection, and malignancy. An elevated D-dimer level should be further evaluated with one of the other tests. A single duplex ultrasound has a positive predictive value for DVT of 94 percent, and a positive impedance plethysmography (IPG) has 83 percent positive predictive value. Contrast venography is the traditional gold standard test, but it is invasive, painful, and sometimes causes iatrogenic venous thrombus. MRI is highly accurate and can visualize parts of the venous system not usually accessible, such as the calves and the pelvic veins. However, it is expensive, lacks portability, and many patients are excluded because of prosthetic implants.

65. **The answer is D.** *(Chapter 56)* Renal insufficiency is a common side effect of cyclosporine immunosuppressive therapy. Although rejection can be entirely asymptomatic, a variety of symptoms are possible. They include all of the classic signs and symptoms of CHF, nausea, vomiting, ascites, any type of dysrhythmia, and even circulatory collapse. Accelerated coronary artery disease in the transplanted heart is also thought to represent rejection, and it frequently leads to ischemia or infarction. Chest pain is an extremely uncommon symptom and does not correlate with myocardial ischemia.

66. **The answer is B.** *(Chapter 245)*   Although an increased pulse is worrisome, a "normal" HR does not rule out a serious disease process. The normal tachycardic response to pain and hypovolemia may be blunted or absent due to medications such as β blockers. Also, the heart becomes less sensitive to catecholamines with advancing age. Due to cerebral atrophy, increased space within the skull may delay presentation of intracranial hemorrhages. Although overall cervical spine fractures are less common with age, the incidence of C1 and C2 fractures increases.

67. **The answer is C.** *(Chapter 50)*   Despite widespread treatment of streptoccocal pharyngitis with antibiotics, rheumatic heart disease remains the most common cause of MVS. As in most valvular diseases, symptoms present in the fourth and fifth decades, and dyspnea on exertion is the most frequent presenting complaint. Associated syncope is uncommon, although it can be the presenting symptom for aortic stenosis or idiopathic hypertrophic subaortic stenosis (IHSS). Hemoptysis is the second most common presenting symptom for MVS, and usually manifests as pink frothy sputum, but sometimes as frank blood from dilated bronchial veins that rupture as back pressure from the stenosis increases. Longstanding MVS leads to a dilated left atrium and almost inevitably to atrial fibrillation if the stenosis is not corrected.

68. **The answer is C.** *(Chapter 50)*   The increased incidence of TIA in patients younger than 45 years who have MVP is thought to be secondary to sterile emboli from platelet and fibrin deposits on the defective valve. Sudden death is very rare in MVP, but is more likely if the patient presents with syncope or near syncope and ECG abnormalities. Only about 20 percent of patients with MVP have the classic mid-systolic click. Although most patients are asymptomatic, the incidence of MVP in the general population is 3 to 10 percent.

69. **The answer is D.** *(Chapter 50)*   The incidence of endocarditis in patients with isolated AS is only about 2 percent. Congenital bicuspid valve is the leading cause of AS, with rheumatic heart disease being the second, followed by degenerative calcification in patients older than 70 years. Dyspnea is the most common presenting symptom, followed by paroxysmal nocturnal dyspnea, syncope on exertion, angina, and MI. The angina experienced with AS is often due to a perfusion pressure phenomenon, with inadequate perfusion from the coronary vessels across the myocardium to the endocardium. LVH is the most common ECG finding.

70. **The answer is D.** *(Chapter 50)*   Patients with valvular heart disease are at increased risk for developing endocarditis. Prophylactic antibiotics should be administered before abscess drainage, urethral catheter placement (if there is a suspicion of infected urine), dental procedures, nasal packing, rigid bronchoscopy, cytoscopy, anoscopy, vaginal delivery, and abortion. Endotracheal intubation does not require prophylaxis.

71. **The answer is C.** *(Chapter 50)*   IHSS presents clinically about 10 years earlier than other valvular diseases and is a cause of sudden death among young athletes. Symptoms of IHSS may be decreased with squatting. MVP is a rare cause of sudden death.

72. **The answer is C.** *(Chapter 50)*   Afterload reduction is an important therapeutic intervention for most valvular emergencies. Its effect is to optimize forward-moving pressure gradients. In AS, however, vasodilating agents must be used with caution because they can decrease perfusion pressure across the thickened myocardium. Rate control is more important in these patients to maximize ventricular outflow and diastolic perfusion time.

73. **The answer is B.** *(Chapter 50)*   This is the typical presentation of a patient with hypertrophic cardiomyopathy: a familial disorder with asymmetric hypertrophy of the left ventricle, in particular the septal wall. The ECG shows Q waves with upright septal T waves, typical of the "pseudo-infarction" pattern. Chest pain is usually due to an imbalance between the oxygen demand of the hypertrophied myocardium and the available blood

flow. Tachycardia worsens the symptoms by decreasing diastolic coronary perfusion time, increasing the end diastolic intraventricular pressure. β Blockers are the intervention of choice. Nitroglycerin and CPAP would not be indicated because they decrease venous return and further compromise filling of the noncompliant ventricle. Dopamine would increase the incidence of dysrhythmias after a ventricular fibrillatory arrest.

74. **The answer is D.** *(Chapter 51)* Blind or ECG-guided percardiocentesis is associated with a 7 to 15 percent incidence of complications. These include tension pneumothorax, liver laceration, AV fistula, and laceration of the coronary or internal mammary vessels leading to MI or hemopericardium. Echocardiography is the guidance technique of choice in performing emergent pericardiocentesis because it helps identify the largest pocket of effusion. Left-to-right subxyphoid approach lowers the incidence of coronary artery laceration.

75. **The answer is E.** *(Chapter 51)* The patient's presentation is classic for acute percardial tamponade. He displays Beck's triad (hypotension, JVD, and muffled heart sounds), and electrical alternans, created by the heart swinging in the pericardial fluid. Differential diagnosis includes pulmonary embolism (PE), tension pneumothorax, AMI, myocardial contusion, and air embolism. Echocardiography is the diagnostic modality of choice because it can rule out constricting pericardial effusion, show increased right-sided pressures suggestive of PE, and detect wall-motion abnormalities associated with myocardial compromise. Treatment of pericardial tamponade includes intravenous fluids, oxygen, and pericardiocentesis. Dopamine may be helpful as a temporizing measure to elevate BP. Intubation and other forms of positive pressure ventilation are not recommended because they decrease venous return.

76. **The answer is C.** *(Chapter 51)* Although most cases of CM are idiopathic, patients should have a thorough work-up for all known causes. A history of hypertension, alcohol use, valvular disease, chemotherapy, or heavy metal exposure should be elicited. Treatment for dilated and restrictive CM is the same, but caution should be used in patients with amyloidosis because they may be prone to digoxin toxicity due to amyloid fibril binding of digoxin. The presence of fever and myalgias supports a diagnosis of myocarditis rather than CM.

77. **The answer is C.** *(Chapter 51)* Enteroviruses, especially cocksackie B, predominate as the causal agent in acute myocarditis. Adenovirus, influenza B, parainfluenza, mumps, CMV, hepatitis B, herpes, varicella, EBV, and HIV have also been implicated. Myocarditis is detected in 10 percent of routine autopsies and in up to 50 percent of AIDS patients' autopsies. Up to 40 percent of patients with acute cardiomyopathy and up to 63 percent of patients with chronic cardiomyopathy have histologic evidence of myocarditis. Histologic evidence includes myocardial necrosis, vacuolization, and lymphocytic infiltration. Cardiac function returns to baseline level in the majority of patients within weeks to months of the acute illness. Long-term prognosis is variable.

78. **The answer is C.** *(Chapter 51)* Acute myocarditis presents in previously healthy patients as a viral prodrome followed by dyspnea and tachycardia out of proportion to the fever. Other possible diagnoses in the described setting include PE, hyperthyroidism, toxins, and myocardial ischemia. Anxiety is a diagnosis of exclusion. Although all of the listed interventions should be considered, nitroglycerin is contraindicated in PE because it decreases needed preload, and β blockers or lorazepam could precipitate hypotension in a patient with acute myocarditis. Echocardiography would be the next diagnostic modality of choice in the work-up of this patient.

79. **The answer is A.** *(Chapter 51)* Acute pericarditis is not associated with dysrhythmias. If dysrhythmias are present, the patient should be assessed for underlying heart disease. Aspirin or nonsteroidal anti-inflammatory medications at high doses are the

treatments of choice for pericarditis, except in cases of uremic pericarditis with co-existing coagulopathy. Steroids and colchicine may also be used, but not as first-line agents. Echocardiogram should be performed in patients with evidence of pericardial effusion (electrical alternans or low-voltage ECG) to rule out impending tamponade or underlying myocarditis. Sixty percent of all patients experience complete recovery within 1 week and another 18 percent within 3 weeks. Pericarditis recurs in 20 percent of patients.

80. **The answer is C.** *(Chapter 51)* The ECG changes suggestive of acute pericarditis are uncommon in uremic patients because the epicardium is rarely involved. Pericardial friction rubs and pericardial effusions occur frequently. Uremic pericarditis is one of the most common causes of cardiac tamponade. Treatment consists of daily hemodialysis for 2 to 6 weeks. Hemodialysis-associated pericarditis requires a work-up for viral, bacterial, and tubercular causes. Aspirin and nonsteroidal anti-inflammatory medications should be used with caution.

81. **The answer is B.** *(Chapter 51)* ECG changes in acute pericarditis classically occur in three phases. In the first few days, diffuse concave ST elevation predominates, usually no greater than 5 mm, and is most prominent in the limb leads and in leads V_5 and V_6. In contrast to the changes seen with early repolarization, with acute pericarditis, the ST segments are usually greater than or equal to one-fourth of the amplitude of the T wave. PR segment depression is not associated with early repolarization. The ST elevations seen in acute pericarditis can be distinguished from those seen with AMI in that they are usually diffuse, concave, less than 5 mm, and unassociated with T-wave inversions. The second and third phases of ECG changes consist of normalization of the ECG followed by T-wave inversion with normal ST segments. In some cases, T-wave inversions persist indefinitely.

82. **The answer is C.** *(Chapter 50)* The correct combinations are 1 + 8, 2 + 7, 3 + 9, 4 + 6, and 5 + 10. MS spares the left ventricle, but inevitably causes left atrial enlargement, seen on ECG as biphasic P waves, especially in leads II and V_1. As disease progresses, pulmonary hypertension and right-sided failure develop and manifest as right-axis deviation. AS leads to LVH, often with left or right bundle branch blocks. Mitral valve prolapse is usually associated with a normal ECG. Acute inferior MI can cause ischemia of the papillary muscle and thus acute mitral insufficiency. Flash pulmonary edema in a patient with acute inferior MI should raise the suspicion of mitral insufficiency. IHSS usually involves asymmetric hypertrophy of the left ventricle and can show septal Q waves, with upright T waves and poor R-wave progression across the precordium on ECG. These changes are not related to coronary insufficiency and are known as a "pseudoinfarction" pattern.

83. **The answer is E.** *(Chapter 50)* Intraaortic balloon pumps are contraindicated in AI because they force blood back down into the open ventricle and cause further cardiac decompensation. Thrombolytics may be helpful in acute mitral insufficiency secondary to papillary muscle ischemia, as can be seen in inferior MI secondary to right coronary occlusion. Emergent surgery is the appropriate therapeutic intervention for acute left-sided valve insufficiency causing cardiac failure. Syncope secondary to aortic stenosis with minimal exertion usually indicates a critical valve stenosis (diameter < 0.5 cm) and merits recommendation for urgent surgical correction. Cardioversion should not be attempted for atrial fibrillation with MS because the dysrhythmia is usually longstanding and associated with a high thromboembolic risk.

84. **The answer is B.** *(Chapter 50)* This patient has pulmonary edema secondary to acute aortic insufficiency with the characteristic clinical findings of a wide pulse pressure and short upsweeping pulses. The most likely cause for acute cardiac failure in this febrile intravenous drug user is infective endocarditis leading to valve rupture. Concurrent with resuscitation, the most important action is to call a cardiac surgeon to perform

emergency valve repair. Furosemide and nitrates are helpful temporizing measures to reduce afterload and improve cardiac output. Blood cultures and empiric antibiotics are also indicated. Emergent echocardiography would be helpful to confirm the diagnosis while preparations for surgery are underway. Naloxone has no role, and an intraaortic counterpulsation balloon is contraindicated.

85. **The answer is B.** *(Chapter 50)* Fatality rates for left-sided disease are greater than those for right-sided disease because of the increased incidence of cardiac failure and neurologic complications. *Streptococcus viridans* is the most common organism implicated in left-sided endocarditis, with *Staphylococcus aureus* increasing in incidence. Enterococcal and fungal infections are also seen. Right-sided endocarditis is caused by *S. aureus* in more than 75 percent of cases, followed by *S. viridans* and gram-negative rods. Blood cultures should be drawn from three different venous sites and sent for aerobic, anaerobic, and fungal cultures. Antifungal agents should be considered in patients with HIV or other immunocompromised states or in patients with indwelling catheters. Murmurs are heard in only 35 to 50 percent of patients with right-sided disease but in up to 80 percent of patients with left-sided disease.

86. **The answer is B.** *(Chapter 50)* Because patients frequently present with nonspecific complaints, the diagnosis of subacute bacterial endocarditis is often missed. Malaise (95 percent) and intermittent fever (80 percent) are the most common complaints, followed by anorexia, weakness, and weight loss. Neurologic symptoms such as headache, personality change, altered level of consciousness, and focal deficits are seen in 35 to 40 percent of cases. Peripheral vascular lesions (e.g., splinter hemorrhages, Osler nodes, Roth spots, Janeway lesions, or petechia) are found in more than 50 percent of patients. Splenomegaly is seen in 25 percent of patients. Almost all patients have a murmur at some point during the disease. Subacute endocarditis is predominantly left sided.

87. **The answer is D.** *(Chapter 49)* The Framingham heart study reported a 50 percent mortality in 5 years for CHF patients, with half the population dying within the first year. ACE inhibitors have been shown to slow the progression of disease and improve function in CHF patients, but they have not decreased the frequency of sudden death. β Blockers are a useful adjunct in selected patients because they counteract the hyperadrenergic neurohumoral feedback seen in congestive failure.

88. **The answer is E.** *(Chapter 49)* This patient's most likely diagnosis is acute pulmonary edema (APE) status post anterior MI. He should receive aspirin, but β blockers should be avoided because the patient is in cardiogenic shock. Positive pressure ventilation by face mask (CPAP or BiPAP) or by endotracheal intubation enhances oxygenation of the compromised myocardium and helps decrease preload. Too much positive pressure must be avoided to not compromise cardiac output. Nitroglycerin decreases preload, relaxes the pulmonary vasculature, and augments coronary perfusion. Furosemide also helps decrease preload and afterload. Dopamine may be needed to maintain adequate SBP. Historically, morphine was thought to decrease afterload and pulmonary hypertension (through central sympatholytic mechanisms) but is now thought to work primarily through its sedative and anxiolytic effects to decrease cardiac demand. APE showing cephalization on chest x-ray is associated with a pulmonary wedge pressure (PWP) greater than 15 mm Hg; the presence of interstitial edema (Kerly B lines) correlates with a PWP of 19 to 25 mm Hg; and alveolar edema is associated with a PWP greater than 25 mm Hg.

89. **The answer is C.** *(Chapter 49)* Dobutamine produces a more favorable balance between myocardial oxygen supply and demand than does dopamine and is the drug of choice in normotensive patients with APE. Dopamine may be more useful in hypotensive patients. Nitroglycerin sublingual for the relief of APE symptoms is usually given at twice the dose of that given for angina (0.8 vs. 0.4 mg). Loop diuretics at doses of 1 mg/kg

should be administered to hypertensive patients with APE. Nitroprusside can induce ischemia in patients with coronary artery disease, and thus nitroglycerin is the vasodilator of choice, having both veno- and vasodilatory effects.

90. **The answer is D.** *(Chapter 52)* Pregnancy is considered a hypercoagulable state and thus a risk factor for DVT and PE. PE is the most common cause of nonsurgical maternal death in the peripartum period. Women older than age 40 years and of African descent are at highest risk. Thrombolytic therapy is indicated for treatment of massive PE with refractory hypoxemia and circulatory collapse. The use of thrombolytic agents has largely replaced thrombectomy, except in cases in which thrombolytic therapy is contraindicated. This patient is at risk for uterine bleeding because she is 4 days postpartum. Urokinase and streptokinase are less effective than r-tPA in improving symptoms. Heparin and LMWH are possible treatments for hemodynamically stable PE patients but would not be indicated in this scenario. Intrapulmonary artery infusion is no more effective than peripheral intravenous administration, and the risk of bleeding at the pulmonary catheter placement site is high.

91. **The answer is A.** *(Chapter 52)* Overall, $\dot{V}/\dot{Q}$ scanning is 98 percent sensitive but only 10 percent specific for the diagnosis of PE. A normal $\dot{V}/\dot{Q}$ can reliably rule out the diagnosis of PE. A low-probability scan with a low clinical suspicion has a predictive value of 96 percent for exclusion of PE, whereas a high-probability scan with a high clinical suspicion has a 96 percent positive predictive value. The difficulty in using $\dot{V}/\dot{Q}$ scan findings for the diagnosis of PE is the lack of a universal definition of "clinical suspicion." D-dimers are highly dependent on the assay used to measure them; some clinical trials have shown a high negative predictive value, but they have not yet become the standard of care.

92. **The answer is B.** *(Chapter 52)* PE is more common in men than in women before the age of 50 years, but this sex difference disappears with age. An intermediate $\dot{V}/\dot{Q}$ scan in conjunction with this high index of suspicion would merit anticoagulation. Risk of bleeding in this postsurgical trauma patient would need to be weighed against the benefits of heparinization. With this clinical presentation, a low-probability $\dot{V}/\dot{Q}$ scan does not obviate the need for further work-up. In addition to surgery as a PE risk factor, if the patient had an indwelling central venous catheter in the intensive care unit, he is at risk for upper extremity DVT. The next diagnostic test would be spiral CT, magnetic resonance angiography, or pulmonary arteriography. PE can induce the release of chemical mediators that cause bronchoconstriction.

93. **The answer is D.** *(Chapter 52)* PE presents with a syncopal episode up to 15 percent of the time. Altered mental status and generalized seizures may also be the presenting complaint, especially in the elderly. The most common presenting symptoms are chest pain and dyspnea (up to 85 percent); anxiety occurs in more than 50 percent of PE patients. Tachypnea (RR > 16) is seen in more than 98 percent of all cases, and tachycardia (resting HR > 100) is seen in up to 44 percent of all patients. Other signs are variable. The risk for embolism from proximal DVT is highest in the first week of its formation.

94. **The answer is A.** *(Chapter 52)* PE can be categorized as "massive" or "submassive." Massive PE presents with hypotension and hypoxemia, accounts for 5 percent of all cases, and is associated with a 40 percent mortality rate. Submassive PE presents with normal hemodynamics and hypoxemia. It carries a 2 percent mortality rate if treated appropriately; mortality rates increase to 20 percent if untreated. Only 40 to 50 percent of the pulmonary vasculature must be occluded for hypoxia and hypotension to manifest. However, patients with preexisting cardiac or pulmonary disease show signs of massive PE with lesser degrees of occlusion. ECG changes are seen in about 40 percent of patients with PE, most commonly nonspecific ST and T-wave changes. Other ECG changes include inverted T waves in the precordial leads, mimicking subendocardial infarct, new right-axis deviation or right bundle branch block, and an $S_1Q_3T_3$ pattern.

95. The answer is D. *(Chapter 255)* The correct combinations are: 1 + 9, 2 + 7, 3 + 8, 4 + 6, and 5 + 10. Doppler flow studies are a useful adjunct for ED evaluation of peripheral vascular integrity and disease. Normal arteries have a biphasic or triphasic waveform. Monophasic waveforms with each pulse indicate poor arterial flow and probable proximal arterial stenosis. These patients present clinically with a history of claudication. Monophasic flow that changes with respiration suggests detection of venous flow, and the probe should be repositioned to assess arterial flow. Flow during diastole heralds an arteriovenous fistula. Normal ankle brachial indices (ABIs) are greater than or equal to 1.0. ABIs less than 0.9 indicate arterial injury. With rest ischemia, ABIs are less than 0.5 and a vascular surgeon should be consulted. If the ABI is less than 0.3, a vascular emergency exists.

96. The answer is C. *(Chapter 57)* The role of nuclear imaging in risk stratification of patients with equivocal presentations is evolving. The two radioisotopes most widely used are thallium 201 and technetium-99m sestamibi (T99). Thallium 201 is a potassium cation analog that is taken up by active well-perfused myocytes during exercise. It redistributes to less well-perfused myocardium during rest and shows "cold spots" on imaging. T99 has higher energy photon emission and shows better contrast than does thallium, but does not redistribute and requires a second injection for the rest study. A nuclear study is an excellent diagnostic modality for patients with ECG changes that limit the usefulness of an ECG stress test (e.g., left bundle branch block, LVH, and concurrent digitalis therapy). The sensitivity of nuclear stress testing for coronary ischemia is greater than 85 percent versus only 60 to 70 percent for the ECG stress test.

97. The answer is B. *(Chapter 57)* Despite two sets of negative cardiac enzymes and a prolonged pain-free period, this patient needs to be risk-stratified for evidence of coronary ischemia. In patients with LVH and a possible strain pattern, ECG stress tests can be nondiagnostic. An echocardiogram can show wall-motion abnormalities in patients with nonspecific ECG changes but is unlikely to show a wall-motion abnormality in this patient in the absence of chest pain. A Holter monitor might pick up dysrhythmias but would not be the best test to evaluate for ischemia. Angiography is invasive and not generally used as the first line to evaluate for coronary ischemia in a pain-free patient.

98. The answer is B. *(Chapter 57)* Echocardiography is a useful adjunct in evaluating patients presenting to the ED with chest pain. The echocardiogram can detect wall-motion abnormalities indicative of ischemia or infarct, even in the presence of nonspecific ECG changes. Echo findings change the diagnosis of up to 18 percent of patients with nonspecific ECG changes. Normal left ventricular wall motion during chest pain suggests a noncardiac origin of the chest pain. Cardiac ultrasound is superior to clinical assessment of Killip classification and more accurate than ECG in predicting death and major complications. It may also detect areas of prior infarct, valvular abnormalities, intraventricular thrombi, signs of right-heart strain, and pericardial effusion.

DERMATOLOGIC EMERGENCIES

QUESTIONS

DIRECTIONS: Each question below contains five suggested responses. Select the **one best** response to each question.

99. All of the following have been associated with the development of Stevens-Johnson syndrome EXCEPT

(A) systemic steroids
(B) mycoplasma
(C) herpes simplex virus
(D) anticonvulsants
(E) a seasonal profile

100. Which one of the following statements is true about erythema multiforme?

(A) Steroids shorten the course of the disease
(B) Bullous skin lesions cause denudement of the skin
(C) Prophylactic antibiotics reduce the risk of infection
(D) Mucosal lesions can be maculopapular, urticarial, or target shaped
(E) Patients must be instructed to have a follow-up visit in 1 week

101. All of the following can be found in association with allergic contact (toxicodendron) dermatitis EXCEPT

(A) urticaria
(B) vesicles and bullae
(C) sparing of the palmar aspects and web spaces of the hands
(D) a linear pattern of erythema and papules
(E) a 3- to 5-day course for dermatologic manifestation

102. Clinical features of a disseminated gonococcal infection include all of the following EXCEPT

(A) an association with menses
(B) an association with pregnancy
(C) fever and multiple papular, vesicular or pustular lesions
(D) arthralgias
(E) treatment with oral ciprofloxacin is replacing the traditional use of intravenous ceftriaxone

103. All of the following are true about erysipelas EXCEPT

(A) facial and scalp manifestations occur in infants and the elderly
(B) it progresses to skin desquamation
(C) bacteremia common in the lower extremity manifestations
(D) fever
(E) a sharp well-demarcated edge

104. All the following statements are true about black widow spider bites EXCEPT

(A) Benzodiazepines are very effective in relieving symptoms
(B) The spider is not always black
(C) Antivenin is very effective in relieving symptoms
(D) The classic round ulceration with raised edges appears within 1 to 2 days after the bite
(E) The neurotoxin can cause a rigid painful abdomen, hypertension, shock, coma and muscle paralysis

105. All of the following have been associated with brown recluse spider bites EXCEPT

(A) a poor response to dapsone
(B) myalgias and arthralgias
(C) seizures
(D) hemolysis
(E) renal failure

106. All of the following are indicated in the treatment of scabies infestations in pregnancy and young children EXCEPT

(A) premethrin (Elemite)
(B) lindane
(C) calamine lotion
(D) 5 percent sulfur solution
(E) two or three applications 24 or 12 h apart, respectively

107. All the following statements are true about tinea capitis infections EXCEPT

(A) Topical antifungal therapy is ineffective
(B) Adenopathy is a common presenting complaint
(C) Antibiotics are required when a pustular "kerion" develops
(D) It is most common in children
(E) It requires a minimum of 6 weeks of therapy

DERMATOLOGIC EMERGENCIES

ANSWERS

99. The answer is A. *(Chapter 241)* Steroids have not been associated with Stevens-Johnson syndrome (SJS). Nearly 50 percent of cases of SJS are considered to be idiopathic. Implicated agents include mycoplasma, herpes simplex viruses, malignancies, and medications. Those medications include anticonvulsants and antibiotics. Cases commonly appear in the fall and spring.

100. The answer is B. *(Chapter 241)* Bullous skin lesions can be found in erythema multiforme. They cause denudement of the skin. Lesions are typically maculopapular, urticarial, target shaped, vesicular, or bullous. Mucosal lesions are typically vesiculobullous. Systemic steroids are controversial. They may provide symptomatic relief. However, they do not shorten the course of the disease. Antibiotic prophylaxis is not proven to be effective and can result in colonization by drug-resistant bacteria. Follow-up in less than 1 week is essential to monitor for the potential development of SJS. Topical steroids are used for symptomatic relief.

101. The answer is E. *(Chapter 239)* A 3- to 5-day course for the dermatologic manifestation is not typical of the disease. Mild cases typically last 7 to 10 days, whereas severe ones can require more than 3 weeks of therapy. Urticarial eruptions result from systemic absorption. Common manifestations include linear patterns, erythema, papules, vesicles, and bullae. Target lesions of erythema multiforme have been reported. Lesions on the hands typically are dorsal and spare the palmar aspect and web spaces.

102. The answer is E. *(Chapter 241)* Disseminated gonococcal infections should be treated with intravenous ceftriaxone or ciprofloxacin for 7 days. Oral outpatient management with ciprofloxacin is not an accepted standard of care for complicated cases of gonococcal infections. An association with menses, late pregnancy, and the immediate postpartum period is common. Fever, arthralgias, and multiple (10 to 20) papular, vesicular, or pustular lesions are classic features of the disease.

103. The answer is C. *(Chapter 238)* Erysipelas is a distinct *Streptococcus A* cellulitis. High fever is common. Bacteremia is also typically common except in lower extremity manifestations. Facial and scalp manifestations are predominately in infants and in the elderly. It progresses to skin desquamation during convalescence. A sharp well-demarcated advancing edge is distinctive.

104. The answer is D. *(Chapter 242)* The "bull's eye" pattern is found in cases of brown recluse spider bites and is not consistent with black widow spider bites. Erythema and swelling typically appear within 20 to 60 min after the bite. Pain and cramps begin 20 to 40 min later, locally and then generally. Symptoms typically resolve 2 to 3 days after the bite. Antivenin (Lyovac), benzodiazepines, and opiates are all very effective in relieving symptoms. However, antivenin is typically reserved for complicated cases, pregnancy, children, the cardiac patient, and the elderly. Being a horse serum preparation, antivenin therapy carries risks such as anaphylaxis and serum sickness. The spider is not always black; it has a classic orange-red hourglass-shaped marking. A rigid abdomen that mimics peritonitis occurs when abdominal wall muscles are involved. In severe envenomations, the powerful neurotoxin can cause hypertension, shock, coma, and muscle paralysis.

105. **The answer is A.** *(Chapter 242)* The venom in brown recluse spider bites includes proteases, hemolytic enzymes, and substances that affect coagulation and the complement system. Pain, myalgias, arthralgias, vomiting, seizures, hemolysis, and renal failure all have been described as manifestations of the bite. Dapsone is a leukocyte inhibitor and has been associated with preventing the progression of tissue necrosis. Patients must be closely monitored for side effects such as hemolysis and agranulocytosis.

106. **The answer is B.** *(Chapter 242)* Lindane and cromatiton are two scabicides with potential toxicity that should be avoided in pregnancy and young children. Premethrin (Elemite) and a 5 percent sulfur solution are used typically in two applications 24 h apart. A third application 12 h later can be also used. Calamine lotion is used after the treatment to alleviate the itching that may last a few more days.

107. **The answer is C.** *(Chapter 238)* Tinea capitis infections of the scalp require up to 6 weeks of oral antifungal therapy. Patients then should be reevaluated to assess the need for a longer course of therapy. Topical antifungal therapy is ineffective. Posterior cervical adenopathy, hair loss, and itching are common presenting complaints. A pustular "kerion" may develop and does not indicate a need for antibiotics. The disease is most common in children.

EMERGENCY MEDICAL SERVICES AND DISASTER MEDICINE

QUESTIONS

DIRECTIONS: Each question below contains five suggested responses. Select the **one best** response to each question.

108. Which of the following acts of Congress authorized the U.S. Department of Transportation to fund ambulances, communications, and training programs for prehospital medical services?

(A) 1966 National Highway Safety Act
(B) 1973 National Highway Safety Act
(C) 1966 Public Law 93-154
(D) 1973 Public Law 93-154
(E) 1965 EMS Act

109. Which of the following is NOT a component of "off-line" medical control?

(A) Protocol development
(B) Quality assurance
(C) Budget development
(D) Provider education
(E) Approval of medical devices used in out-of-hospital care

110. Approximately what percentage of an EMS system's volume deals with children 16 years or younger?

(A) 0 to 5
(B) 5 to 10
(C) 10 to 15
(D) 15 to 20
(E) < 2

111. Which of the following is a contraindication to the application of a femoral traction splint?

(A) Angulated tibia fracture
(B) Femur fracture
(C) Pelvic fracture
(D) Ankle fracture
(E) Severe head trauma

112. Which of the following statements regarding a two-member crew configuration of a prehospital helicopter is TRUE?

(A) The crew should consist of individuals with the same level of training so that scope and limitations of practice are clearly understood by each member
(B) Patient outcome is improved by using crews with a higher level of formal training
(C) A paramedic–paramedic configuration is the best choice because paramedics are most familiar with the prehospital environment
(D) A physician crew member is desirable but often impossible because of budget constraints
(E) Using a physician as one member of the crew has not been shown to improve patient outcome

113. Which of the following is FALSE regarding the use of helicopters in EMS?

(A) Ideally, the pilot should decide whether it is safe to fly before being told the nature of the mission
(B) Interfacility transfers are more than twice as frequent as scene responses
(C) Patients with injuries that could be exacerbated by low barometric pressure (with resultant barotrauma) are poor candidates for helicopter transport
(D) A helicopter needs a minimum of a 60-ft^2 landing zone
(E) Per patient mile, helicopters are safer than ground ambulances

114. You are asked to give a lecture to the paramedics about what they should consider when performing inter-facility transfers of neonates to a higher level of care. All of the following mechanisms for conserving body temperature are LESS effective in neonates than in adults EXCEPT

(A) shunting blood from the skin and periphery to the core
(B) increasing basal metabolic rate
(C) voluntary muscle activity
(D) shivering
(E) nonshivering thermogenesis

115. During the same lecture described in question 114, what fluid type would you advise the paramedics to use during transport of a neonate with a birth weight greater than 1000 g?

(A) Normal saline
(B) Half normal saline
(C) Lactated ringers
(D) 5 percent dextrose in water
(E) 10 percent dextrose in water

116. In preparation for interfacility transport, you decide to prophylactically intubate a critically ill child. Cuffed endotracheal tubes should NOT be used in children younger than which age?

(A) 15 years
(B) 10 years
(C) 7 years
(D) 5 years
(E) 3 years

117. Which of the following are phases to a disaster response according to the ACEP classification system?

(A) Activation
(B) Triage
(C) Recovery
(D) A and C
(E) All of the above

118. Which of the following is NOT one of the seven key functions of the Incident Command System (ICS)?

(A) Information officer
(B) Liaison officer
(C) Safety officer
(D) Finance section chief
(E) Triage officer

119. Which of the following statements is TRUE regarding the National Disaster Medical System (NDMS)?

(A) It deals strictly with civilian, not wartime, casualties
(B) It is a partnership between four federal agencies
(C) It was created in the early 1960s when policy makers realized the United States did not have a hospital bed system that could accommodate mass casualties
(D) It is an organizational arm of the United States Red Cross
(E) Patients are triaged to different hospitals under the direction of the state EMS medical director

120. What is the MOST common presenting complaint by patients at a mass gathering?

(A) Dermal injury
(B) Musculoskeletal injury
(C) Headache
(D) Abdominal pain
(E) Chest pain

121. Above which gestational age should premature infants generally be aggressively resuscitated?

(A) 24 weeks
(B) 25 weeks
(C) 26 weeks
(D) 27 weeks
(E) 28 weeks

122. Which of the following is TRUE regarding out-of-hospital cardiac arrest?

(A) The annual incidence of out-of-hospital cardiac arrest is about 1 per 100,000 in the United States
(B) Sudden cardiac death is the number one cause of out-of-hospital death in the United States
(C) Ventricular tachycardia is a positive predictor for survival of out-of-hospital cardiac arrest
(D) Cardiac arrest makes up approximately 20 percent of an urban EMS system's call volume
(E) Prehospital thrombolytic therapy after successful return of spontaneous circulation in a patient with ECG changes consistent with myocardial infarction improves patient outcome

EMERGENCY MEDICAL SERVICES AND DISASTER MEDICINE

ANSWERS

108. The answer is A. *(Chapter 1)* The 1966 National Highway Safety Act authorized the U.S. Department of Transportation to fund ambulances, communications, and training programs for prehospital medical services. In 1973, Public Law 93-154 was passed with the goal to improve emergency care and EMS on a national scale. This law identified 15 essential elements of an EMS system: (1) personnel, (2) training, (3) communications, (4) transportation, (5) facilities, (6) critical care units, (7) public safety agencies, (8) consumer participation, (9) access to care, (10) standardization of patients' records, (12) public information and education, (13) independent review and evaluation, (14) disaster linkage, and (15) mutual aid agreements.

109. The answer is C. *(Chapter 1)* The medical director is responsible for off-line (indirect) medical control. The major components of off-line medical control are (1) development of protocols for drugs and devices, (2) development of medical accountability (quality assurance), and (3) development of ongoing education. Budget development may be an administrative task of the service medical director, but it is not considered an off-line *medical* control component.

110. The answer is B. *(Chapter 4)* It is estimated that 5 to 10 percent of a system's volume consists of pediatric patients. The most common pediatric emergencies are trauma, respiratory emergencies, and seizures. Cardiac arrest in children is rare (approximately 1 per 10,000 children per year in the United States).

111. The answer is C. *(Chapter 2)* The femoral traction splint is the preferred device for immobilization of femur fractures. Traction is applied by using a hitch on the ankle that encounters resistance when the splint impinges proximally on the pelvis. These splints cannot be used if a pelvic fracture is suspected because pressure on the pelvis may further displace the fracture and increase bleeding. A hip dislocation is another contraindication to using a femoral traction splint.

112. The answer is E. *(Chapter 3)* Multiple configurations are possible for a helicopter medical crew. The most frequently used pairing is a nurse with a paramedic because of their complementary clinical skills. The literature does not support the belief that the addition of a physician to the crew leads to better patient outcomes.

113. The answer is C. *(Chapter 3)* Because helicopters generally transport patients at altitudes less than 3500 ft, low barometric pressure with barotrauma is usually not a factor. Mission patterns differ widely among flight programs, with the national average in 1997 for scene and interfacility flights being 30 and 70 percent, respectively. Although EMS helicopters have a crash rate exceeding that of non-EMS helicopters, it is probably true that, per patient mile, EMS helicopters are safer than ground ambulances. Pilots should assess the weather and other safety hazards independent of the nature of the mission so that they are not pressured to risk unsafe flights out of concern for the patient's condition.

114. The answer is E. *(Chapter 4)* Mechanisms for conserving body temperature include (1) shunting blood from the skin and periphery to the core, (2) increasing basal metabolic rate, (3) voluntary muscle activity, (4) shivering, and (5) nonshivering thermogenesis. Neonates have limited ability to maintain normal body temperature and should be transported in a "neutral thermal environment." Of the mechanisms listed, nonshivering thermogenesis is the only one that is as effective in neonates as in adults.

115. **The answer is E.** *(Chapter 4)*   Because of the risk of hypoglycemia, all neonates should receive glucose-containing fluids in preparation for and during transport. Ten percent dextrose should be used in infants with a birth weight greater than 1000 g. Five percent glucose is safer in smaller infants because of the risk of hyperglycemia with the more concentrated solution.

116. **The answer is C.** *(Chapter 4)*   Because the narrowest anatomic portion of the airway is below the cords in children younger than 7 years, cuffed endotracheal tubes should not be used in this population. In addition, the distance between the thoracic inlet and carina is extremely short in small children, so care must be taken to avoid a right mainstem intubation.

117. **The answer is D.** *(Chapter 5)*   The American College of Emergency Physicians (ACEP) describes three phases of a disaster response: activation, implementation, and recovery. The first phase, the "activation phase," has two components: notification and initial response, and establishment of an incident command post. The second phase is the "implementation phase" and consists of three components: search and rescue, triage with stabilization and transport, and definitive scene management. The third and final stage is the "recovery phase." *Recovery* refers to withdrawal from the scene and return to normal operations.

118. **The answer is E.** *(Chapter 5)*   The ICS is a nationally accepted management structure used to organize a disaster response. It was first used to respond to a series of wildfires in Southern California in 1970. There are seven key functions that the incident commander must manage. The typical organization of the seven functions is an information officer, liaison officer, and safety officer, all attached to the incident commander, plus four section chiefs for finance, logistics, operations, and planning. The triage officer would be located in a subfunction rather than in one of the seven top areas. ICS has the flexibility to expand or contract depending on the nature and magnitude of the disaster.

119. **The answer is B.** *(Chapter 5)*   The NDMS is a partnership between four federal agencies: the Department of Health and Human Services, Department of Defense, Federal Emergency Management Agency, and Veterans Administration. It was established in 1984 to address the need for a national system to provide hospital beds in the event of mass casualties resulting from war or a civilian disaster. The NDMS links the federal government with state and local agencies and private sector hospitals to address health and medical care needs after a catastrophic disaster. Part of its medical response component consists of disaster medical assistance teams comprised of civilian volunteers.

120. **The answer is A.** *(Chapter 6)*   Mass gatherings present unique challenges to emergency responders. Large numbers of people are located at a single site, making treatment and transportation difficult. The most common presenting complaint at mass gatherings is dermal injury, followed by headache, musculoskeletal complaints, and gastrointestinal complaints.

121. **The answer is A.** *(Chapter 4)*   Although the legal age of viability differs by state, an infant born at a gestational age of less than 24 weeks, weighing less than 500 g, and who has gelatinous skin and fused eyes is generally not viable. By contrast, infants born after 24 weeks of gestation are likely to have a relatively good outcome and should be aggressively resuscitated.

122.   **The answer is B.**   *(Chapter 1)*   Sudden cardiac death is the number one cause of out-of-hospital death in the United States. The annual incidence of out-of-hospital cardiac arrest is 1 per 1000. Ventricular fibrillation, not tachycardia, is a positive predictor for survival of cardiac arrest. Cardiac arrest comprises about 5 percent of the volume of calls in an EMS system. Studies of field administration of thrombolytic agents by paramedics have shown that it is feasible but does not improve outcome. However, equipping ambulances with 12-lead ECGs can decrease the time to ED treatment of thrombolytic candidates.

ENVIRONMENTAL EMERGENCIES

QUESTIONS

DIRECTIONS: Each question below contains five suggested responses. Select the **one best** response to each question.

123. All of the following are predisposing factors for hypothermia EXCEPT

(A) Wernicke's disease
(B) alcoholism
(C) hyperglycemia
(D) severe burns
(E) extremes of age

124. Which of the following statements regarding heat-related illness is FALSE?

(A) Adult patients with a core temperature of 40°C (104°F) require aggressive cooling measures
(B) Salicylate ingestion may induce hyperpyrexia
(C) Elderly and psychiatric patients are at increased risk for heat stroke
(D) The body acclimatizes to heat exposure by gradually decreasing the sodium and chloride concentration in sweat
(E) Oral rehydration inadequately compensates for fluid losses

125. All of the following are true of chemical burns EXCEPT

(A) acids cause deeper tissue injury than do alkalis
(B) most chemical burns should be copiously irrigated with water
(C) calcium gluconate is a specific antidote for hydrofluoric acid burns
(D) Neosporin ointment is useful for removing tar from skin
(E) time of exposure is the most important factor in determining the extent of tissue damage

126. Which of the following types of electrical injury is correctly paired with its resultant complication?

(A) Low-voltage alternating current (AC) and ventricular fibrillation
(B) lightning and ventricular fibrillation
(C) high-voltage AC and superficial burns
(D) lightning and compartment syndrome
(E) high-voltage AC and tetanic contraction

127. All of the following statements are true regarding cold-related injury EXCEPT

(A) chilbains (pernio) is more common in women
(B) dry heat is the best method for rewarming frostbite
(C) early surgical intervention is contraindicated for severe frostbite
(D) body parts affected by cold injury are more sensitive to reinjury
(E) trench foot may result in irreversible damage

128. What is the MOST common finding in a patient with a brown recluse spider bite?

(A) Severe itching
(B) Severe muscle cramps
(C) Anaphylaxis
(D) Local tissue necrosis
(E) Respiratory failure

129. A 25-year-old man complains of pain and swelling in the hand and forearm, perioral numbness, and vomiting after trying to catch a rattlesnake. Blood pressure is 90/60 mm Hg. All of the following are appropriate therapies EXCEPT

(A) fluid resuscitation
(B) administration of 10 vials of antivenin
(C) measurement of coagulation factors and platelets
(D) immediate fasciotomy of the arm
(E) pain medication

130. All of the following are signs and symptoms of acute altitude mountain sickness EXCEPT

(A) headache
(B) ataxia
(C) vomiting
(D) fatigue
(E) peripheral edema

131. A 22-year-old otherwise healthy diver sustains a wound while diving in the Gulf of Mexico and presents with a temperature of 100.6°F and a draining leg wound with surrounding warmth, redness, tenderness, and swelling. Which of the following antibiotics is LEAST appropriate?

(A) Ciprofloxacin
(B) Ceftriaxone
(C) Cefazolin
(D) Trimethoprim-sulfamethoxazole
(E) Cefuroxime

132. A 55-year-old male diver begins complaining of back pain and urinary retention 1 h after a dive. What is the MOST likely diagnosis?

(A) Barotrauma to the bladder
(B) Lumbar strain
(C) Neurotoxin from a marine envenomation
(D) Nitrogen narcosis
(E) Decompression sickness

133. Which of the following is LEAST important in the initial evaluation of a near-drowning victim?

(A) Arterial blood gas (ABG)
(B) Core temperature
(C) Chest x-ray (CXR)
(D) C-spine precautions
(E) Electrolytes

134. Which of the following patients require admission to a burn-care facility?

(A) A 35-year-old man with extensive partial-thickness burns on the back, shoulders, and buttocks
(B) A 60-year-old diabetic with a full-thickness burn of the entire forearm
(C) A 25-year-old woman with full-thickness burns of both hands and lower arms
(D) A 40-year-old house-fire victim with multiple, small partial-thickness burns and wheezing
(E) All of the above

135. All of the following are useful in determining the severity of radiation exposure EXCEPT

(A) time to development of nausea and vomiting
(B) lymphocyte count
(C) type of radiation exposure (e.g., γ vs. β)
(D) presence of skin erythema
(E) severity of symptoms

136. A 35-year-old man presents complaining of headache, weakness, nausea, and vomiting after working with paint remover in an enclosed space. Which of the following statements regarding management of this patient's problem is TRUE?

(A) A special antidote kit is required
(B) Carboxyhemoglobin level is not helpful in this case
(C) Treatment must continue longer in patients with this exposure than from other sources
(D) The patient's oxygen–hemoglobin dissociation curve is shifted to the right
(E) Severe metabolic acidosis may be present

ENVIRONMENTAL EMERGENCIES

ANSWERS

123. **The answer is C.** *(Chapter 186)* Hypoglycemia and Wernicke's disease may lead to hypothermia secondary to hypothalamic dysfunction. Other endocrine disorders such as hypothyroidism and hypoadrenalism predispose to hypothermia because of decreased metabolic rate. Severe burns and other dermal diseases may impair the ability of the skin to thermoregulate or prevent vasoconstriction. Patients at the extremes of age are more vulnerable to hypothermia. The use of any drug, including alcohol, that causes altered sensorium places a patient at higher risk for hypothermia.

124. **The answer is A.** *(Chapter 187)* Heat stroke is defined as a body temperature of greater than 40°C (104°F) accompanied by altered mental status and anhidrosis. Patients with heat stroke should be aggressively cooled to a temperature of 40°C (104°F), at which point cooling measures should stop to avoid overshoot hypothermia. Prognosis is related to the rate of cooling rather than to the initial temperature. Salicylates cause uncoupling of oxidative phosphorylation, which leads to increased heat production. Elderly and psychiatric patients are at increased risk for heat stroke because they are less likely to remove themselves from hot environments. Ingestion of psychiatric medications also increases susceptibility to heat stroke. The body is able to acclimatize to hot temperatures over time by various mechanisms including decreasing the concentration of sodium and chloride in sweat. In the acute situation however, the body is not accurately able to assess fluid losses and cannot compensate by oral rehydration. Athletes given free access to water when exercising in the heat will only drink 50 percent of their fluid losses.

125. **The answer is A.** *(Chapter 195)* Acids generally cause protein denaturation and coagulation necrosis that create a tough eschar, limiting the spread of the toxic compound. Alkalis cause liquifaction necrosis, allowing the agent to penetrate more deeply into the tissue and cause more extensive damage. The mainstay of therapy for all chemical burns is reducing the length of time of exposure to the compound by immediate copious irrigation with water. In addition, hydrofluoric acid burns should be treated with calcium gluconate. Neosporin contains plyuoxylene sorbitan, an emulsifying agent that is useful for removing tar.

126. **The answer is A.** *(Chapters 196 and 197)* The type of injury pattern from an electrical burn depends on the source: high-voltage AC, low-voltage AC, or lightning. The most common initial rhythm in cardiac arrest is asystole from lightning strikes and ventricular fibrillation from low-voltage AC. Low-voltage AC causes tetanic contraction of muscle and may cause victims to pull themselves closer to the source secondary by flexor muscle contraction. The immediate cause of death from high-voltage AC and lightning is apnea. Lightning causes superficial burns and a ferning pattern, whereas AC results in deep tissue burns and injury. Although minimal external signs of damage are present after this deep tissue injury, compartment syndrome requiring fasciotomy may develop. High-voltage AC is usually a single blast that throws the victim from the source. Lightning can also cause a blast effect.

127. **The answer is B.** *(Chapter 185)* Rapid rewarming is the primary therapy for frostbite. The injured part should be immersed in warm water (40–42°C). Dry heat from fires or car exhaust should be avoided because it may cause thermal damage in addition to the cold injury. Early surgical intervention is not indicated because the extent of injury is difficult to assess initially and areas of eschar may be protective to underlying healing tissue. Once affected by chilbains, frostnip, or other cold injury, the body part involved becomes more susceptible to reinjury. Trench foot develops from exposure to wet, cold, but nonfreezing conditions over hours to days. Early on, tissue damage is reversible but can become permanent if the foot is not removed from the cold environment.

128. **The answer is D.** *(Chapter 188)*   The brown recluse species (*Loxosceles reclusa*) is one of the most common types of spider in the United States. A necrotic wound that may take weeks or months to heal often follows a bite. Wounds may be resistant to treatment and result in long-term disability. Severe muscle cramping, particularly of the abdominal musculature, is the hallmark of black widow spider envenomation. Anaphylaxis may result from insect stings, the most common being from yellow jackets. Respiratory failure may result from anaphylaxis and rarely from black widow spider envenomation, but it is not common after brown recluse spider bite.

129. **The answer is D.** *(Chapter 189)*   The mainstay of treatment after rattlesnake bites is neutralization of the venom with antivenin. Large amounts of antivenin may be required. Coagulation factors and platelets should be checked in all snake-bite victims to help determine the severity of envenomation. Supportive care, including fluid resuscitation, is important for all patients with pit viper envenomation. If compartment syndrome is suspected, pressures should be measured. Fasciotomy should only be performed when compartment pressures remain above 30 mm Hg after medical treatment.

130. **The answer is B.** *(Chapter 191)*   Acute mountain sickness can occur at altitudes as low as 6900 ft (2100 m). Susceptibility differs by individual and is also influenced by rate of ascent, altitude of usual residence, and sleeping altitude. Signs and symptoms resemble those of an alcohol hangover and include headache, nausea, and fatigue or weakness. Patients may exhibit fluid retention and mild peripheral edema. The presence of ataxia suggests a more serious condition, high altitude cerebral edema (HACE). HACE may progress to coma and death if the patient does not descend quickly to a lower altitude.

131. **The answer is C.** *(Chapter 190)*   Infections from marine-acquired wounds require special care. The wound should be cultured for both aerobic and anaerobic bacteria, and antibiotic treatment should be initiated to include coverage for *Vibrio* species. This requires a second- or third-generation cephalosporin, ciprofloxacin, trimethoprim-sulfamethoxazole, or tetracycline. Fresh-water wound infections should be treated with antistaphylococcal and antistreptococcal antibiotics along with an aminoglycoside to cover *Aeromonas* species.

132. **The answer is E.** *(Chapter 192)*   Barotrauma is the most common affliction of divers and usually affects the ears, sinuses, lungs, and, rarely, the gastrointestinal tract. The bladder is not involved. Decompression sickness (DCS) is caused by formation of gas bubbles in tissues after ascent from a dive and results in vascular occlusion, usually in the venous circulation. DCS may have cutaneous manifestations including rash and pruritus. It classically causes joint and back pain and may be associated with neurologic symptoms secondary to spinal cord involvement. Patients with neurologic or other severe forms of DCS should be referred for hyperbaric oxygen therapy. Nitrogen narcosis is due to the anesthetic effects of breathing nitrogen at high partial pressures and causes divers to become altered on deep dives.

133. **The answer is E.** *(Chapter 193)*   Near-drowning victims require aggressive resuscitation and evaluation. A core temperature must be obtained because near-drowning patients are frequently hypothermic and require rewarming. Furthermore, hypothermic

patients in cardiac arrest should continue to be resuscitated until the core temperature reaches at least 30°C. CXR may demonstrate pulmonary edema but may be initially normal. Patients with a normal CXR may still be hypoxic, and oxygenation should be measured by ABG or pulse oximetry. Because many near-drownings occur secondary to trauma, all victims need their C-spines evaluated for injury. Electrolytes are rarely abnormal in near-drowning victims unless a large amount of salt-water has been aspirated.

134. **The answer is E.** *(Chapter 194)* Burn-center admission criteria include: patients 10 to 50 years old with partial-thickness burns over an area greater than 15 percent of total body surface area (TBSA) or full-thickness burns greater than 5 percent TBSA; any patient younger than 10 years or older than 50 years with partial-thickness burns greater than 10 percent TBSA or full-thickness burns greater than 3 percent TBSA; any patient with partial- or full-thickness burns to the face, hands, feet or perineum, or circumferential limb burns; a patient with burns and inhalation injury; and any patient with burns and underlying medical problems. Percentage of TBSA can be calculated in adults by the rule of nines by using the size of the back of the patient's hand as 1 percent or a Lund and Browder burn diagram. Children have a relatively larger head size and smaller legs.

135. **The answer is E.** *(Chapter 199)* Although severity of symptoms does not correlate with dose of radiation received, time to onset of symptoms does. Skin erythema indicates skin exposure greater than 300 rem (3 Sv); seizures occur with central nervous system exposure greater than 2000 rem (20 Sv). Lymphocyte counts greater than 1200/µL 48 h after exposure suggest good prognosis, counts between 300 and 1200 indicate fair prognosis, and counts less than 300 indicate poor prognosis. The type of radiation exposure is important in determining the severity of injury. γ Rays readily penetrate body tissues. α Particles do not penetrate skin, and β particles only barely penetrate the skin. Both α and β particles can cause damage if inhaled or ingested.

136. **The answer is C.** *(Chapter 198)* Carbon monoxide (CO) exposure occurs from many sources including fires, engines, home furnaces, and heaters. Methylene chloride, a chemical found in many paint removers, is inhaled and then converted to CO when metabolized by the liver. The elimination half-life of CO from methylene chloride is about twice that of inhaled CO because it is stored in tissues and gradually released. Carboxyhemoglobin levels guide therapy and may indicate severity of exposure. CO binds hemoglobin with a 250 times greater affinity than does oxygen. Therefore, all patients should be treated with 100 percent oxygen therapy. Once bound, CO causes the hemoglobin molecule to hold more tightly to oxygen at the other binding sites, thus shifting the oxygen–hemoglobin dissociation curve to the left. The presence of a high carboxyhemoglobin level and a severe metabolic acidosis should suggest concomitant intoxication with cyanide, as can commonly occur in house or industrial fires. CO alone does not cause a severe metabolic acidosis.

EYE, EAR, NOSE, THROAT, AND MAXILLOFACIAL EMERGENCIES

QUESTIONS

DIRECTIONS: Each question below contains five suggested responses. Select the **one best** response to each question.

137. A 23-year-old female presents to the ED complaining of 24 h of left eye irritation and redness. Physical examination shows normal visual acuity, pupillary action, and motor function. There are several patches of dark red blood scattered across the sclera. The patient denies any history of trauma. All of the following are important considerations in this setting EXCEPT

(A) hypertension
(B) coagulopathy
(C) ruptured globe
(D) incidental ocular trauma
(E) domestic violence

Questions 138–139.

138. A 30-year-old contact-lens wearer complains of 2 days of left eye pain and discharge with blurred vision. She immediately stopped using the contact lens at the onset of symptoms and began antibiotic drops left over from a previous eye infection. There is moderate conjunctival injection and a pinhole-corrected visual acuity of 20/40 on the left. Slit lamp shows an oval-shaped corneal abrasion with dense fluorescein uptake and a halo of white stromal infiltrate. The most likely infective organism associated with this disorder is

(A) *Herpes zoster*
(B) *Herpes simplex*
(C) *Pseudomonas*
(D) *Staphylococcus*
(E) *Candida albicans*

139. Appropriate management for the above patient may include all of the following EXCEPT

(A) culture of the corneal lesion
(B) frequent topical antibiotic therapy (every 12 h)
(C) cycloplegic drops
(D) pain control
(E) eye patch

140. A 65-year-old female arrives via ambulance minutes after accidentally instilling several drops of cyanoacrylate (SuperGlue) into the left eye. She mistook the tube of glue for the artificial tears she uses for dry eyes. The upper and lower lids are joined medially, and there is a large concretion of glue on the lateral corneal surface. All of the following are accepted treatments EXCEPT

(A) immediate copious water irrigation
(B) acetone soaks
(C) mineral oil
(D) mechanical debridement
(E) surgical debridement

141. A 15-year-old boy presents to the ED with a blunt injury to the right eye sustained in a brawl during school recess. He describes watery, clear discharge, photophobia, and a dull ache in the injured right eye. Physical examination shows 20/80 visual acuity correcting to 20/40 with pinhole. The right pupil is dilated and sluggishly reactive, but extraocular movements are intact. There is scleral and ciliary injection with moderate cell and flare in the anterior chamber on slit lamp examination. The MOST likely diagnosis is

(A) traumatic cranial nerve III palsy
(B) traumatic mydriasis with iritis
(C) conjunctivitis with traumatic lens dislocation
(D) conjunctivitis with iris sphincter rupture
(E) conjunctivitis with ruptured globe

Questions 142–143.

142. A patient presents to the ED complaining of mild pain with markedly decreased vision after blunt eye trauma. Physical examination shows 20/100 vision with pinhole, an afferent pupillary defect, and a meniscus of red cells in the lower portion of the anterior chamber. Treatment of this condition may include all of the following EXCEPT

(A) hospitalization for rest and elevation of the head
(B) atropine 1 percent topical eye drops
(C) topical prednisolone
(D) aminocaproic acid
(E) surgical wash out of the anterior chamber

143. Potential complications of the above disorder include all of the following EXCEPT

(A) rebleed in 2 to 5 days
(B) acute glaucoma
(C) cataract
(D) corneal staining
(E) optic atrophy

144. A 25-year-old male presents to the ED after being struck in the right eye with a fist. On examination of extraocular movement, you notice entrapment of upward gaze with diplopia. You make a clinical diagnosis of an orbital blowout fracture. While awaiting radiographic confirmation, each of the following physical findings could be anticipated EXCEPT

(A) anesthesia to the right anterior cheek
(B) orbital emphysema
(C) enophthalmos
(D) subconjunctival hemorrhage
(E) CSF rhinorrhea

145. Which of the following statements is TRUE regarding acute traumatic retinal detachments?

(A) Most detachments can be visualized on standard fundoscopy
(B) Eighty percent of detachments occur within 24 h of the traumatic event
(C) Most detachments originate in the inferotemporal quadrant
(D) Visual outcome depends on the extent of involvement of the optic disc
(E) Sudden onset of pain is a prominent feature

Questions 146–147.

146. A 62-year-old female with a medical history of hypertension, diabetes, and glaucoma complains of 1 day of sudden, painless loss of vision to the right eye. Physical examination shows only hand-motion visual acuity to the affected side. There is an afferent pupillary defect and absent red reflex on the right. You are unable to visualize the fundus. Slit lamp examination is normal. The MOST likely diagnosis is

(A) acute open-angle glaucoma
(B) optic neuritis
(C) vitreous hemorrhage
(D) central retinal artery occlusion
(E) central retinal vein occlusion

147. Which of the following would constitute the most appropriate management of this patient's condition?

(A) Pilocarpine, intravenous diamox, and urgent laser iridectomy
(B) Intravenous prednisolone
(C) Expectant management with delayed phototherapy
(D) Ocular massage
(E) Anterior chamber paracentesis

148. A victim of an assault with a baseball bat presents to the ED for evaluation. Assessment shows an obvious mid-face fracture and unstable mandible. The left eye is noted to be mildly proptotic with severe conjunctival swelling and a subconjunctival hemorrhage. The pupil is fixed and mid-point. Visual acuity is to count fingers only. Appropriate initial management would include all of the following EXCEPT

(A) broad-spectrum antibiotic coverage
(B) sedation and analgesia
(C) radiographic imaging via CT
(D) antibiotic ointment and gauze eye patch
(E) immediate ophthalmologic consultation

149. A 35-year-old mother of four children presents complaining of bilateral eye irritation, redness, and decreased vision of 2 weeks. She describes worsening symptoms despite having self-treated with over-the-counter eye drops. All four children are developing symptoms. Physical examination shows injected conjunctiva, tender preauricular nodes, and keratitis with subepithelial infiltrates. The MOST likely diagnosis is

(A) corneal ulcer
(B) *Herpes simplex* conjunctivitis
(C) *Herpes zoster* conjunctivitis
(D) *Staphylococcal* conjunctivitis
(E) epidemic keratoconjunctivitis

150. A 62-year-old male seeks medical attention for 5 days of unilateral eye redness, irritation, and decreased vision. On review of systems, the patient denies fever, weight loss, myalgias, or headache. Physical examination is notable for 20/100 vision on the affected side, injected conjunctiva, and more than one cell in the anterior chamber. Intraocular pressure is measured at 15 bilaterally. There is a small vesicle present at the tip of the nose. All of the following therapies are appropriate EXCEPT

(A) cyclopentolate drops
(B) acyclovir drops
(C) prednisolone drops
(D) Viroptic (trifluridine) drops
(E) ophthalmologic consultation

Questions 151–152.

151. A 75-year-old female with diabetes and hypertension complains of abrupt onset of right eye pain, blurred vision, unilateral headache, and mild nausea. Physical examination is notable for 20/200 vision on the right, conjunctival injection, and a cloudy, edematous cornea. Vision does not correct with pinhole. The pupil is midpoint and nonreactive to light. Slit lamp examination is negative for corneal staining. Which of the following tests would be MOST appropriate at this point?

(A) Erythrocyte sedimentation rate (ESR)
(B) Pupillary dilation and direct fundoscopy
(C) Orbital CT with 3-mm cuts
(D) Schiotz tonometry
(E) Intraocular ultrasound

152. The MOST appropriate initial therapy for this patient would include

(A) parenteral steroid therapy
(B) anterior chamber paracentesis
(C) pilocarpine ophthalmologic drops
(D) tropicamide ophthalmologic drops
(E) phenylephrine ophthalmologic drops

153. A 43-year-old African-American male presents with complaints of 2 weeks of progressive left eye pain, redness, and photophobia. He states that he has had several similar episodes in the past, all of which spontaneously resolved. Review of systems is positive for a recent diagnosis of restrictive lung disease but negative for joint pains, headache, or dysuria. Physical examination shows mildly decreased visual acuity and scleral injection greatest at the limbus. Slit lamp examination is notable for moderate anterior chamber cell and flare, a small hypopion, but no corneal uptake. The MOST likely underlying diagnosis in this patient is

(A) Reiter's syndrome
(B) rheumatoid arthritis
(C) HLA-B27
(D) sarcoidosis
(E) tuberculosis

154. A 25-year-old hockey player complains of 2 days of right eye blurred vision after catching an elbow to the face during a match. Physical examination shows a resolving periorbital ecchymosis. Visual acuity is 20/200 OD and 20/20 OS correcting to 20/20 bilaterally with pinhole. Fundoscopy and visual field examinations are normal. Which of the following conditions do you suspect?

(A) Acute posttraumatic cataract
(B) Retinal detachment
(C) Lens dislocation
(D) Hyphema
(E) Preexisting myopia

Questions 155–156.

155. A 71-year-old hypertensive male reports sudden painless loss of vision to the right eye beginning 20 min before. He experienced no headache, dizziness, chest pain, or syncope. Since his arrival to the ED, his vision has returned to normal. Physical examination shows 20/30 visual acuity bilaterally, normal intraocular pressure, and a quiet anterior chamber on slit lamp examination. Fundoscopy shows copperwire changes with few flame hemorrhages. The MOST likely etiology of this patient's disorder is

(A) central retinal artery occlusion
(B) central retinal vein occlusion
(C) temporal arteritis
(D) amaurosis fugax
(E) retinal detachment

156. Appropriate initial management for the patient above can include which of the following treatments?

(A) Ocular massage
(B) Parenteral steroids
(C) Anterior chamber paracentesis
(D) Antiplatelet therapy
(E) Laser retinal surgery

157. A 59-year-old male presents 4 h after experiencing an abrupt, painless loss of vision in the left eye. Physical examination shows severe visual impairment on the left, with light perception only, and an afferent pupillary defect. Fundoscopy is notable for a pale retina and a cherry-red–appearing macula. You make a diagnosis of central retinal artery occlusion. Regarding this patient, all of the following statements are true EXCEPT

(A) The cherry-red spot depicts localized retinal hemorrhage
(B) Urgent anticoagulation may be indicated
(C) Open angle glaucoma has been associated with this disorder
(D) Anterior chamber paracentesis may dislodge intraarteriole clot
(E) This patient has a poor prognosis, with a less than 10 percent chance for return of vision

158. A 47-year-old female presents with a 6-h history of sudden, painless visual loss to the left eye. Vital signs show a heart rate of 85 beats per minute, blood pressure of 180/110 mm Hg, and respiratory rate of 16 breaths per minute. Corrected visual acuity is 20/25 OD and 20/200 OS. There is an afferent pupillary defect on the left. The conjunctiva, sclera, cornea, and anterior chamber are normal. Fundoscopy shows macular edema and marked venous dilation with retinal hemorrhages in all four quadrants. The MOST likely etiology of this presentation is

(A) central retinal artery occlusion
(B) central retinal vein occlusion
(C) amaurosis fugax
(D) temporal arteritis
(E) malignant hypertension

159. A 22-year-old female complains of 1 day of dull right eye pain and blurry vision. Review of systems is positive for occasional double vision, and one episode of right-hand numbness the previous year which spontaneously resolved. The patient denies fevers, weight loss, or rash. Visual acuity is 20/100 OD and 20/20 OS. There is pain on range of motion in the affected eye. Conjunctiva, sclera, and slit lamp examinations are normal. Fundoscopy shows a swollen, hyperemic optic disc on the right side. What is the MOST likely cause of this disorder?

(A) Intracranial mass lesion
(B) Multiple sclerosis (MS)
(C) Orbital cellulitis
(D) Acute angle closure glaucoma
(E) Iridocyclitis

160. A 15-year-old male presents with no significant medical history and complains of right-sided headache, nausea, and fatigue. Before the onset of the headache, the patient experienced a large dark "hole" in his right visual field with adjacent bright flashing lights. All visual symptoms resolved with the onset of headache. Physical examination is notable for bilateral photophobia, normal visual acuity, and normal external eye and slit lamp examinations. The patient has a supple neck and nonfocal neurologic examination. The MOST likely etiology of the patient's symptoms is

(A) amaurosis fugax
(B) TIA
(C) subarachnoid hemorrhage
(D) retinal detachment
(E) ocular migraine

161. An 18-year-old male presents to the ED with his mother complaining of right-sided monocular blindness after being struck in the face by a younger sibling. Examination of the head and neck shows no obvious signs of trauma. Visual acuity is "no light perception" OD and 20/20 OS. Pupillary response is normal, and there is no afferent pupillary defect. Slit lamp examination and fundoscopy are normal. Neurologic examination is nonfocal. The most likely etiology of this patient's disorder is

(A) cortical blindness
(B) functional blindness
(C) retinal detachment with macular involvement
(D) vitreous hemorrhage
(E) traumatic lens dislocation

162. A patient presents with a bilateral homonymous quadranopsia involving the right upper visual field. Which of the following represents the MOST likely anatomic location of the abnormality?

(A) Prechiasmal, right side
(B) Optic chiasm
(C) Postchiasmal, prethalamic, left side
(D) Occipital lobe, right side
(E) Occipital lobe, left side

163. All of the following statements regarding acute angle closure glaucoma are true EXCEPT

(A) It is the most common form of glaucoma
(B) It may be precipitated by emotional upset
(C) It has been associated with certain over-the-counter medications
(D) It may be treated with laser iridectomy
(E) It may result in abdominal pain, nausea and vomiting

164. All of the following statements regarding the ED use of topical ophthalmic steroids are true EXCEPT that topical steroids

(A) can exacerbate ocular *Herpes simplex* infections
(B) are often prescribed for ocular *Herpes zoster* infections
(C) improve symptoms in cases of traumatic iritis
(D) may result in cataract formation
(E) are therapeutic in cases of allergic conjunctivitis

165. All of the following patients are at risk for necrotizing external otitis EXCEPT

(A) AIDS patients
(B) cancer patients
(C) diabetics
(D) elderly patients
(E) swimmers

166. Bullous myringitis is commonly related to which organism?

(A) *Haemophilus influenzae*
(B) *Moraxella catarrhalis*
(C) *Mycobacterium tuberculosis*
(D) *Mycoplasma pneumoniae*
(E) *Pseudomonas aeruginosa*

167. Which of the following is NOT associated with acute mastoiditis?

(A) Bezold abscess
(B) Facial palsies
(C) Hearing loss
(D) Meningitis
(E) Normal tympanic membrane in 30 percent of cases

168. Which of the following is the most likely pathogen in a patient with mastoiditis of more than 3 months?

(A) *Haemophilus influenzae*
(B) *Bacteroides* species
(C) *Mycoplasma pneumoniae*
(D) *Moraxella catarrhalis*
(E) *Pseudomonas* species

169. What is the most common cause of hearing loss in a previously healthy patient?

(A) Barotrauma
(B) Cerumen impaction
(C) Neuronitis
(D) Otitis media
(E) Tympanic membrane perforation

170. In the absence of a foreign body in the external auditory canal, which of the following is the most common cause of unilateral sensory hearing loss?

(A) Acoustic neuroma
(B) Autoimmune disorders
(C) Meniere's disease
(D) Pharmacologic ototoxicity
(E) Viral neuronitis

171. Tympanic membrane perforations occur in all of the following conditions EXCEPT

(A) barotrauma
(B) direct trauma
(C) lightning strike
(D) mandible fracture
(E) otitis media

172. What is the most common form of barotrauma in recreational scuba divers?

(A) Barotitis media
(B) Canal squeeze
(C) Eustachian barotrauma
(D) Inner ear barotrauma
(E) Auricular barotrauma

173. Which of the following is NOT a predisposing factor for epistaxis?

(A) Cocaine use
(B) Hypertension
(C) Infection
(D) Peptic ulcer disease
(E) Uremia

174. All of the following are important questions to ask a patient with acute epistaxis EXCEPT

(A) Is there a history of drug use?
(B) How long has there been bleeding?
(C) Is there ear pain?
(D) Is there a history of liver disease?
(E) Is there a sensation of blood in the back of the throat?

175. All of the following are accepted methods of controlling anterior epistaxis EXCEPT

(A) direct cautery of a bleeding vessel
(B) nasal packing
(C) embolization
(D) direct pressure
(E) application of vasoconstrictive agents

176. Complications of epistaxis controlled with anterior nasal packing include all of the following EXCEPT

(A) anemia
(B) dislodgment
(C) sinusitis
(D) toxic shock syndrome
(E) vertigo

177. A posterior source of epistaxis should be suspected in all of the following conditions EXCEPT

(A) bleeding from both nares
(B) epistaxis with associated presyncope or syncope
(C) presence of foreign body
(D) no anterior source
(E) sensation of blood down back of throat

178. Which type of force is most likely to cause a nasal bone fracture?

(A) Barotrauma
(B) Frontal
(C) Inferior to superior
(D) Lateral
(E) Superior to inferior

179. Complications of nasal trauma include all of the following EXCEPT

(A) avascular necrosis of the nasal septum
(B) extraocular movement dysfunction
(C) fracture of the cribriform plate
(D) saddle deformity
(E) septal hematoma

180. Clinical features suggestive of nasal foreign body in children include all of the following EXCEPT

(A) persistent foul-smelling rhinorrhea
(B) persistent unilateral epistaxis
(C) recurrent unilateral epistaxis
(D) recurrent unilateral otitis media
(E) unilateral sensation of nasal obstruction

181. Common bacterial pathogens that produce acute sinusitis include all of the following EXCEPT

(A) *Haemophilus* species
(B) *Bacteroides* species
(C) *Moraxella* species
(D) *Streptococcal* species
(E) *Staphylococcal* species

182. All of the following are complications of sinusitis EXCEPT

(A) facial cellulitis
(B) mastoiditis
(C) periorbital cellulitis
(D) Pott's Puffy tumor
(E) subdural empyema

183. Signs and symptoms associated with mandibular fractures include all of the following EXCEPT

(A) deformity of the dental arch
(B) limited range of motion
(C) mental nerve anesthesia
(D) subconjunctival hemorrhage
(E) sublingual hematoma

184. Which area of the mandible is MOST commonly fractured?

(A) Angle
(B) Condyle
(C) Molar
(D) Mental
(E) Symphysis

185. Which of the following is the LEAST likely clinical feature of a zygomatic–maxillary complex (ZMC) fracture?

(A) Diplopia
(B) Epistaxis
(C) Facial emphysema
(D) Mental nerve anesthesia
(E) Subconjunctival hemorrhage

186. What is the MOST common finding after orbital floor fracture?

(A) Corneal abrasion
(B) Diplopia
(C) Epistaxis
(D) Retinal detachment
(E) Sinusitis

187. Which of the following maxillofacial fractures extends bilaterally through the frontozygomatic suture lines?

(A) LeForte I
(B) LeForte II
(C) LeForte III
(D) Mandibular fracture
(E) Pyramidal fracture

188. Which of the following fractures is MOST commonly associated with CSF rhinorrhea?

(A) LeForte I
(B) LeForte II
(C) LeForte III
(D) Pyramidal fracture
(E) ZMC fracture

189. After a mandible dislocation, in which direction is the condyle of the mandible MOST commonly displaced relative to the temporomandibular joint (TMJ) fossa?

(A) Anteriorly
(B) Laterally
(C) Medially
(D) Posteriorly
(E) Posterolaterally

190. Symptoms of TMJ syndrome (myofascial pain dysfunction) include all of the following EXCEPT

(A) bruxism
(B) crepitus
(C) dysphonia
(D) earache
(E) tinnitus

191. All of the following are causes of sialoadenitis EXCEPT

(A) diabetes
(B) irradiation
(C) paramyxovirus
(D) phenothiazines
(E) uremia

192. In which of the following glands does sialolithiasis (salivary calculi) MOST frequently occur?

(A) Lacrimal
(B) Meibomian
(C) Parotid
(D) Sublingual
(E) Submandibular

193. Classic symptoms of peritonsillar abscess (PTA) include all of the following EXCEPT

(A) drooling
(B) muffled voice
(C) sore throat
(D) stridor
(E) trismus

194. In which age group is retropharyngeal abscess MOST likely to occur?

(A) in those 1 to 5 years old
(B) in those 5 to 10 years old
(C) in those 10 to 15 years old
(D) in those 15 to 25 years old
(E) in those older than 60 years

195. All of the following are commonly seen in Ludwig's angina EXCEPT

(A) decreased neck motion
(B) drooling
(C) dysphagia
(D) palpable fluctuance
(E) trismus

196. Each of the following is associated with Ludwig's angina EXCEPT

(A) age between 20 and 60 years
(B) chronic alcoholism
(C) diabetes mellitus
(D) female sex
(E) systemic lupus erythematosus (SLE)

EYE, EAR, NOSE, THROAT, AND MAXILLOFACIAL EMERGENCIES

ANSWERS

137. **The answer is C.** *(Chapter 230)* This patient has a subconjunctival hemorrhage. Symptoms are typically limited to minor irritation and eye watering, with an otherwise normal physical examination. The cause is usually minor ocular trauma that may have been inconsequential to the patient. Domestic violence is always a concern. Sneezing and violent coughing are also associated with this disorder. More serious nontraumatic causes include hypertension and coagulation disorders. Ruptured globe often presents with a subconjunctival hemorrhage, but other features such as decreased visual acuity, pain, and abnormal intraocular pressure dominate the clinical picture.

138–139. **The answers are C and E, respectively.** *(Chapter 230)* Contact-lens–related disorders can range from simple conjunctivitis to keratitis, corneal abrasion, and even corneal ulcer. This patient presents with eye pain, redness, and decreased visual acuity. The white haze around the abrasion represents white cell infiltration and confirms the diagnosis of corneal ulcer. *Pseudomonas* is the leading organism in contact-lens–related bacterial ulcers and can devastate a cornea in 24–48 h. Treatment includes all of the stated items except an eye patch, which is contraindicated because it may worsen the underlying infection or retard healing.

140. **The answer is B.** *(Chapter 230)* Cyanoacrylate-based glues form strong tissue bonds within seconds of application. The small tubular dispensers resemble many ophthalmologic medications, leading to accidental exposures. Physician use of tissue adhesives for wound closure may become a new source of risk. Although acetone and ethanol/water mixtures can dissolve glue on normal skin, these substances are extremely toxic to the eye and must be avoided. Mineral oil may soften the glue enough to allow separation of the lids. Mechanical or surgical debridement is usually necessary to remove glue from the cornea. A corneal abrasion typically results, which can be treated in the usual fashion.

141. **The answer is B.** *(Chapter 230)* There are a number of potential consequences to blunt eye trauma. The constellation of eye pain, photophobia, ciliary injection, and anterior chamber cell and flare is strongly suggestive of traumatic iritis. Furthermore, the ciliary body may respond to blunt trauma with either spasm and constriction (traumatic miosis) or dilation and cycloplegia (traumatic mydriasis), as demonstrated in this case. Cranial nerve III palsy is an unlikely result of blunt eye trauma, particularly if extraocular movements are intact. *Iris sphincter rupture* refers to small rents in the margin of the iris, resulting in a triangular notch in the border of the pupil.

142–143. **The answers are A and C, respectively.** *(Chapter 230)* The condition described is a hyphema: blood in the anterior chamber resulting from a rupture of one or more iris stromal vessels. Severity of the bleed can vary from minor hemorrhage visible only on slit lamp to the "8-ball" hyphemas in which the anterior chamber is filled with clot. Between 8 and 33 percent of patients experience a rebleed usually after 2 to 5 days, which is invariably worse than the original event. Potential complications include acute and chronic glaucoma related to occlusion of the trabeculae, corneal staining, and optic atrophy. Cataracts may occur after blunt eye trauma, but this is independent of the hyphema. Treatment centers on the prevention of rebleeding (bed rest and aminocaproic acid) and patient comfort (cycloplegics, prednisolone). Studies have debunked the practice of routine hospitalization after finding no difference in outcome between treatment and control groups. Daily intraocular pressure monitoring is nevertheless recommended to assess for developing glaucoma.

144. The answer is E. *(Chapter 230)* The orbital blowout fracture results from the transmission of a sudden rise in intraorbital pressure downward through the thin orbital floor into the maxillary sinus. Subsequent prolapse of the inferior rectus muscle, orbital fat, and connective tissue may result in enophthalmos and diplopia because of the restricted upward gaze. There can be compression of the infraorbital branch of cranial nerve V-2, resulting in anesthesia to the cheek and upper lip. Communication with the air-containing maxillary sinus permits the development of orbital emphysema, particularly after a sneeze or blowing one's nose. Subconjunctival hemorrhage is common, but cerebrospinal fluid (CSF) rhinorrhea has not been described with this fracture.

145. The answer is C. *(Chapter 230)* The typical retinal detachment is heralded by painless flashes of light, floaters, and a shade across the visual field. Interestingly, most detachments follow a latent period, up to 8 months posttrauma in 50 percent of cases. Detachments begin as small tears in the ora serrata (called dialysis), most frequently affecting the inferotemporal quadrant, followed by the superonasal quadrant. Because most detachments are very peripherally situated on the retina, standard fundoscopy is typically inadequate for visualization. Although a number of techniques have been developed to correct the detachment, visual outcome remains largely determined by the degree of macular involvement.

146–147. The answers are C and C, respectively. *(Chapter 230)* Diabetic retinopathy carries a risk of spontaneous vitreous hemorrhage. The bleed may range from minor, with symptoms limited to a few floaters, to severe, with painless loss of vision, a dark pupil, and absent red reflex. This latter finding and absence of pain are the keys to diagnosing this condition and would not be expected in any of the other disease processes listed. Treatment is expectant. Once the vitreous clears, the patient can undergo photocoagulation therapy to prevent future hemorrhage.

148. The answer is D. *(Chapter 230)* This case scenario should suggest two likely diagnoses: ruptured globe and retroorbital hematoma. The differentiation between these two entities may be difficult on purely clinical grounds. Both are characterized by pain, visual and pupillary defects, marked conjunctival swelling (chemosis), and occasionally proptosis. The management keys are to provide comfort for the patient, advance the work up (CT, computed tomography), and avoid worsening the condition through secondary trauma. This last comment is particularly directed at ruptured globes, where all pressure on the eye must be meticulously avoided to prevent extrusion of intraocular contents and permanent loss of vision. A metallic shield should be placed over the eye instead of the usual compressive two-gauze eye patch.

149. The answer is E. *(Chapter 230)* Epidemic keratoconjunctivitis is a highly contagious form of viral conjunctivitis. It is characterized by rapid spread through contact groups, tender preauricular adenopathy, keratitis with subepithelial infiltrates, and an unusually long course (2–3 weeks). Differential diagnosis includes contact conjunctivitis, episcleritis, and atypical viral conjunctivitis. Treatment is symptomatic, but occasionally antibiotics are given to avoid secondary infection.

150. The answer is D. *(Chapter 230)* The presence of a nasal vesicle and eye pain strongly suggest *Herpes zoster* with ocular involvement via the shared nasociliary branch of the trigeminal nerve. Virtually any part of the eye may be affected including the lids, conjunctiva, cornea, ciliary body, or extraocular muscles. Treatment is directed at control of symptoms: topical prednisolone to decrease inflammation, cycloplegic drops to reduce spasm, and acyclovir to reduce the length and severity of infection. Viroptic, which is typically used for *Herpes simplex* infections, is ineffective against *Herpes zoster*.

151–152.   The answers are D and C, respectively.   *(Chapter 230)*   The constellation of signs and symptoms demonstrated by this patient is highly suggestive of acute angle closure glaucoma. These patients typically present with eye pain, headache, a fixed midpoint pupil, an edematous cornea, and decreased vision. Elevated intraocular pressure as measured by Schiotz tonometer, a TonoPen, or an applanation tonometric device secures the diagnosis. This disorder occurs in anatomically susceptible patients who have small or shallow anterior chambers. There is an increased resistance to the flow of aqueous humor from the posterior to the anterior chamber, resulting in intraocular hypertension. Attacks are often precipitated by conditions that result in pupillary dilatation: prolonged exposure to dim light or the use of anticholinergic or sympathomimetic agents.

Therapy of acute angle closure is two pronged: (1) increase the flow of aqueous through the trabecular meshwork and (2) decrease the overall production of aqueous. Cholinergic agents such as pilocarpine cause miosis that in turn creates a more favorable angle for aqueous flow. β-Adrenergic agents (timolol) decrease aqueous production, and acetazolamide and mannitol, both diuretic agents, decrease total intraocular volume. Mydriatic agents must be avoided because they may worsen already compromised flow through the narrowed angle.

153.   The answer is D.   *(Chapter 230)*   The patient's ophthalmologic disorder is most consistent with anterior uveitis, also known as iritis. Pain and photophobia with an active anterior chamber sediment (cell, flare, or hypopion) is characteristic of this disorder. Uveitis is often a response to some underlying inflammatory condition, and a major goal of management is to explore the broad differential. All of the listed items have been associated with uveitis. However, based on the patient's sex, race, and recent diagnosis of restrictive lung disease, sarcoidosis is the most likely culprit.

154.   The answer is C.   *(Chapter 230)*   The key to this problem is realizing that the patient's poor visual acuity resolves with pinhole, implying a pure refractive error. This leaves essentially two possibilities: lens dislocation and myopia. The acute onset of symptoms and severity of the visual impairment support the diagnosis of lens dislocation. Partial lens dislocation may also occur, resulting in the unusual symptom of unilateral diplopia. Surgery is required for lens removal and replacement with an implant.

155–156.   The answer is D for both questions.   *(Chapter 230)*   Amaurosis fugax describes a condition of transient, monocular, graying or blurring of all or part of the visual field. The pathophysiology is similar to transient ischemic attacks (TIAs) of the cerebral circulation and involves the obstruction of retinal arterioles by cholesterol or fibrin platelet emboli. Cholesterol emboli, also called Hollenhorst plaques, typically arise from atherosclerotic disease of the carotid artery and may presage future strokes. They are occasionally visible on fundoscopy as small refractile bodies within a retinal vessel. The key to diagnosis is the transient nature of the symptoms. Management should focus on investigation and remedy of the source of the emboli and stroke prevention, typically with antiplatelet drugs.

157.   The answer is A.   *(Chapter 230)*   Central retinal artery occlusion (CRAO) is a true ophthalmologic emergency relating to obstructed blood supply to the retina. Reestablishment of retinal circulation must be accomplished within 90 min of symptom onset. Persistent visual loss beyond 2 h offers little hope for recovery. Therapeutic interventions focus on dislodging and dissolving the clot and include (1) anterior chamber paracentesis, which may decompress the eye and dislodge the clot, (2) intermittent (on and off) ocular massage, (3) inhalation of carbon dioxide, which causes retinal artery dilation and an improved perfusion gradient, and (4) acute anticoagulation. CRAO has been associated with hypertension, diabetes, vascular disease, sickle cell anemia, and glaucoma. The *cherry-red spot* refers to the macula, which has an alternate blood supply and appears bright red against the pale background of the ischemic retina.

158. The answer is B. *(Chapter 230)* Central retinal vein occlusion distinguishes itself from other causes of painless monocular vision loss with its characteristic fundoscopic findings. Retinal vein dilation and diffuse hemorrhages, sometimes described as "blood and thunder," contrast markedly with the pale retina of central artery occlusion or the relatively normal-appearing fundi of temporal arteritis and amaurosis fugax. Malignant hypertension can produce similar appearing flame hemorrhages, but the process is invariably bilateral, and the visual impact tends to be less marked.

159. The answer is B. *(Chapter 230)* This patient has optic neuritis, defined as inflammation or demyelination of any portion of the optic nerve. Classic signs and symptoms include visual loss of variable severity and dull eye pain that typically is worse with eye movement. Patients also describe a dimness to their vision and a loss of color intensity. When the optic disc is involved, it appears swollen and hypervascular. Causes include MS, Lyme disease, lupus, sarcoid, syphilis, and toxin exposure. Optic neuritis is a classic first presentation of MS as is diplopia because of lesions of the medial lateral fasciculus. This patient's age and prior neurologic symptoms support the diagnosis of MS.

160. The answer is E. *(Chapter 230)* This patient is describing a classic, prodromal aura of migraine headaches. Typical aura symptoms precede the headache, last 10–15 min, and consist of a wide range of photoimagery: scotomas, scintillations, flashing lights, and even visual hallucinations. Although amaurosis fugax and TIA can present with scotoma, these are unlikely to occur in this age group or in association with headache. Retinal detachment would not resolve with time, and subarachnoid hemorrhage, although still a consideration, should have meningismus and no aura.

161. The answer is B. *(Chapter 230)* Patients with functional blindness fall into two categories: hysterical conversion reaction and malingering. "No light perception" vision in the setting of a normal pupillary response and an absent afferent pupillary defect strongly suggest functional blindness. Cortical visual tracts can be tested by eliciting optokinetic nystagmus. This is an involuntary reflex in which the affected eye tracks objects moving in a horizontal direction, e.g., a tape measure moving back and forth or a spinning top with painted vertical lines. Cortical blindness can occur with bilateral occipital infarction (unlikely in this patient).

162. The answer is E. *(Chapter 230)* Homonymous visual field cuts imply a postchiasmal location of the abnormality because this is the first point where fibers from the same visual field of both eyes join. Fibers further divide between the thalamus and occipital lobe into upper and lower quadrant visual fields. The most common location for quadranopsia defects is the occipital lobe. Stroke, tumor, and atypical migraine may present with quadranopsia. Visual fields are named from the perspective of the patient, i.e., the right visual field corresponds to the left side of the retina. Therefore, a right-sided visual field cut involves the left-sided neurologic tracks.

163. The answer is A. *(Chapter 230)* Primary open angle glaucoma is the most common form of glaucoma, accounting for more than 90 percent of cases. It is currently the leading cause of blindness in the United States. Attacks of closed angle glaucoma are precipitated by events resulting in prolonged pupillary dilatation: dimly lit rooms, anticholinergic and sympathomimetic medications, and emotional upset that can produce increased adrenergic outflow. Headache, nausea, and abdominal pain may be more pronounced in presenting symptoms than eye complaints. Laser iridectomy represents definitive therapy.

164. The answer is D. *(Chapter 230)* Cataract formation is a complication of prolonged steroid use. The short-term limited use of topical steroids in the ED does not pose a risk for cataracts. Use of steroids in *Herpes simplex* infections must be avoided all costs. However, their use in a variety of inflammatory conditions such as iritis, *Herpes zoster* reactivations, or allergic conjunctivitis can be highly beneficial.

165. The answer is E. *(Chapter 231)* Necrotizing external otitis, also called malignant external otitis, is a dreaded progression of otitis externa. This disease requires aggressive treatment with anti-pseudomonal antibiotics. Eighty to ninety percent of cases occur in elderly, diabetic patients, with the remainder in debilitated or immunocompromised hosts. Swimmers commonly contract a benign, self-limited form of otitis externa.

166. The answer is D. *(Chapter 231)* Bullous myringitis is commonly associated with *Mycoplasma pneumoniae* infection. It is a variant of acute otitis media, in which bullae or vesicles are visualized on the tympanic membrane. These blebs resolve spontaneously and require no specific therapy. Therapy of acute otitis media with bullous myringitis consists of antipyretics, analgesics, and antibiotics directed at *Mycoplasma* species.

167. The answer is E. *(Chapter 231)* Acute mastoiditis is a serious complication of acute otitis media. Symptoms of mastoiditis include otalgia, otorrhea, headache, and hearing loss. Serious complications include osteitis, subperiosteal abscess, meningitis, facial nerve palsies, and extension of the abscess into the neck (Bezold abscess). The tympanic membrane may show erythema, opacity, perforation with drainage, or loss of landmarks. A normal ear examination is present in fewer than 10 percent of cases.

168. The answer is E. *(Chapter 231)* In chronic mastoiditis, defined as lasting longer than 3 months, mixed infections are the most common. *P. aeruginosa* is the predominant organism through *Bacteroides* species are also commonly found. Other causes of chronic mastoiditis include *Mycobacterium tuberculosis* and sterile infection.

169. The answer is B. *(Chapter 231)* Although barotrauma, perforation, and otitis media can cause hearing loss, cerumen impaction is the most likely cause. The resultant loss of conductive hearing would lead to an abnormal Weber test, with lateralization to the affected ear. The Rinne test would demonstrate bone conduction greater than air conduction.

170. The answer is E. *(Chapter 231)* Unilateral sensory loss presents with a normal Rinne test (air conduction greater than bone conduction) and a Weber test that lateralizes to the unaffected ear. Viral neuronitis is the most common cause, with mumps as the most frequent agent in children. Acoustic neuromas and Meniere's disease present less frequently with hearing loss. Other uncommon etiologies of unilateral hearing loss include autoimmune disorders, blood dyscrasias, and idiopathic causes.

171. The answer is D. *(Chapter 231)* Tympanic membrane rupture commonly occurs after direct trauma and blast injuries with changes in air or water pressure. Otitis media, lightning strikes, and caustic exposure can also cause perforation. Whereas temporal bone fracture can cause rupture, isolated mandible fracture does not.

172. The answer is A. *(Chapter 231)* Barotitis media (middle ear squeeze) is the most common form of barotrauma in scuba divers. On descent, pressure on middle ear gas increases. With eustachian tube dysfunction (due to anatomic abnormality or respiratory infection), the tympanic membrane retracts, resulting in mucosal engorgement, hemorrhage, and often tympanic membrane perforation. The resultant cold water in the middle ear commonly produces vertigo, nausea, and vomiting. Divers may also complain of acute pain and diminished hearing secondary to conductive hearing loss.

173. The answer is D. *(Chapter 233)* Both infection and cocaine use can cause mucosal erosions in the nose, resulting in epistaxis. Lowering blood pressure in a hypertensive patient may aid in control of epistaxis after pain is controlled. Uremia-induced dysfunction in the normal clotting cascade may also contribute to epistaxis. Peptic ulcer disease by itself does not cause epistaxis, and it is not a predisposing factor unless the patient takes nonsteroidal antiinflammatory drugs.

174. **The answer is C.** *(Chapter 233)* History of drug use, both illicit and prescribed, is important to ascertain in a patient presenting with epistaxis. Cocaine and medications that interfere with the normal clotting cascade may predispose to bleeding. In addition, liver disease or hemophilia can make achieving hemostasis challenging. A sensation of blood in the back of the throat suggests a more serious posterior bleed. Ear pain does not by itself aid in the evaluation of epistaxis.

175. **The answer is C.** *(Chapter 233)* Direct pressure applied for 5 to 10 min is the initial means of managing epistaxis. If a bleeding vessel is identified and the bleeding is temporarily controlled, cautery with a silver nitrate stick often provides definitive treatment. Nasal packing with a sponge or petroleum gauze is also efficacious, but the packing is uncomfortable and it must remain in place. Topical vasoconstrictive agents such as cocaine have been described to aid in the control of anterior epistaxis, but these agents must be used with caution in elderly patients. Embolization may play a role in the management of posterior, but not anterior, hemorrhage.

176. **The answer is E.** *(Chapter 233)* The failure rate of anterior nasal packing is about 25 percent. Anemia may result when anterior nasal packing fails to control the bleeding. Posterior dislodgment of nasal packing may occur but was more common in the past when physicians made their own packing material. Sinusitis and toxic shock syndrome have both been described as complications. Vertigo should not be attributed to nasal packing.

177. **The answer is C.** *(Chapter 233)* Bleeding from both nares is more often associated with a posterior source because the site of hemorrhage is closer to the choanae and blood may cross the midline. The sensation of blood in the oropharynx is also more common with a posterior bleed. Anterior bleeding usually remains unilateral and rarely flows down the throat unless the patient is supine. Epistaxis-associated syncope suggests a large blood loss, making a posterior source more likely. A nasal foreign body is more likely to cause an anterior bleed secondary to erosion or irritation of the nasal mucosa.

178. **The answer is D.** *(Chapter 233)* The nasal bones are protected to some extent by surrounding cartilaginous tissue. Blows to cartilage are less likely to produce fractures than are strikes directly to bone. Lateral forces are more likely to produce fractures because there is no cartilaginous padding. Barotrauma has little role in nasal fractures. A simple nasal fracture is a clinical diagnosis and does not require x-ray confirmation.

179. **The answer is B.** *(Chapter 233)* The main complications of nasal fractures are fractures to the cribriform plate and nasoseptal hematoma. Patients with nasal fractures must always be assessed for the presence of septal hematoma. Untreated septal hematomas often become infected and can result in avascular necrosis. Cartilaginous destruction occurs from compromised blood flow and may cause a cosmetic deformity known as the saddle deformity. Extraocular movements are typically unaffected by simple nasal trauma. If impaired, an orbital wall fracture must be sought.

180. **The answer is D.** *(Chapter 233)* Diagnosing nasal foreign bodies in small children requires a high degree of clinical suspicion. Older children are less likely to place objects into their noses. Clinicians should suspect a foreign body when a young child presents with persistent nasal drainage, sinusitis, or epistaxis. Although common in children, recurrent otitis media has not been associated with the presence of a nasal foreign body.

181. **The answer is B.** *(Chapter 233)* Sinusitis can be debilitating for patients and difficult for clinicians to treat. Acutely, the major causes of sinusitis tend to be aerobic bacteria.

Anaerobes should be suspected with persistent symptoms. *Bacteroides* species are more often implicated in chronic than in acute sinusitis.

182. **The answer is B.** *(Chapter 233)* Sinusitis can have grave consequences if left untreated. Local infiltration into the surrounding bone and soft tissues causes spreading infection. Cellulitis, both periorbital and facial, is a well-documented complication. In addition, sinusitis can lead to facial abscesses or subdural empyemas. Pott's Puffy tumor results from destruction of the anterior table of the frontal bone, with local abscess formation. Mastoiditis is not commonly seen after sinusitis.

183. **The answer is D.** *(Chapter 249)* Mandibular fractures produce a variety of signs and symptoms. Limited range of motion of the jaw, deformity of the dental arch, and malocclusion are prominent features. Mental nerve anesthesia and sublingual hematomas are often overlooked. Subconjunctival hemorrhage, although seen in mid-face fractures, does not commonly occur with mandible fractures.

184. **The answer is A.** *(Chapter 249)* The angle of the mandible is the most commonly fractured portion. This is closely followed by the condyle, molar, and mental regions. With angle fractures, the proximal segment is often displaced superiorly to the distal segment. This is caused by the pterygomasseteric sling pulling the proximal segment upward. Most mandible fractures heal well with intermaxillary fixation (wiring the upper and lower teeth in occlusion).

185. **The answer is D.** *(Chapter 249)* Symptoms of ZMC fractures include epistaxis, diplopia from disrupted and entrapped extraocular muscles, and facial emphysema (from fracture of the maxillary sinus causing air in the local tissues). In addition, subconjunctival hemorrhage can occur from blood tracking from fracture sites along the maxilla. Mental nerve anesthesia is often seen in mandibular fractures but less commonly in ZMC fractures.

186. **The answer is B.** *(Chapter 249)* Orbital floor fractures occur from direct blows to the globe that cause transmitted forces to the orbital encasement. The orbital floor is the weakest structure and is most commonly fractured. Extraocular muscles or the surrounding fat may become trapped in an orbital floor fracture, leading to diplopia. Sinusitis may be a complication if the orbital floor fracture extends into the maxillary sinus. As the sinus fills with blood, a fertile culture medium for bacteria is produced. Corneal abrasions, epistaxis, and traumatic retinal detachment may also be seen after facial trauma.

187. **The answer is C.** *(Chapter 249)* LeForte III fractures extend through the frontozygomatic suture lines, across the orbits, and through the base of the nose. The LeForte II fracture, also known as the pyramidal fracture because of its extension in a pyramidal fashion through the maxilla, does not involve the zygomatic suture lines. The LeForte I fracture is even more limited and involves only the maxilla. All the LeForte-type fractures produce a free-floating jaw in which the body of the maxilla is separated from the base of the skull superior to the palate. Mandibular fractures tend not to involve the suture lines.

188. **The answer is C.** *(Chapter 249)* A patient who presents with clear nasal discharge after a facial injury must be suspected of having CSF rhinorrhea. Of the fractures listed, this is most commonly a complication of a LeForte III injury that extends through the cribriform plate of the ethmoid bone. CSF leaks through the torn meninges, providing a direct communication with the subarachnoid space. If a CSF leak is undetected and untreated, brain abscess or encephalitis may develop.

189. **The answer is A.** *(Chapter 232)* In most mandible dislocations, the condyle of the mandible is displaced anteriorly as the condyle slips out of the TMJ fossa. The muscles of the mandible may spasm, causing trismus and making reduction more difficult. Reduction consists of downward pressure on the mandible while the jaw is opened wide to free the

condyle from its dislocated position anterior to the eminence. After relocation, the chin is pressed backward to allow the mandible to return to the fossa as the jaw is closed.

190. **The answer is C.** *(Chapter 232)* TMJ syndrome is a common and debilitating problem. Symptoms include bruxism (grinding of teeth), crepitus over the joint, earache, and tinnitus from proximity to the facial nerves. Dysphonia is not a common presenting symptom of TMJ syndrome because word enunciation does not typically involve much mandible movement. TMJ treatment includes analgesics, muscle relaxants, warm compresses, dental occlusions to limit bruxism, and stress reduction.

191. **The answer is A.** *(Chapter 232)* Although diabetes can place a patient at risk by causing dehydration, it is not a primary cause of sialoadenitis. Causes of acute salivary gland dysfunction include irradiation, paramyxovirus (mumps), phenothiazines, and uremia. Systemic diseases such as tuberculosis, actinomycoses, and sarcoidosis may present with chronic sialoadenitis. Squamous carcinomas and lymphomas are also in the differential of enlarged salivary glands. Treatment is directed at the underlying disease.

192. **The answer is E.** *(Chapter 232)* More than 80 percent of salivary calculi are found in the submandibular gland. Five to twenty percent occur in the parotid gland, with only rare formation in the sublingual gland. Lacrimal glands do not contain salivary calculi. Meibomian glands are located on the eyelid, and obstruction may lead to chalazion formation.

193. **The answer is D.** *(Chapter 235)* Stridor occurs when there is a narrowing of the hypopharynx. It is classically seen with advanced epiglottitis, as air traverses through a narrowed opening. PTAs tend to not produce enough airway compromise to produce stridor. Drooling, muffled voice, sore throat, and trismus all occur frequently.

194. **The answer is A.** *(Chapter 235)* Retropharyngeal abscesses occur predominately in children younger than 5 years. Complications include mediastinitis secondary to spread via contiguous fascial planes, airway obstruction, empyema, and erosion into the carotid artery. A lateral soft tissue x-ray of the neck is diagnostic in up to 88 percent of cases and should be performed at the bedside if there is any concern for impending airway obstruction.

195. **The answer is D.** *(Chapter 234)* Ludwig's angina is a potentially life-threatening infection of the submandibular space involving the connective tissue, fascia, and muscles, but not the glands. Patients frequently give a history of recent odontogenic infection. Ludwig's angina often produces trismus, dysphonia, and dysphagia. The infected tissues are often indurated (described as "brawny" edema) but not fluctuant. In addition to assessing for airway compromise, broad-spectrum antibiotics and emergent consultation for possible surgical drainage are the mainstays of treatment.

196. **The answer is D.** *(Chapter 234)* Ludwig's angina occurs most frequently in previously healthy males age 20 to 60 years. Alcoholism, diabetes, and SLE may also be predisposing factors. Because one-third of patients ultimately require tracheostomy or intubation, airway equipment should be at the bedside of any patient suspected of having this diagnosis.

GASTROENTEROLOGIC EMERGENCIES

QUESTIONS

DIRECTIONS: Each question below contains five suggested responses. Choose the **one best** response to each question.

197. All of the following are contraindications to passing a nasogastric tube EXCEPT

(A) suspected perforation of the esophagus
(B) confirmed perforation of the esophagus
(C) history of esophageal varices
(D) nearly complete obstruction of the esophagus due to benign or malignant strictures
(E) presence of an esophageal foreign body

198. A 5-year-old male presents to the ED 3 h after a possible button battery ingestion. The patient is in no acute distress, vital signs are stable, and examination is benign. A chest x-ray shows what appears to be a small button battery in the stomach. Which of the following is the MOST appropriate next action?

(A) Upper GI series to further delineate the exact location of the foreign body
(B) Attempt battery removal by the Foley balloon catheter technique
(C) Immediate GI consultation for endoscopic removal
(D) Immediate surgical consultation
(E) Discharge to home with parental observation and weekly radiographs

199. Which of the following statements is TRUE regarding PUD?

(A) Cigarette smoking is not a predisposing factor
(B) NSAIDs destroy gastric mucosa by increasing secretion of hydrochloric acid
(C) There is an association with infection with *Helicobacter pylori*
(D) Patients classically complain of burning epigastric pain that occurs immediately after eating a spicy meal
(E) Broad-spectrum antibiotics to treat *H. pylori* are considered first-line therapy

200. A 44-year-old male with a long history of alcohol use and presumptive gastritis presents to the ED complaining of sudden onset of severe abdominal pain and vomiting. Vital signs are blood pressure (BP) of 110/60 mm Hg, heart rate of 110 beats per minute, temperature of 101°F, and respiratory rate of 30 breaths per minute. Examination is remarkable for diaphoresis and epigastric tenderness with mild guarding. Laboratory work-up is within normal limits except for a white blood cell count (WBC) of 30,000 and an amylase level of 2,000. Chest x-ray shows a small amount of free air under the diaphragm. What is the MOST likely diagnosis?

(A) Acute pancreatitis with associated Mallory-Weiss syndrome
(B) Acute pancreatitis with associated Boerhaave's syndrome
(C) Acute pancreatitis with associated enzymatic destruction of bowel wall
(D) Acute pancreatitis secondary to anterior duodenal ulcer perforation
(E) Acute pancreatitis secondary to posterior duodenal ulcer perforation

201. When assessing a patient for acute appendicitis, which of the following describes the obturator sign?

(A) Pain produced by internal rotation of the fixed right thigh with the patient supine
(B) Pain produced by external rotation of the fixed right thigh with the patient supine
(C) Pain produced by extension of the right thigh with the patient in the left lateral decubitus position
(D) Pain sensation in the right lower quadrant with palpation of the left lower quadrant
(E) Cutaneous hyperesthesia in the T10, T11, and T12 dermatomes

202. Which of the following statements is TRUE regarding radiographic differences in appearance between the small and large bowels?

(A) Transverse linear densities that arise from the bowel wall and extend part way into the lumen are characteristically seen in the small intestine

(B) Haustrae are the transverse linear densities found in the small intestine

(C) Transverse linear densities that extend completely across the bowel lumen are found in the colon

(D) Plicae circulares are the transverse linear densities found in the colon

(E) Haustrae are less numerous and situated farther apart than plicae circulares

203. Which of the following is NOT a predisposing factor for the development of a hernia?

(A) Ascites

(B) Obesity

(C) Cystic fibrosis

(D) Chronic obstructive pulmonary disease

(E) Peritoneal dialysis

204. All of the following are TRUE regarding Crohn's disease EXCEPT

(A) it is characterized by segmental involvement of the intestinal tract

(B) there is an associated 10- to 30-fold increase in the development of carcinoma of the colon

(C) approximately 90 percent of patients develop perianal fissures, fistulas, abscesses, or rectal prolapse

(D) extraintestinal manifestations include arthritis, dermatitis, and hepatobiliary disease

(E) peak incidence occurs between ages 15 and 22 years

205. A 55-year-old male without significant medical history presents to the ED with the complaint of left lower quadrant pain and constipation. Vital signs are temperature of 100.5°F, pulse of 85, BP of 150/80, and respiratory rate of 12. The patient's physical examination is unremarkable except for mild left lower quadrant tenderness without guarding and rebound. Rectal examination shows heme-negative stool and no tenderness. Laboratory examinations, including a chemistry panel, are within normal limits except for a WBC of 13,000 with a left shift. Which of the following would be the MOST appropriate management for this patient?

(A) Prompt surgical evaluation in the ED

(B) Emergent upper GI series

(C) Emergent barium enema

(D) Discharge to home with bowel rest and oral antibiotics

(E) Discharge home with repeat abdominal examination in 12 h or sooner if worse

206. Which of the following is the MOST common cause of painful rectal bleeding?

(A) Internal hemorrhoids

(B) External hemorrhoids

(C) Diverticulitis

(D) Anal fissure

(E) Rectal foreign body

207. Which one of the following infectious etiologies of diarrhea accounts for the highest percentage of cases?

(A) Bacterial

(B) Parasitic

(C) Undetermined

(D) Viral

(E) Fungal

208. All of the following are TRUE regarding acalculous cholecystitis EXCEPT

(A) it occurs in 5 to 10 percent of patients with acute cholecystitis

(B) patients are frequently elderly and have a history of diabetes

(C) it often occurs as a complication of another process

(D) diagnosis is difficult due to the subtle clinical presentation

(E) gallstones are absent

209. All of the following statements regarding hepatitis are TRUE EXCEPT

(A) the incubation period for hepatitis A is 15 to 50 days

(B) hepatitis B is primarily spread through blood and body fluids

(C) although the clinical course of hepatitis C is milder than that of hepatitis B, there is more risk for later development of cirrhosis and hepatocellular carcinoma with hepatitis C

(D) hepatitis D can cause both acute and chronic hepatitis

(E) although the clinical course is similar, there is a lower rate of fulminant liver failure and death from hepatitis E than from hepatitis A.

210. Which of the following drugs is NOT associated with acute pancreatitis?

(A) Heparin

(B) Furosemide

(C) Rifampin

(D) Salicylates

(E) Warfarin

211. Which of the following etiologic agents is the MOST common cause of infection in liver transplant patients?

(A) *Candida*

(B) *Cytomegalovirus*

(C) *Herpes simplex* virus

(D) *P. carinii*

(E) *L. monocytogenes*

212. In working up a patient with acute abdominal pain, which of the following etiologies is LEAST likely to represent an immediate life threat?

(A) Myocardial infarction

(B) Splenic rupture

(C) Abdominal aortic aneurysm

(D) Perforated duodenal ulcer

(E) Ruptured ectopic pregnancy

213. Which of the following statements is TRUE regarding acute abdominal pain?

(A) Peritonitis causes a visceral type of pain and is secondary to peritoneal inflammation from an irritant

(B) Obstruction of a hollow viscus produces a colicky, diffuse visceral pain associated with nausea and vomiting

(C) Intraabdominal causes of pain include bacterial peritonitis, bowel ischemia, and tuboovarian abscess

(D) Referred pain from the abdomen may radiate to the back or groin, but not into the thorax

(E) Metabolic disorders are rarely a significant source of acute abdominal pain

214. All of the following are TRUE regarding the evaluation of a patient with acute abdominal pain EXCEPT

(A) the onset, location, and severity of pain are useful differentiating factors

(B) the most important physical examination modality is palpation

(C) the WBC may be normal even in inflammatory conditions such as appendicitis

(D) ultrasonography is a valuable imaging tool increasingly available to emergency physicians

(E) analgesic medications should be withheld until a surgeon evaluates the patient because they may obscure the diagnosis

215. Which of the following is the MOST common cause of upper GI bleeding?

(A) Esophageal varices

(B) Mallory-Weiss tear

(C) PUD

(D) Erosive gastritis

(E) Arteriovenous malformations

216. A patient presents with what appears to be massive lower GI hemorrhage. Which one of the following is the LEAST likely etiology?

(A) Diverticulosis

(B) Angiodysplasia

(C) Gastric varices

(D) Duodenal ulcer

(E) Hemorrhoids

217. A 56-year-old male with a history of heavy alcohol use presents to the ED complaining of vomiting blood for several hours. Vital signs are BP of 90/60, pulse of 110, respiratory rate of 16, and temperature of 98°F. Primary resuscitative measures are begun, and placement of an NGT shows active bright red bleeding. Which of the following is the treatment of choice?

(A) Tamponade with a Sengstaken-Blakemore tube
(B) Therapeutic upper GI endoscopy
(C) Octreotide infusion
(D) Vasopressin infusion
(E) Immediate referral for surgical intervention

218. Which of the following is a mechanical or obstructive cause of dysphagia?

(A) Aortic aneurysm
(B) *Candida* esophagitis
(C) Multiple sclerosis
(D) Scleroderma
(E) Gastroesophageal reflux

219. Which one of the following statements regarding esophageal trauma is TRUE?

(A) Ingestion of lye causes a partial-thickness burn to the mucosa
(B) Contrast studies are contraindicated if a perforation is suspected
(C) Swallowed foreign bodies may cause a partial-thickness laceration that leads to severe bleeding
(D) Mallory-Weiss syndrome involves a laceration of the otherwise normal esophagus after repeated emesis
(E) Boerhaave's syndrome is a full-thickness perforation, usually leading to severe mediastinitis

220. Which one of the following patients who swallowed a foreign body is MOST likely to require endoscopy or surgery for definitive treatment?

(A) An asymptomatic child with a button battery shown to be in the stomach on x-ray
(B) A 34-year-old male with an impacted piece of steak, who is tolerating his secretions well
(C) A 6-year-old male who swallowed a penny that appears to be in the esophagus on x-ray
(D) An adult psychiatric patient who swallowed a razor blade
(E) A 22-year-old male who swallowed heavily wrapped cocaine that appears to have passed the pylorus

221. Which of the following is TRUE regarding meat impaction in the esophagus?

(A) Endoscopy should be performed within 6 h, even in patients who are handling their own secretions
(B) Esophageal pathology is present in up to 50 percent of patients
(C) Glucagon, nifedipine, and meat tenderizer should all be tried before endoscopy
(D) After the patient feels the bolus has passed, a barium swallow should be performed
(E) Patients without airway compromise can be observed as outpatients and scheduled for a 24-h follow-up

222. In a young, otherwise healthy patient with a newly suspected diagnosis of PUD, what would be the MOST appropriate course of action in the ED?

(A) Begin symptomatic and therapeutic treatment with cimetidine
(B) Immediate referral for endoscopy
(C) Begin empiric treatment of *H. pylori* with a triple antibiotic regimen
(D) Begin combination therapy with an H_2 receptor antagonist, proton pump inhibitor, and antacids
(E) Begin therapy with sucralfate and order an *H. pylori* breath test

223. In a patient with PUD, all of the following clinical signs or symptoms should raise concern of a complication EXCEPT

(A) passage of melanotic stool
(B) burning epigastric pain occurring every night
(C) abrupt onset of mid-back pain
(D) repeated episodes of vomiting over the previous 12 h
(E) severe, diffuse abdominal pain

224. A 25-year-old male presents to the ED with abdominal pain. His pain is vague, periumbilical, and associated with anorexia and nausea. He is afebrile with normal vital signs. Physical examination is normal except for mild umbilical discomfort, without guarding or rebound. Initial work-up includes a normal CBC and urinalysis. Which one of the following would be the LEAST appropriate course of action?

(A) Abdominal computed tomography (CT) to evaluate for appendicitis

(B) Abdominal ultrasound to evaluate for appendicitis

(C) Coverage with broad-spectrum antibiotics for acute appendicitis

(D) Observation with surgical consultation if symptoms progress

(E) Observation and discharge home with close follow-up if symptoms resolve

225. Which of the following scenarios may represent acute appendicitis?

(A) A 4-year-old male with vomiting and lethargy

(B) A 75-year-old female with fever and abdominal pain

(C) A 26-year-old female who is 32 weeks pregnant with right upper quadrant pain

(D) A 45-year-old male with AIDS and who has vomiting and diarrhea

(E) All of the above

226. What is the MOST common cause of large bowel obstruction?

(A) Adhesions

(B) Incarcerated hernia

(C) Diverticulitis

(D) Neoplasm

(E) Sigmoid volvulus

227. Which of the following is TRUE regarding small bowel obstruction?

(A) It is rarely associated with abdominal pain

(B) It usually presents with clear, nonbilious vomiting

(C) Diffuse, severe abdominal tenderness indicates secondary peritonitis

(D) X-ray shows air-filled bowel with prominent haustrae

(E) Nasogastric tube decompression is generally ineffective

228. Which of the following is MOST accurate regarding hernias in children?

(A) All umbilical hernias should be referred for immediate surgical repair

(B) Inguinal hernias usually resolve spontaneously

(C) Umbilical hernias are highly prone to incarceration

(D) Indirect inguinal hernias are caused by congenital failure of the processus vaginalis to close

(E) Umbilical hernias are caused by congenital weakness of the linea albus of the rectus sheath

229. All of the following statements are TRUE regarding hernias EXCEPT

(A) indirect inguinal hernias result from congenital defects and frequently incarcerate

(B) direct inguinal hernias result from acquired defects in the transversalis fascia and rarely incarcerate

(C) femoral hernias occur more commonly in males and frequently incarcerate

(D) acquired umbilical hernias are associated with obesity and pregnancy and frequently incarcerate

(E) pelvic hernias are extremely rare but may occur through the sciatic and obturator foramina

230. All the following are TRUE regarding Crohn's disease EXCEPT

(A) up to 50 percent of patients have involvement of both small bowel and colon

(B) extraintestinal manifestations are common and include arthritis, uveitis, and liver disease

(C) abscesses and fistulas are frequent complications

(D) Up to 10 percent of patients develop perianal complications

(E) Obstruction can occur as a result of stricture formation and bowel-wall edema

231. A healthy 25-year-old male complains of constant throbbing rectal pain that worsens immediately before defecation. Examination is remarkable for a temperature of 101.5°F and a tender, fluctuant, erythematous mass in the perianal region. Fullness and induration are appreciated on rectal examination. What would be the MOST appropriate course of action?

(A) Discharge home with instructions for sitz baths and bulk laxatives

(B) Discharge home with instructions for sitz baths and topical steroid cream

(C) Incision and drainage in the ED using local anesthetic

(D) Anoscopy to evaluate for internal hemorrhoids or cryptitis

(E) Surgical consultation for incision and drainage in the operating room

232. Which of the following is TRUE regarding hemorrhoids?

(A) Internal hemorrhoids are usually painful and associated with heavy bleeding

(B) External hemorrhoids are relatively painless and rarely thrombose

(C) Internal hemorrhoids are usually nonpalpable and best evaluated with anoscopy

(D) Both internal and external hemorrhoids require prompt surgical referral for treatment

(E) Thrombosed internal hemorrhoids may be treated with excision of the clots in the ED

233. Which of the following causes of constipation may NOT be safely managed on an outpatient basis?

(A) Hypothyroidism

(B) Fecal impaction

(C) Hyperparathyroidism

(D) Lead poisoning

(E) Sigmoid volvulus

234. Which of the following is the MOST common presentation of gallstones?

(A) Acute pancreatitis

(B) Acute cholecystitis

(C) Biliary colic

(D) Ascending cholangitis

(E) Gallbladder empyema

235. A 40-year-old female with known gallstones presents with colicky right upper quadrant pain and vomiting. She has a history of similar episodes that usually resolve after 3 to 4 h. Vital signs are BP of 110/60, pulse of 78, respiratory rate of 16, and temperature of 98.4°F. Physical examination shows a mildly tender right upper quadrant without signs of peritonitis. Which one of the following would be LEAST appropriate in her ED management?

(A) Intravenous fluid administration

(B) Pain control with opiate analgesics

(C) Pain control with ketorolac

(D) Antiemetic administration

(E) Immediate surgical consultation

236. All of the following are TRUE regarding acute rejection in liver transplant patients EXCEPT

(A) acute rejection is most commonly seen 7 to 14 days posttransplant

(B) clinical presentation is easily differentiated from postoperative complications

(C) it may be triggered at any time by tapering of immunosuppressive agents

(D) diagnosis can only be made with certainty by ultrasound with biopsy

(E) acute rejection is managed primarily by high-dose glucocorticoids

237. All of the following are causes of unconjugated hyperbilirubinemia EXCEPT

(A) acetaminophen poisoning

(B) hemolytic anemia

(C) transfusion reaction

(D) congestive heart failure

(E) sickle cell anemia

238. A 35-year-old male who was exposed to hepatitis A presents with new-onset jaundice and vomiting. Vital signs are normal, and physical examination shows mild hepatomegaly with right upper quadrant tenderness. Laboratory studies show an ALT of 300 U/L; total bilirubin of 9 mg/dL; prothrombin time of 16.0 s (normal = 10.0–12.0 s), and glucose of 75 mg/dL. After intravenous fluid administration, vomiting resolves, and he is able to tolerate oral hydration. Which of the following would indicate that the patient should be admitted to the hospital?

(A) Elevated ALT, indicating hepatocellular damage

(B) Hyperglycemia

(C) Symptomatic vomiting

(D) Prolonged prothrombin time

(E) Age > 30 years

239. What is the MOST common cause of pancreatitis in an urban hospital setting?

(A) Cholelithiasis
(B) Alcoholism
(C) Abdominal trauma
(D) Penetrating peptic ulcer
(E) Salicylate poisoning

240. Which of the following is NOT a complication of acute pancreatitis?

(A) Adult respiratory distress syndrome (ARDS)
(B) Myocardial depression
(C) Disseminated intravascular coagulopathy (DIC)
(D) Malabsorption
(E) Pancreatic pseudocyst

241. A 55-year-old female presents to the ED with a fever 4 days after undergoing a laparoscopic cholecystectomy. What is the MOST likely cause of the fever?

(A) Pneumonia
(B) Thrombophlebitis
(C) Urinary tract infection
(D) Wound infection
(E) Deep venous thrombosis

242. A patient who has recently undergone gastrointestinal surgery presents to the ED with abdominal pain and vomiting. Which of the following would be the LEAST likely surgical complication?

(A) Intestinal obstruction
(B) Intraabdominal abscess
(C) Pancreatitis
(D) Cholecystitis
(E) Pseudomembranous colitis

243. A patient with suspected cholelithiasis presents to the ED. What is the initial imaging study of choice?

(A) Abdominal plain film
(B) Abdominal ultrasound
(C) Abdominal CT
(D) Radionuclide scan (HIDA)
(E) Barium contrast radiography

GASTROENTEROLOGIC
EMERGENCIES

ANSWERS

197. **The answer is C.** *(Chapter 71)* A nasogastric tube (NGT) is useful for diagnostic purposes in the setting of gastrointestinal (GI) bleeding; most cases of esophageal injuries are due to ingestion, intestinal obstruction, and multisystem trauma. An NGT should not be attempted in patients with actual or suspected perforations of the esophagus, nearly complete obstruction of the esophagus due to benign or malignant strictures, or the presence of an esophageal foreign body. Patients with esophageal varices may be bleeding from another GI source. If bleeding is profuse, the source should be confirmed by endoscopy. For patients with severe facial trauma, an orogastric tube should be placed instead of an NGT.

198. **The answer is E.** *(Chapter 72)* Button batteries lodged in the esophagus require emergency removal to avoid esophageal burns and perforation. If the button battery has passed the esophagus and the patient is asymptomatic, home observation with serial x-rays to ensure passage through the pylorus is the appropriate course of action. Most button batteries that have passed the esophagus will transit through the entire body within 24 to 48 h without difficulty. If the battery is of large diameter and the patient is younger than 6 years, the battery is less likely to pass, and endoscopic retrieval is the preferred treatment.

199. **The answer is C.** *(Chapter 73)* Cigarette smoking is a predisposing factor for peptic ulcer disease (PUD), possibly due to an inhibition of bicarbonate ion production or to increased gastric emptying. Nonsteroidal antiinflammatory drugs (NSAIDs) inhibit prostaglandin synthesis and thus bicarbonate production and mucosal blood flow, allowing ulcer formation. Although *H. pylori* infection is associated with PUD, treatment is not necessarily associated with resolution of the symptoms. Patients with PUD typically complain of burning epigastric pain that occurs 1 to 3 h after a meal or wakes them in the middle of the night. Elderly patients with PUD are less likely to experience pain than their younger counterparts.

200. **The answer is E.** *(Chapter 83)* Because the pancreas adheres to the posterior duodenum, ruptured posterior duodenal ulcers generally penetrate into the pancreas rather than perforate into the free peritoneum. Anterior ulcers are more likely to perforate into the peritoneal cavity. A Mallory-Weiss tear of the esophageal wall usually presents with symptoms similar to reflux esophagitis and causes moderate, self-limited bleeding. Patients with Boerhaave's syndrome rapidly deteriorate to a state of shock and septicemia due to a malignant mediastinitis.

201. **The answer is A.** *(Chapter 74)* An inflamed appendix may irritate the obturator muscle. The obturator sign is present when a supine patient complains of right lower quadrant pain during passive internal rotation of the flexed right thigh, a motion that stretches the obturator muscle. Other clinical signs of acute appendicitis include the psoas sign (right lower quadrant pain on thigh extension with the patient in the left lateral decubitus position), Rovsing's sign (right lower quadrant pain with palpation on the left), and cutaneous hyperesthesia in the T10, T11, and T12 dermatomes.

202. **The answer is E.** *(Chapter 75)* Large and small bowel obstructions can be distinguished radiographically by differences in appearance between the small intestine and the colon. Plicae circulares are transverse linear densities found in the small intestine. They extend completely across the bowel lumen. Haustrae are thicker, less numerous projections located in the colon. They extend only partly into the lumen.

203. **The answer is B.** *(Chapter 76)* Ascites, peritoneal dialysis, ventriculoperitoneal shunt, cystic fibrosis, and chronic obstructive pulmonary disease all predispose patients to hernia formation because they increase intraabdominal pressure. Other risk factors include a positive family history, undescended testis, and genitourinary abnormalities.

204. **The answer is B.** *(Chapter 77)* There is a 10- to 30-fold increase in the development of colon cancer in patients with ulcerative colitis (UC), not Crohn's disease. First-degree relatives of patients with UC have a 3.5-fold increased risk of developing Crohn's disease and a 15-fold increased risk of developing UC. Crohn's disease is a chronic inflammatory disease of the GI tract of unknown cause characterized by segmental involvement of the intestinal tract. *Regional enteritis* and *terminal ileitis* are other terms used to describe the same disease.

205. **The answer is D.** *(Chapter 77)* The patient described in the scenario most likely has diverticulitis. Patients with localized pain and no signs and symptoms of peritonitis or systemic infection do not require hospitalization. Outpatient management consists of bowel rest, broad-spectrum oral antibiotic therapy, and close follow-up.

206. **The answer is D.** *(Chapter 78)* Anal fissures result from a linear tear of the anal canal beginning at or just below the dentate line and extending distally along the anal canal. Patients complain of sharp, cutting pain, most severe during and immediately after a bowel movement. Bleeding is scant and bright red. Anal fissures are especially painful because of the rich supply of somatic sensory nerve fibers located in the anoderm.

207. **The answer is D.** *(Chapter 79)* Viruses cause the vast majority of infectious diarrheas. The most common agents are Rotavirus, Calicivirus, Astrovirus, and Norwalk agent. Bacteria cause about 20 percent of cases of diarrhea by either direct invasion or secondary to enterotoxin production. Parasites are next most common etiologic agents.

208. **The answer is D.** *(Chapter 81)* Acalculous cholecystitis occurs in 5 to 10 percent of patients with acute cholecystitis. Patients frequently are elderly and have a history of diabetes mellitus. There are two distinguishing features of acalculous cholecystitis: (1) it frequently occurs as a complication of another process and (2) patients frequently are gravely ill on initial presentation.

209. **The answer is E.** *(Chapter 82)* Although hepatitis B is spread primarily through blood and body fluids, up to 50 percent of cases have no clear etiology. The clinical course of hepatitis C is milder than that for hepatitis B, but there is a greater risk for long-term adverse complications. Hepatitis D is a cause of both acute and chronic hepatitis. Despite a similar clinical course, fulminant liver failure and death are more common after infection with hepatitis E than with hepatitis A.

210. **The answer is A.** *(Chapter 83)* Drugs and toxins are major causes of acute pancreatitis. Some of the medications associated with the occurrence of acute pancreatitis are oral contraceptives, estrogens, phenformin, glucocorticoids, rifampin, tetracycline, isoniazid, thiazide diuretics, furosemide, salicylates, indomethacin, calcium, warfarin, and acetaminophen. Other etiologic factors contributing to the development of pancreatitis include infection, collagen vascular disease, metabolic disturbances, and trauma.

211. **The answer is B.** *(Chapter 86)* Complications of infections in liver transplant patients account for nearly 90 percent of deaths. The most common infectious agent after transplantation is *Cytomegalovirus* (CMV), a herpes virus. Reported occurrence ranges from 23 to 85 percent of all liver transplant patients. Fortunately, CMV is rarely fatal.

212. **The answer is D.** *(Chapter 68)* When approaching a patient with acute abdominal pain, the clinician must consider conditions that can be an immediate threat to the patient's life. Splenic rupture, ruptured ectopic pregnancy, and abdominal aortic aneurysm can all be associated with massive bleeding and rapid decline. Extraabdominal conditions that present with abdominal pain such as myocardial infarction can also be life threatening. Perforated duodenal ulcers are serious but almost never result in significant hemorrhage, and thus are not usually an immediate threat to life.

213. **The answer is B.** *(Chapter 68)* Three types of pain responses are possible with acute abdominal pain. Peritonitis is a somatic pain and is usually sharper, more constant, and more localized than visceral pain. Obstruction of a hollow viscus is a common cause of visceral pain and is colicky, intermittent, and usually mid-line. Referred pain is often felt in the back, groin, or thighs. Patients may also complain of pain in the supraclavicular region, especially if the diaphragm is irritated by collections of blood or pus. Abdominal pain can arise from intraabdominal, extraabdominal, metabolic, or neurogenic origins. Intraabdominal origins of pain are divided into three categories: peritoneal inflammation, obstruction of a hollow viscus, and vascular etiologies. Extraabdominal sources can arise from the abdominal wall, thorax, or pelvis (as in the case of tubo-ovarian abscess). Metabolic disorders such as diabetic ketoacidosis and sickle cell crisis often present with diffuse abdominal pain.

214. **The answer is E.** *(Chapter 68)* The evaluation of abdominal pain should begin with a detailed history. The onset, severity, location, and character of pain and the presence of associated symptoms guide work-up and treatment. Although a complete physical examination is necessary, palpation of the abdomen is the most important modality for diagnosis. Laboratory tests are useful adjuncts, but the limitations of a complete blood count (CBC) must be recognized. Helpful imaging modalities include standard radiographs, ultrasonography, barium contrast studies, and computed tomography. Intravenous opiate analgesia is humane and may actually assist in diagnosis by facilitating physical examination in a patient who could otherwise not tolerate it.

215. **The answer is C.** *(Chapter 70)* Upper GI bleeding is defined as bleeding that originates proximal to the ligament of Treitz. PUD, including gastric, duodenal, and stomachal ulcers, is the most common cause of upper GI bleeding, accounting for nearly 60 percent of cases. The next most common etiologies for upper GI bleeding are erosive gastritis, esophagitis, and duodenitis, together representing 15 percent of all cases. Gastric irritants such as alcohol, salicylates, and NSAIDs predispose patients to upper GI bleeding. Esophageal and gastric varices account for only 6 percent of upper GI bleeding but carry a high mortality rate. They result from portal hypertension and are seen most commonly in patients with alcoholic liver disease. Mallory-Weiss syndrome is due to a mucosal tear in the esophagus and is classically associated with repeated bouts of retching. Arteriovenous malformations are an uncommon cause of upper GI bleeding.

216. **The answer is E.** *(Chapter 70)* The most common cause of what initially appears to be lower GI bleeding is actually bleeding from an upper GI source. Brisk bleeding from either varices or PUD can be the cause of apparent lower GI hemorrhage. Diverticulosis and angiodysplasia are the most common causes of confirmed lower GI bleeding. Both occur more commonly in the elderly, are painless, and may be massive. Although hemorrhoids are a common etiology of minor lower GI bleeding, they do not usually cause significant hemorrhage. Other less frequent sources of lower GI bleeding include malignancies, inflammatory bowel disease, polyps, infectious gastroenteritis, and Meckel's diverticulum.

217. **The answer is B.** *(Chapter 70)* GI bleeding is a common problem seen in the ED and is potentially life threatening. For patients with significant active bleeding, emergency endoscopy is the treatment of choice. Esophageal varices can be treated endoscopically with either band ligation or sclerotherapy, resulting in control of acute bleeding in up to 90 percent of patients. Hemostasis can be achieved with nonvariceal sources of bleeding as well. Drug therapy with both octreotide and somatostatin reduces bleeding from both varices and PUD and is a useful adjunct to endoscopy. Vasopressin therapy has largely been discontinued due to a high rate of adverse effects including hypertension, arrhythmias, myocardial ischemia, and decreased cardiac output. Balloon tamponade can be used as a temporizing measure to control bleeding by placing direct pressure on the gastric and esophageal mucosa. However, it is frequently associated with complications, including mucosal ulceration, esophageal or gastric rupture, asphyxiation from dislodged balloons, and aspiration pneumonia. Although it is appropriate to make a surgeon aware of a critical patient, emergency surgical intervention is indicated only in those patients who fail endoscopic hemostasis and medical therapy.

218. **The answer is A.** *(Chapter 71)* Dysphagia is an awareness of something wrong with the smooth pattern of swallowing. Its presence, with or without odynophagia (pain on swallowing), almost always indicates an esophageal problem. The two basic causes of dysphagia are mechanical (narrowing or obstruction of the lumen) and nonobstructive. Mechanical problems may arise from within the esophageal lumen, the wall, or from sources outside the esophagus that compress extrinsically, such as the thyroid or cardiovascular structures. Mechanical etiologies include swallowed foreign bodies, esophageal tumors, hiatal hernias or compression from a goiter, enlarged lymph nodes, or thoracic aortic aneurysm. Nonobstructive dysphagia can be either motility related (from intrinsic muscular or nervous disorders) or nonmotility related (from reflux or inflammation). Etiologies of nonobstructive dysphagia include scleroderma, esophageal spasm, stroke, reflux esophagitis, multiple sclerosis, and infection, especially in immunocompromised patients.

219. **The answer is E.** *(Chapter 71)* Injuries to the esophagus may be classified as partial thickness (involving the mucosa or submucosa) or full thickness (involving the muscle layers). The esophagus has no serosa, so complete perforation tends to extend into the mediastinum. Partial tears are often caused by swallowed objects and tend to heal spontaneously with some dysphagia, odynophagia, and mild upper GI bleeding. Ingestion of caustic substances such as lye causes a more severe full-thickness injury, usually without complete perforation. Mallory-Weiss syndrome is a type of partial-thickness laceration that occurs in a weakened esophageal wall. It is caused by increased abdominal pressure, usually from violent, repeated emesis. Boerhaave's syndrome is a full-thickness perforation, also associated with violent emesis. Forceful expulsion of fluid through the perforation leads to a rapidly progressive mediastinitis. If perforation is suspected, water-soluble contrast should be used in an imaging study to confirm the diagnosis.

220. **The answer is D.** *(Chapter 72)* Swallowed foreign bodies can be innocuous or life threatening. Most objects pass spontaneously and can be managed expectantly. Adults with meat impaction who are tolerating secretions can be watched for up to 12 h and will usually pass the bolus with the aid of sedation and other adjunctive therapies. Children with a coin lodged in the esophagus must have it removed but do not always need endoscopy. Children who have ingested a button battery must have it removed if it lodges in the esophagus. However, asymptomatic children with a battery in the stomach can be observed. Cocaine ingestion is becoming increasingly common and can pose a problem when the cocaine is loosely wrapped or fails to pass the pylorus. If a tightly wrapped packet appears to be passing through the intestinal tract, observation is appropriate. Ingestion of sharp objects is more concerning. Large objects and those with extremely sharp edges such as razor blades should be removed before they pass the stomach because they are associated with a high perforation rate once past the pylorus.

221. **The answer is D.** *(Chapter 72)* Patients who are managing their own secretions after meat impaction can be treated expectantly. However, the impaction should not be allowed to remain longer than 12 h. Endoscopy is the preferred method for removal, but alternatives may be tried if it is not available. Glucagon, nifedipine, and sedation have all been reported to work. Meat tenderizer has been advocated in the past but is not currently recommended because of the risk of complications from enzymatic action on the esophagus. Up to 97 percent of patients with meat impaction have underlying esophageal pathology, and a barium swallow should be performed to confirm passage and evaluate pathologic conditions.

222. **The answer is A.** *(Chapter 73)* There are several approaches to the patient with suspected PUD. Traditional therapeutic regimens heal the ulcer, relieve pain, and prevent complications, but do not prevent recurrence. Therapy with an H_2 receptor antagonist, proton pump inhibitor, sucralfate, or antacids would be appropriate. They have all been shown to heal ulcers equally well when used alone, and combination therapy is rarely necessary. Treatment of *H. pylori* infections is usually reserved for patients with documented infection. Serologic testing is used to detect *H. pylori*, and the breath test (using carbon-labeled urea) is used primarily after treatment to confirm eradication of infection. Immediate referral for definitive diagnosis by endoscopy may be indicated with concerning symptoms but is not necessary in an otherwise healthy patient.

223. **The answer is B.** *(Chapter 73)* PUD is characterized by burning epigastric pain that is relieved by food. Pain typically recurs as the gastric contents empty, usually at night. Complications of ulcer disease include hemorrhage, perforation, and gastric outlet obstruction from scarring or edema at the pylorus. Signs and symptoms that should alert the clinician to hemorrhage are the vomiting of bright red blood, coffee-ground emesis, melena, or hematochezia. Perforation usually manifests with sudden, generalized abdominal pain due to peritonitis that results from leakage of gastric or duodenal contents. Perforation with posterior extension into the pancreas presents as abrupt back pain. Gastric outlet obstruction typically leads to persistent nonbilious vomiting. Patients with any of these complications require immediate resuscitation and specialty consultation.

224. **The answer is C.** *(Chapter 74)* The approach to a patient with possible appendicitis can be difficult given the wide spectrum of presentations. Early in the course, pain may not be localized to the right lower quadrant, and the patient is often afebrile. Diagnostic imaging may be useful in suspicious, but atypical cases. Both CT and ultrasound have been widely used, and local availability may determine which test is selected. Clinical observation with serial examinations for 4 to 6 h is an alternative approach to imaging. Patients whose examination progresses should have early surgical consultation. If the clinical condition remains benign, a 12- to 24-h follow-up with instructions to return sooner if the condition worsens is appropriate. Broad-spectrum antibiotics play an important role in the management of patients with appendicitis who are awaiting surgery. However, they should not be given to patients with undiagnosed abdominal pain because the antibiotics may obscure the diagnosis.

225. **The answer is E.** *(Chapter 74)* Certain groups of patients have atypical presentations and are at risk for delayed diagnosis of acute appendicitis. Children younger than age 6 years have a rate of misdiagnosis approaching 57 percent and up to 90 percent perforation rates. Confounding factors include communication difficulties and atypical symptoms of peritonitis such as lethargy. Elderly patients also have a high incidence of perforation, and symptoms may be subtle, even late in the course. Pregnant patients pose difficulty because the gravid uterus changes the position of the appendix in the abdomen, and pain may be in an unusual location. An ultrasound can aid in distinguishing a pelvic from an abdominal etiology for the pain. Patients who are immunocompromised are susceptible to delayed diagnosis because of their frequent unrelated GI symptoms. CT is helpful in differentiating surgical from nonsurgical conditions.

226. **The answer is D.** *(Chapter 75)* It is important to distinguish between large and small bowel obstruction because treatment differs by the site of the obstruction. The most common cause of colonic obstruction is neoplasm, and anyone with symptoms of large bowel obstruction should be evaluated for carcinoma. The next most frequent cause is diverticulitis, followed by sigmoid volvulus and, less commonly, cecal volvulus. Surgical adhesions are the most frequent cause of small bowel obstruction, followed by incarcerated hernias and primary small bowel lesions.

227. **The answer is C.** *(Chapter 75)* Although the site and nature of the bowel obstruction determines the clinical presentation, almost all patients complain of pain. Vomiting is also uniformly present and is typically bilious with proximal obstruction and fecal with distal obstruction. The presence of severe abdominal tenderness indicates a course complicated by peritonitis secondary to impending or actual perforation and requires immediate surgical consultation. Abdominal x-ray can confirm the diagnosis of bowel obstruction, identify free air from a perforation, and localize the site of obstruction. Transverse linear densities (plicae circulares) that extend completely across the bowel lumen characterize the small bowel. Haustrae are found in large bowel. Although surgical intervention is usually required for confirmed mechanical obstruction, an NGT should be placed for decompression of bowel contents and air.

228. **The answer is D.** *(Chapter 76)* Hernias are extremely common in children, with indirect inguinal and umbilical hernias being the most prevalent types. Failure of the processus vaginalis to close after the testis and spermatic cord (round ligament in females) descend through the inguinal canal results in an indirect inguinal hernia. Inguinal hernias are prone to incarceration and strangulation in the first year of life. Thus, they require timely surgical consultation after ED reduction and are usually repaired electively shortly after diagnosis. Umbilical hernias are more common in females and result from weakness or incomplete development of the fibromuscular ring surrounding the umbilical cord. Umbilical hernias rarely incarcerate, and more than 80 percent close spontaneously by the age of 3 or 4 years. After age 4, children should be referred for surgical closure.

229. **The answer is C.** *(Chapter 76)* Hernias are extremely common but most often are asymptomatic. Inguinal hernias occur more commonly in males, and femoral and umbilical hernias are more frequent in females. Indirect inguinal hernias result from congenital failure of the peritoneal evagination to close and frequently incarcerate and strangulate. Direct inguinal hernias are acquired defects that do not involve passage through the inguinal canal and rarely incarcerate. Femoral hernias are protrusions through the femoral canal, and they frequently incarcerate. Umbilical hernias in adults are acquired defects, usually resulting from increased abdominal distention secondary to obesity, pregnancy, or ascites. In contrast to the defect in young children, umbilical hernias in adults frequently incarcerate. Rare types of hernias include pelvic and lumbar types. These often present atypically and with intermittent bouts of obstruction.

230. **The answer is D.** *(Chapter 77)* Crohn's disease is a chronic inflammatory bowel disease characterized by segmental involvement of both the small and large intestines, with the ileum being most commonly affected. In addition to GI symptoms of abdominal pain, anorexia, diarrhea, and weight loss, approximately one-third of patients have extraintestinal manifestations. These associated symptoms may be arthritic, dermatologic, hepatobiliary, or vascular in nature. Complications of Crohn's disease occur frequently, and 75 percent of patients require surgery within 20 years of onset of symptoms. Intraabdominal abscesses, fistulas, and bowel obstructions are common conditions necessitating surgical intervention. Perianal complications are the most frequent, seen in up to 90 percent of patients, and include perianal abscesses, fissures, fistulas, and rectal prolapse.

231. **The answer is E.** *(Chapter 78)* Abscesses are common in the perianal and perirectal region and usually begin with infection of an anal crypt and gland. Infection can progress

to involve areas of potential space surrounding the anorectum, including the perianal, perirectal, ischiorectal, intersphincteric, and supralevator spaces. Because of inadequate drainage, there is up to a 32 percent recurrence rate in patients who have a simple incision and drainage performed in the ED with local anesthetic. In addition, deep abscesses have the potential to spread insidiously and extensively through the communicating submucosal tissues and may point some distance away from the anal verge. Hence, all but the most superficial, isolated perianal abscesses should be drained in the operating room.

232.   **The answer is C.**   *(Chapter 78)*   Hemorrhoids are one of the most common problems afflicting human beings, and they may be internal or external in origin. Internal hemorrhoids arise above the dentate line, are not readily visible or palpable, and are best visualized through an anoscope. They are typically painless and present with self-limited bleeding accompanying defecation. Unless a complication occurs, treatment is local and nonsurgical, with relief of symptoms by sitz baths and bulk laxatives. Complications such as thrombosis and strangulation are usually painful, accompanied by significant edema, and require surgical evaluation. In contrast, external hemorrhoids are typically painful, easily visualized and palpated at the anal verge, and frequently thrombose. Treatment is also with sitz baths and laxatives, but local excision of clot is also appropriate and can provide significant relief.

233.   **The answer is E.**   *(Chapter 79)*   Constipation is the most common digestive complaint in the United States, and the differential diagnosis is broad. Determining the rapidity of onset is important because acute constipation mandates evaluation for intestinal obstruction. Disorders causing obstruction such as volvulus, tumor, hernia or adhesions require surgical consultation and admission. Other causes of constipation can usually be managed on an outpatient basis with medications and instruction on behavior modification. Patients with fecal impaction may be discharged home after manual disimpaction has been performed. If an organic cause such as hypothyroidism, hyperparathyroidism, or heavy metal poisoning is suspected, work-up may be initiated in the ED if close follow-up is arranged with the patient's primary physician.

234.   **The answer is C.**   *(Chapter 81)*   Patients with gallstones present in a variety of ways, and biliary colic (or symptomatic cholelithiasis) is the most common. The pain is colicky in nature, occurs after meals, and typically lasts from 1 to 6 h. Pain lasting longer than 6 h that is accompanied by fever or leukocytosis suggests a diagnosis of cholecystitis. Biliary colic and acute cholecystitis are by far the most common manifestations of gallstone disease. Complications from gallstones may be life threatening. Acute pancreatitis, ascending cholangitis, gallbladder empyema, and emphysematous cholecystitis all require aggressive patient resuscitation and prompt surgical consultation.

235.   **The answer is E.**   *(Chapter 81)*   Patients with uncomplicated symptomatic cholelithiasis do not require immediate surgical intervention. ED intervention is geared toward pain relief and correction of volume deficits. Pain control can be achieved with administration of opiate analgesics or ketorolac. Antiemetics and gastric decompression with an NGT may be necessary for treatment of protracted vomiting. If the patient's symptoms resolve within 4 to 6 h and she tolerates oral fluids, discharge to home with outpatient follow-up is appropriate.

236.   **The answer is B.**   *(Chapter 86)*   Liver transplantation is becoming more common, and patients will be seen in the ED for a variety of associated conditions. Allograft rejection occurs in two syndromes, acute and chronic. Acute rejection usually occurs at 7 to 14 days posttransplant, at a frequency varying from 40 to 80 percent. The incidence declines after several months but may be triggered by tapering of immunosuppressive drugs. Clinical presentation is subtle and difficult to distinguish from complications such as infection, hepatic artery thrombosis, and biliary obstruction. Diagnosis can only be made with certainty by hepatic ultrasound and biopsy. Management is with high-dose glucocorticoids and subsequent taper and is best done at a transplant center. Chronic rejection occurs in 5 percent of cases and is the major cause of late graft failure.

237. **The answer is A.** *(Chapter 80)* Hyperbilirubinemia can be conjugated or unconjugated depending on whether the defect occurs before or after the conjugation phase in the hepatocyte. If increased production of bilirubin exceeds the ability of the hepatocytes to conjugate it, unconjugated hyperbilirubinemia occurs. This is the case in hemolysis from transfusion reactions, hemolytic anemia, and sickle cell anemia. With congestive heart failure, the liver is unable to take up and conjugate bilirubin. In patients with conjugated hyperbilirubinemia, the cause may be either intrahepatic or extrahepatic. Intrahepatic cholestasis results from an inability of the hepatocyte to excrete conjugated bilirubin due to damage of the biliary endothelium or hepatocyte damage, as in toxic hepatitis from acetaminophen poisoning. In extrahepatic cholestasis, there is obstruction of outflow in the biliary tree, as occurs with gallstones.

238. **The answer is D.** *(Chapter 82)* Hepatitis A, spread primarily by the fecal-to-oral route, is most common in children and adolescents. Adults tend to have a more severe or prolonged course but only rarely develop fulminant hepatic failure. Symptom onset is abrupt, and jaundice and hepatomegaly are usually mild. Outpatient management is generally sufficient, with emphasis on rest, adequate oral intake, and avoidance of hepatic toxins. Indications for admission include encephalopathy, prothrombin time prolonged more than 3 s, intractable vomiting, hypoglycemia, bilirubin greater than 20 mg/dL, age older than 45 years, and immunosuppression. Elevated liver enzymes alone are not an indication for admission and are not reliable indicators of disease severity.

239. **The answer is B.** *(Chapter 83)* Acute pancreatitis is a common cause of abdominal pain, with a prevalence estimated at 0.5 percent. In the United States, cholelithiasis and alcoholism account for up to 90 percent of cases. Alcohol-related disease is more common in the urban hospital setting and typically affects males between the ages of 35 and 45. Biliary disease is more frequent in the community hospital setting and typically affects females older than age 50. After biliary and alcohol disease, drugs account for up to half of the remaining cases.

240. **The answer is D.** *(Chapter 83)* Acute pancreatitis is unique compared with other intraabdominal processes because of its propensity to cause remote systemic effects. Pancreatitis evokes a generalized systemic inflammatory response that may lead to shock, ARDS, DIC, and eventually multisystem organ failure. Local complications include phlegmons, abscesses, and pseudocysts, usually in the first 2 to 3 weeks after onset of disease. Malabsorption may be seen with chronic pancreatitis but does not occur until more than 90 percent of glandular function is lost.

241. **The answer is C.** *(Chapter 84)* Laparoscopic procedures and early postsurgical discharge are becoming increasingly common cost-effective alternatives to laparotomy. As a result, more patients are presenting to the ED with postoperative fever. Fever during the first 24 h is usually caused by atelectasis or necrotizing streptococcal infections. In the first 24 to 72 h, respiratory complications such as pneumonia, and intravenous catheter related complications (e.g., thrombophlebitis) are the predominant causes. Urinary tract infections become evident 3 to 5 days postoperatively and are more common in females and patients who have had bladder catheterization or instrumentation. Clinical signs of wound infection usually develop 7 to 10 days postoperatively. Deep venous thrombosis may result in fever at any time but usually not before postoperative day 5.

242. **The answer is E.** *(Chapter 84)* After GI surgery, functional ileus is an expected complication. Small bowel tone usually returns in 24 h and colonic function in 3 to 5 days. Mechanical ileus can be delayed and is usually due to adhesions. Intraabdominal abscesses are often accompanied by fever and tenderness and are most frequently caused

by preoperative contamination or spillage of bowel contents during surgery. Pancreatitis is usually due to direct manipulation of the pancreatic duct and occurs commonly after biliary tract surgery and endoscopic retrograde cholangiopancreatography. The etiology of cholecystitis is unclear, and acalculous cholecystitis is a particular concern. It occurs most commonly in elderly males, and early operative intervention reduces morbidity and mortality. Other postoperative complications include fistula formation and tetanus (reported in GI surgery from intraoperative spillage of *Clostridium tetani* in devitalized tissue). Pseudomembranous colitis is a complication of perioperative courses of antibiotics but typically presents with diarrhea, fever, and occasionally crampy abdominal pain.

243. **The answer is B.**   *(Chapter 87)*   Ultrasound has emerged as a valuable tool for certain conditions in the ED. It is the initial study of choice for evaluation of patients with right upper quadrant pain and can accurately detect cholelithiasis. Plain film radiography is a poor imaging choice to detect gallstones but is useful in evaluating obstruction or suspected perforation. CT is the diagnostic tool of choice for many abdominal conditions, including pancreatitis, some trauma, and selected aortic aneurysms, but is more costly and invasive than ultrasound for evaluating gallstones. Radionuclide scanning is a useful adjunct if ultrasound results are inconclusive or acalculous cholecystitis is suspected. Barium radiography is useful for imaging in some GI conditions, especially suspected intussusception, but not for evaluating the gallbladder.

GERIATRIC EMERGENCIES

QUESTIONS

DIRECTIONS: Each question below contains five suggested responses. Choose the **one best** response to each question.

244. All of the following are true statements about falls in the elderly EXCEPT

(A) most falls occur on steps or other uneven surfaces
(B) most falls result in isolated orthopedic injuries
(C) decreased visual acuity and memory loss make it difficult for elderly patients to avoid environmental hazards
(D) syncope is a frequent cause of falls
(E) falls are the most common accidental injury in patients older than 75 years

245. Which of the following statements is MOST correct regarding abdominal pain in the elderly?

(A) Elderly patients are unlikely to have the problems of younger patients, such as appendicitis or cholecystitis
(B) Given the same underlying diagnosis for an acute abdominal disorder, the elderly have about the same mortality rate as younger patients
(C) The elderly exhibit less pain and tenderness than younger patients, but they are more likely to have fever and leukocytosis than are younger patients
(D) Diagnostic delays and preexisting illnesses lead to a higher mortality in elderly patients than in younger patients
(E) The elderly are more likely than younger patients to seek early medical attention for abdominal pain

246. A 75-year-old male is brought to the ED by his son-in-law for evaluation of altered level of consciousness. The patient has reportedly been bedridden for 2 days. Examination shows advanced sacral decubitus ulcers and bilateral ecchymoses of the upper arms. The son-in-law and the daughter both live with the patient. The son-in-law reports that the patient has been increasingly paranoid in recent weeks, with delusions of poisoning. What is the MOST likely diagnosis?

(A) Urosepsis
(B) Elder abuse
(C) Dementia
(D) Alcohol withdrawal
(E) Medication side effect

247. All of the following are true about elder abuse EXCEPT

(A) physical abuse, neglect, and chronic verbal aggression are all forms of elder abuse
(B) the abuser is often dependent on the victim for financial and emotional support
(C) dementia increases the risk of abuse
(D) abuse correlates with personality problems of the caretaker
(E) a majority of abuse cases can be diagnosed by patient history alone

248. An 80-year-old male is brought by ambulance from church for evaluation of a syncopal episode. The patient denies chest pain or palpitations and has no history of cardiac or cerebrovascular disease. Witnesses report no seizure activity. They loosened his shirt and tie immediately after the event, and the patient regained consciousness quickly. The patient has had several previous similar episodes for which he did not seek medical attention. One occurred while shaving and another occurred while dressing for church. Of the following, what is the MOST likely diagnosis?

(A) Gastrointestinal hemorrhage
(B) Psychogenic syncope
(C) Carotid sinus hypersensitivity
(D) Transient ischemic attack (TIA)
(E) Pulmonary embolism

249. All of the following are true of lacerations and wound care in the elderly EXCEPT

(A) the elderly have about the same response to a tetanus toxoid booster as younger patients
(B) the incidence of tetanus increases with age
(C) aging skin tears with minor friction
(D) in the elderly, skin tears usually present as epidermal flaps
(E) with aging, there is a decrease in cellular growth rate and a degeneration of collagen and elastic fibers

GERIATRIC EMERGENCIES

ANSWERS

244. The answer is A. *(Chapter 245)* Most elderly individuals who fall do so on a level surface, and most sustain isolated orthopedic injuries. Age-related changes in postural stability, balance, motor strength, and coordination make the elderly more prone to tripping and falling. Decreased visual acuity and increased memory loss can cause the patient difficulty in recognizing and avoiding environmental hazards. Syncope has been implicated in many cases of elderly patients who fall.

245. The answer is D. *(Chapter 69)* The elderly are at risk for acute appendicitis, acute cholecystitis, peptic ulcer disease, and intestinal obstruction. Diagnosis is challenging because elderly patients often lack classic signs and symptoms of an acute abdomen such as abdominal rigidity, fever and other abnormal vital signs, and leukocytosis. They may fail to seek early medical attention, and their many preexisting illnesses contribute to a higher mortality rate.

246. The answer is B. *(Chapter 292)* Certain injuries and historical features are characteristic of abuse. Bilateral upper arm bruises are suggestive of holding or shaking, and advanced decubitus ulcers are inconsistent with a history of being bedridden for only 2 days. Abuse is often dismissed as paranoia or dementia. Although any of the other diagnoses may be present, the underlying problem is elder abuse. Social services must be immediately involved in the case management.

247. The answer is E. *(Chapter 292)* Only about one-third of cases can be diagnosed by the victim's statements; another 6 percent are revealed by other informants. More cases are diagnosed by physical examination (43 percent) and social service assessment in the hospital (19 percent). Abuse correlates best with dependency and behavior problems of the caretaker/abuser, but dementia is also a significant risk factor.

248. The answer is C. *(Chapter 46)* The diagnosis of carotid sinus hypersensitivity should be suspected in elderly patients whose immediately presyncopal state is suggestive of carotid sinus stimulation, e.g., wearing a tight collar, shaving, or head turning. Carotid sinus hypersensitivity accounts for as much as 5 percent of syncope in the elderly. The diagnosis may be confirmed by bedside carotid sinus massage with cardiac monitoring and atropine at the bedside. Syncope is a very rare presentation of TIA. A pulmonary embolism large enough to cause syncope is commonly fatal.

249. The answer is A. *(Chapters 40 and 44)* Many elderly patients are inadequately immunized against tetanus, and their response to booster vaccination is diminished. The incidence of tetanus increases with age. A more liberal use of tetanus immune globulin is recommended in the elderly. Collagen and elastic fibers decrease with age, leading to skin tears with only minor friction. Epidermal flaps should be reapproximated with the least possible tension.

HEMATOLOGIC AND ONCOLOGIC EMERGENCIES

QUESTIONS

DIRECTIONS: Each question below contains five suggested responses. Choose the **one best** response to each question.

250. Which one of the following drugs is LEAST likely to result in thrombocytopenia?

(A) Heparin
(B) Quinine
(C) Quinidine
(D) Estrogen
(E) Heroin

251. All of the following statements regarding platelet abnormalities are TRUE EXCEPT

(A) bleeding complications may arise if platelets are < 50,000/μL
(B) patients are at risk for spontaneous bleeding if platelet counts are < 10,000/μL
(C) when platelets drop below 10,000/μL, the patient should receive a platelet transfusion
(D) patients with ITP respond well to platelet transfusion
(E) each unit of platelets transfused should raise the platelet count by about 10,000/μL

252. A suicidal 28-year-old male ingested a handful of rodenticide pellets containing brodifacoum 30 min before ED presentation. Paramedics administered 1 mg/kg of activated charcoal en route to the hospital. The patient is awake and alert, with normal vital signs. There is no evidence of mucosal bleeding, skin bruising, or abdominal pain. A test for occult fecal blood is negative. Laboratory examinations for prothrombin time (PT), partial thromboplastin time (PTT), complete blood count (CBC), and platelets are all normal. What is the MOST appropriate action?

(A) Give additional charcoal, observe for 2 h, and discharge to psychiatry if stable
(B) Admit and request urgent psychiatric consultation
(C) Administer vitamin K 1 mg intravenously, observe for 2 h, and discharge to psychiatry if stable
(D) Administer vitamin K 5 mg subcutaneously, observe for 4 h, and discharge to psychiatry if stable
(E) Admit, mobilize pharmacy resources to assess vitamin K inventory, and obtain psychiatric consultation

253. All of the following antibiotics are associated with drug-induced deficiencies of vitamin K–dependent factors EXCEPT

(A) cefotaxime
(B) trimethoprim
(C) cefoperazone
(D) moxalactam
(E) cefamandole

254. All of the following proteins require vitamin K to function properly EXCEPT

(A) factor II (prothrombin)
(B) factor VII
(C) factor IX
(D) factor X
(E) antithrombin III

255. All of the following statements regarding fresh frozen plasma (FFP) are TRUE EXCEPT

(A) it contains all factors
(B) intravenous administration can lead to volume overload
(C) viral transmission is possible with transfusion
(D) it is a first-line treatment for uremic patients with bleeding
(E) it is a first-line treatment for bleeding patients with a coagulopathy

256. A 50-year-old male presents with a crush injury to the left lower extremity. He underwent a 45-min extrication after an accident at a construction site. Peripheral pulses are intact, but sensorimotor function is diminished. He is hemodynamically stable after standard resuscitation, but the wound site continues to bleed despite a pressure dressing. Available laboratory results include hemoglobin of 12, hematocrit of 32, platelet count of 45,000/μL, PT of 18, and fibrinogen of 80 mg/dL. The surgical team has been called to treat the wound. While awaiting their arrival, all of the following are appropriate interventions EXCEPT

(A) give 2 units of FFP
(B) type and screen 2 units of packed red blood cells
(C) give cryoprecipitate, 10 bags
(D) give platelets, 6 packs
(E) give low-molecular-weight heparin

257. All of the following statements concerning heparin therapy are TRUE EXCEPT

(A) it facilitates antithrombin III binding to activated factors II, IX, XI, and XII
(B) the most common complication is bleeding
(C) one milligram of protamine sulfate neutralizes 1000 units of heparin
(D) thrombocytopenia is a common complication
(E) co-use of cimetidine or NSAIDs increases bleeding risk

258. All of the following statements regarding thrombocytopenia in the setting of heparin use are TRUE EXCEPT

(A) the incidence is lower with low-molecular-weight heparin
(B) the most common form is transient and seldom lowers the platelet count below 100,000/μL
(C) the type with platelet antibody formation can be life threatening and may lower the platelet count below 50,000/μL
(D) arterial thromboses can occur in the more severe form
(E) patients must have a previous exposure to heparin to develop anti-platelet antibodies

259. All of the following statements regarding thrombolytic drugs are TRUE EXCEPT

(A) they are contraindicated if the patient has a history of hemorrhagic stroke
(B) they cannot be used if the patient has active bleeding
(C) they must be avoided if aortic dissection is suspected
(D) they decrease pulmonary artery pressures, improve reperfusion, and increase survival after massive pulmonary embolus
(E) they are indicated for treatment of acute myocardial infarction

260. Which one of the following is the LEAST common hematologic complication of HIV?

(A) Thrombocytopenia
(B) Anemia
(C) ITP
(D) Thrombotic thrombocytopenic purpura (TTP)
(E) Acquired circulating antibodies

261. All of the following statements regarding factor VIII inhibitors are TRUE EXCEPT

(A) PTT is normal, but the PT is prolonged
(B) these inhibitors may develop in patients with previously normal hemostasis
(C) if present, mortality rate approaches 50 percent
(D) these inhibitors may develop in patients with underlying conditions such as pregnancy and autoimmune or lymphoproliferative disorders
(E) these inhibitors can be seen in patients with congenital factor VIII deficiency (hemophilia A)

262. All of the following statements regarding lupus anti-coagulant are TRUE EXCEPT

(A) it is an antiphospholipid antibody that interferes with coagulation
(B) most patients with lupus anticoagulant do not have lupus (SLE) or a clinical bleeding disorder
(C) affected patients are at risk for arterial and venous thrombosis
(D) affected women may have recurrent fetal loss
(E) it is associated with a normal PTT

263. A 15-year-old male with hemophilia A presents with hoarseness, stridor, and anterior neck swelling after an assault in which he sustained a "karate chop" to the throat. What is MOST appropriate sequence of actions?

(A) endotracheal intubation, factor VIII replacement, neck CT
(B) factor VIII replacement, lateral soft-tissue film of the neck
(C) factor VIII replacement, neck CT, close observation for need to intubate
(D) check PTT and factor VIII assay, neck CT, close observation for need to intubate
(E) surgical airway, check factor VIII levels

264. All of the following statements regarding desmo-pressin (DDAVP) are TRUE EXCEPT

(A) it is a beneficial treatment for mild to moderate hemophilia A
(B) it can raise factor VIII activity up to threefold
(C) the usual dose is 0.3 μg/kg of body weight intravenous or subcutaneous every 12 h
(D) a rise in factor VIII levels occurs between 4 and 6 h after administration
(E) common side effects include headache and mild hyponatremia

265. A 22-year-old female with sickle cell anemia (Hb SS) presents with a 2-day history of pleuritic chest pain and mild dyspnea. Vital signs are: temperature 38°C, pulse 90, blood pressure of 126/80 mm Hg, respiration rate of 24 breaths per minute, and room air pulse oximetry of 92 percent. Chest x-ray and electrocardiography are unremarkable. Which one of the following is the LEAST appropriate action?

(A) Give empiric antibiotics, such as cefuroxime and erythromycin
(B) Hydrate the patient with normal saline at 200 cc/h
(C) Treat pain with morphine sulfate boluses of 4 to 6 mg intravenously
(D) Obtain a baseline arterial blood gas and arrange a V̇/Q̇ scan or spiral CT
(E) Give supplemental oxygen

266. A 62-year-old African-American male who received TMP-SMX and pyridium for a urinary tract infection 2 days previously at an outside clinic presents to the ED complaining of dark urine. He denies fever or low back pain. Urinalysis shows a dark yellow urine, positive for blood, leukocytes, nitrites, bilirubin, and urobilinogen and negative for ketones, glucose, and protein. Microscopy shows red blood cells, white blood cells, and bacteria. What is the MOST likely diagnosis?

(A) rhabdomyolysis
(B) side effect of pyridium
(C) gallbladder obstruction
(D) G6PD deficiency
(E) hepatitis

267. A 60-year-old female presents to the ED with a fever of 37.8°C, mild confusion, and headache for the past 2 days. The patient is awake with no nuchal rigidity or lateralizing neurologic signs. CT is negative for mass effect or intracranial bleed. Laboratory findings show a platelet count of 20,000/μL, reticulocytosis, mild leukocytosis with a left shift, schistocytes on peripheral smear, and mild azotemia. Urinalysis shows proteinuria and hematuria. All of the following are appropriate actions EXCEPT

(A) administering FFP
(B) plasma exchange transfusion
(C) prednisone or methylprednisolone intravenously
(D) platelet transfusion
(E) ICU admission

268. A 50-year-old male with known malignancy complains of bilateral lower extremity weakness and acute urinary retention. Ambulation has become increasingly difficult over the past 2 days. Examination is remarkable for percussion tenderness at the thoracolumbar junction. Rectal sphincter tone is preserved. All of the following actions are appropriate EXCEPT

(A) giving decadron 10 mg intravenously
(B) giving solumedrol 30 mg/kg
(C) ordering CT of the thoracolumbar region
(D) calling for emergent neurosurgical consult
(E) placing a Foley catheter with a leg bag and discharging with close urology follow-up

269. A 55-year-old female with previously documented metastatic breast cancer presents to the ED with an altered sensorium. She is afebrile, and there are no focal neurologic signs. Serum calcium is 15 mg/dL. Which of the following is the LEAST appropriate action?

(A) Oncology consultation followed by glucocorticoid administration
(B) Intravenous saline infusion
(C) Intravenous furosemide administration
(D) Oral phosphate administration
(E) Intravenous inorganic phosphate bolus administration

HEMATOLOGIC AND ONCOLOGIC EMERGENCIES

ANSWERS

250. The answer is D. *(Chapters 210–211)* Drugs are commonly responsible for thrombocytopenia. Although all of the listed agents are associated with a reduction in platelet count, there are fewer case reports involving estrogen than those involving heparin, quinine, quinidine, or heroin. Other drugs that cause thrombocytopenia include sulfa-containing antibiotics, amrinone, ethanol, aspirin, valproic acid, indomethacin, thiazide diuretics, phenytoin, cimetidine, penicillin, and interferon.

251. The answer is D. *(Chapter 211)* Patients with idiopathic thrombocytopenic purpura (ITP) have platelet antibodies that increase platelet destruction, thereby limiting the efficacy of transfusion. Patients with hypersplenism are also poor candidates for platelet transfusion because they sequester transfused platelets out of the general circulation. Most patients with platelets fewer than 50,000/μL should receive platelet transfusions to protect against bleeding complications. If platelets drop to less than 10,000/μL, platelet transfusion is strongly advised because of the risk of spontaneous bleeding, including intracranial hemorrhage. Each pack of platelets transfused raises the platelet count by approximately 10,000/μL.

252. The answer is E. *(Chapter 211)* Patients who have ingested significant amounts of brodifacoum require admission and treatment with massive amounts of vitamin K, possibly exceeding the pharmacy's inventory. This type of rat poison is a "superwarfarin" with a long half-life that was created to combat emerging warfarin resistance in rodent pests. Ingestion of "superwarfarin" is associated with a severe, potentially fatal coagulopathy. Profuse mucosal bleeding and internal hemorrhage are common clinical manifestations. Treatment of warfarin overdose depends on the clinical picture, not on the magnitude of PT prolongation. Patients may require large doses of vitamin K (50–100 mg/day) for several weeks. Fresh frozen plasma may also be required. A 10- to 15-mg dose of vitamin K should be administered subcutaneously or intramuscularly to patients who are bleeding. Intravenous vitamin K carries a risk of anaphylaxis, but 1 mg intravenously is considered a safe quantity to give. Patients may be resistant to warfarin therapy for up to 2 weeks after vitamin K administration.

253. The answer is B. *(Chapter 211)* Trimethoprim is a sulfa drug associated with thrombocytopenia, not a coagulopathy secondary to vitamin K deficiency. Drug-induced deficiency of vitamin K–dependent factors is seen with cephalosporins that have an *N*-methylthiotetrazole side chain. These include the second-generation drug cefamandole and the third-generation drugs cefotaxime, cefoperazone, and moxalactam.

254. The answer is E. *(Chapter 211)* Antithrombin III is a protein that forms complexes with factors VII, IX, X, XI, and XII and prothrombin, thereby inhibiting their function. It is not vitamin K–dependent. Factors II, VII, IX, and X, protein C, and protein S are all dependent on vitamin K for proper functioning. Parenchymal liver disease decreases synthesis of factors II, VII, IX, and X. Because vitamin K is fat soluble, malabsorption, hepatic cholestasis, and poor nutrition contribute to vitamin K deficiency.

255. The answer is D. *(Chapter 211)* FFP is not a first-line treatment for patients with uremia and excessive bleeding because of its inability to tolerate the large volume load. Treatment of a bleeding uremic patient should include packed red blood cells, erythropoietin, desmopressin, dialysis, conjugated estrogen, platelet transfusion, or cryoprecipitate infusion. Cryoprecipitate carries a risk of viral transmission and has mostly been replaced by desmopressin. FFP administration also carries a risk of virus transmission. Each unit of FFP contains 200 to 250 units of each coagulation factor. FFP is indicated in the treatment of patients with severe liver disease and bleeding.

256. The answer is E. *(Chapter 211)* In addition to the traumatic injury, this patient has evidence of disseminated intravascular coagulation (DIC), suggested by the prolonged PT, low fibrinogen, and decreased platelets. Clinical manifestations of DIC include bleeding, thrombosis, and purpura fulminans. This patient's continued bleeding and prolonged PT are indications for FFP and cryoprecipitate (to replete fibrinogen). Platelet transfusion is indicated when platelet count is less than $50,000/\mu L$ and there is bleeding, or if platelet count is less than $20,000/\mu L$ regardless of bleeding. Packed red blood cells should be ready in case the hemoglobin and hematocrit continue to drop. Whereas low-dose heparin (5–10 units/kg/h) is used to treat patients with purpura fulminans, low-molecular-weight heparin is not used to treat DIC. Patients with DIC who may benefit from standard heparin therapy include those with carcinoma, acute promyelocytic leukemia, or retained uterine products.

257. The answer is C. *(Chapter 211)* One milligram of protamine sulfate will neutralize 100 units of standard-molecular-weight heparin and is indicated in the setting of severe bleeding after the heparin infusion has been stopped. Bleeding is a common complication of heparin use and occurs in about one-third of patients. One to seven percent of patients will have serious or life-threatening bleeding. Concomitant use of cimetidine, nonsteroidal antiinflammatory drugs (NSAIDs), aspirin, warfarin, and steroids increase a patient's bleeding risk. Underlying conditions that also increase risk of bleeding include history of renal failure, gastrointestinal bleeding, ethanol use, malignancy, recent trauma, and bleeding diatheses. Thrombocytopenia is a common complication of heparin use.

258. The answer is E. *(Chapter 211)* Heparin-associated thrombocytopenia with anti–platelet antibody formation is uncommon but is potentially life threatening. Patients with previous exposure to heparin may have an immediate reaction, whereas patients without previous exposure will more likely develop antibodies over the next 6 to 10 days. Arterial thrombosis is a possible complication. If platelet levels fall below $50,000/\mu L$, heparin transfusion must be stopped; some clinicians have advocated future avoidance of heparin. A more common form of heparin-associated thrombocytopenia without antibody formation occurs in about 25 percent of patients. A transient decrease in platelet count occurs, but seldom below $100,000/\mu L$. The etiology is postulated to be due to platelet aggregation and splenic sequestration.

259. The answer is D. *(Chapters 211, 216)* Thrombolytic drugs have been used to treat massive, acute pulmonary emboli. With treatment, reperfusion is improved and pulmonary artery pressures are decreased. However, clinical trials that conclusively demonstrate improved survival are lacking.

260. The answer is D. *(Chapter 211)* Thrombocytopenia is the most common hematologic complication of HIV infection. Immune platelet destruction, such as that seen with ITP, is also common. Anemia frequently occurs secondary to decreased erythropoiesis and bone marrow suppression from infection or drug therapy. A lupus-type anticoagulant prolongs the PTT and may appear and disappear in concert with the onset and treatment of opportunistic infections. Anti–cardiolipin antibodies, another type of acquired circulating antibody, increase the patient's risk of thrombosis. TTP is an uncommon complication of HIV infection. It may actually herald HIV infection when appearing with a pentad of fever, thrombocytopenia, neurologic symptoms, renal insufficiency, and microangiopathic hemolytic anemia.

261. The answer is A. *(Chapter 211)* Factor VIII inhibitors prolong the PTT (reflecting the intrinsic coagulation cascade), but not the PT (reflecting the extrinsic coagulation cascade). This same pattern is seen in patients with hemophilia A (factor VIII deficiency). The incidence of factor VIII inhibitors is low, estimated at 0.2 to 1.0 per million, but the mortality rate approaches 50 percent. Patients develop massive spontaneous ecchymoses and hematomas. About half of affected people are otherwise healthy and older than 65 years. Associated underlying autoimmune disorders include systemic lupus erythematosus (SLE), rheumatoid arthritis, and ulcerative colitis. Associated lymphoproliferative disorders include multiple myeloma, Waldenström's macroglobulinemia, and benign monoclonal gammopathy. Pregnancy and the immediate postpartum period are also associated. A factor VIII–specific assay shows low or absent factor VIII activity. Treatment involves repletion or supplementation of factor VIII and prothrombin.

262. The answer is E. *(Chapter 211)* Lupus anticoagulant, an antiphospholipid antibody, is often an incidental laboratory finding. Only 5 to 15 percent of patients have SLE, and clinical bleeding is rare unless the patient has an underlying predisposing condition such as hypoprothrombinemia, significant thrombocytopenia, or uremia. Patients with lupus anticoagulant display mild to moderate PTT prolongation and a normal or slightly prolonged PT. Arterial and venous thrombosis occurs in 23 to 53 percent of patients. Recurrent fetal loss is secondary to placental vessel thrombosis and infarction.

263. The answer is A. *(Chapter 211)* This patient has impending airway compromise and should be emergently intubated. After the airway is secured, factor VIII should be replaced and computed tomography (CT) of the neck should be performed. Patients with hemophilia are at risk for spontaneous bleeding and posttraumatic bleeding. Because this patient with hemophilia A has a potentially life-threatening hemorrhage, he requires an initial dose of factor VIII of 50 units/kg. If no factor VIII concentrate is readily available, cryoprecipitate (100 units of factor VIII per bag) or FFP (1 unit of factor VIII/mL) can be administered as a temporizing measure.

264. The answer is D. *(Chapter 212)* DDAVP is a synthetic peptide, not a blood product, so there is no risk of viral transmission. For hemophilia A patients who respond, the rise in factor VIII levels occurs within 1 h of administration. The usual dose is 0.3 μg/kg intravenously or subcutaneously every 12 h for three to four doses, after which temporary tachyphylaxis may occur. DDAVP is postulated to work by causing a release of von Willebrand factor (vWF) from endothelial cells. Increased levels of vWF are able to carry additional factor VIII in the plasma. Mild hyponatremia may occur because of the effect similar to that of anti-diuretic hormone.

265. The answer is B. *(Chapter 213)* Acute chest syndrome, characterized by fever, dyspnea, tachypnea, hypoxia, pleuritic chest pain, leukocytosis, and pulmonary infiltrates, is this patient's most likely diagnosis. Despite the later development of consolidation, initial chest x-ray is often unremarkable. Acute chest syndrome occurs when a pulmonary infarct becomes secondarily infected, and it is seen in 30 percent of patients with sickle cell disease, accounting for 15 percent of adult deaths. It may be difficult to differentiate between acute chest syndrome and pneumonia or pulmonary infarction, and most hematologists recommend empiric antibiotics. If pulmonary embolism is suspected, $\dot{V}/\dot{Q}$ or spiral CT is indicated. Pulmonary angiography carries the risk of further exacerbating pulmonary sickling and should be avoided. Aggressive hydration may precipitate adult respiratory distress syndrome.

266. The answer is D. *(Chapter 213)* Glucose-6-phosphate dehydrogenase (G6PD) deficiency is an inherited enzyme disorder that affects up to 10 percent of the world's population. This deficiency leaves senescent red blood cells vulnerable to oxidative stress and causes hemoglobin to precipitate in the form of Heinz bodies. It is X-linked and manifests in male heterozygotes and female homozygotes. Hemolytic crises occur after bacterial or viral infection, metabolic acidosis, fava bean ingestion, or exposure to oxidant drugs. The most common oxidant drugs are sulfa drugs such as TMP-SMX, chloroquine, pyridium, and nitrofurantoin. With rhabdomyolysis, the urinalysis is positive for blood (myoglobin), but red cells are absent on microscopy. Pyridium will color urine orange. Over a period of several days, a patient with gallbladder obstruction would have pain and might have a urine positive for bilirubin but negative for urobilinogen because the conjugated bilirubin would not reach the intestine.

267. The answer is D. *(Chapter 214)* This patient has thrombotic thrombocytopenic purpura. This disorder is characterized by a microangiopathic hemolytic anemia that results in microthrombi in capillaries and arterioles throughout the body, especially in the brain, heart, kidneys, pancreas, and adrenal glands. Schistocytes are present on peripheral smear. Treatment includes ICU admission, steroids, and plasma exchange transfusion using FFP. Because platelets can exacerbate thrombosis, transfusion should be avoided unless there is uncontrolled hemorrhage.

268. The answer is E. *(Chapter 217)* This patient has evidence of acute spinal cord compression in the thoracic region, demonstrated by bilateral radiculopathy. Aggressive work-up and treatment may help prevent permanent neurologic disability. He requires urgent neurosurgical consultation, high-dose steroids, magnetic resonance imaging, and a Foley catheter. Acute spinal cord compression is common in patients with multiple myeloma, lymphoma, and metastatic breast, lung, and prostate cancers. It can also occur in the setting of epidural hematoma, infection, or fracture.

269. The answer is E. *(Chapter 217)* This patient has severe hypercalcemia that could adversely affect cardiac, neurologic, and muscular function. Saline infusion (1 to 2 L) followed by 80 mg intravenous furosemide are standard initial therapies. Glucocorticoids are efficacious for the treatment of hypercalcemia in the setting of lymphoma, hematologic emergencies, and metastatic lung and breast cancers. Peak effectiveness is not reached for several days. Bisphosphonate and mithramycin are also highly efficacious treatments. One gram of inorganic phosphate, infused over an 8-h period, and never as a bolus, will rapidly reduce serum calcium, but potential adverse effects include accelerated soft-tissue calcifications, hypocalcemia, hypotension, renal failure, and death.

INFECTIOUS DISEASE EMERGENCIES

QUESTIONS

DIRECTIONS: Each question below contains five suggested responses. Choose the **one best** response to each question.

270. A 25-year-old male with a history of recent unprotected sexual intercourse presents with a complaint of urethritis. Gram stain of a urethral smear shows intracellular gram-negative diplococci. All of the following actions are recommended EXCEPT

    (A) administering a single oral dose of cefixime 400 mg
    (B) administering a single oral dose of azithromycin 1 g
    (C) obtaining a serologic test for syphilis
    (D) advising the patient to obtain HIV testing
    (E) administering a single oral dose of metronidazole 2 g

271. Which one of the following is NOT a recommended regimen for the treatment of *N. gonorrhoeae* urethritis or cervicitis?

    (A) Ceftriaxone 125 mg intramuscularly, single dose
    (B) Azithromycin 2 g orally, single dose
    (C) Ciprofloxacin 500 mg orally, single dose
    (D) Ofloxacin 400 mg orally, single dose
    (E) Cefixime 400 mg orally, single dose

272. Which of the following characteristics or findings are suggestive of the secondary stage of syphilis?

    (A) Painless chancre with indurated borders on the penis, vulva, or other areas of sexual contact
    (B) Red papular rash on the trunk and flexor surfaces that spreads to the palms and soles
    (C) Findings that develop about 21 days after initial infection
    (D) Involvement of the cardiovascular and nervous systems
    (E) Symptoms that develop years after initial infection

273. A 19-year-old female presents with painful pustular lesions on the vulva. She recalls having unprotected sexual intercourse approximately 10 days before with a male partner who had a single small lesion on the penis. She also reports dysuria that began when she noticed the lesions. All of the following statements are TRUE regarding the diagnosis EXCEPT

    (A) although direct viral culture is more sensitive for detecting the organism, a smear of these lesions may show large intranuclear inclusions
    (B) infection occurs by direct contact with mucosal surfaces or nonintact skin
    (C) systemic symptoms including fever, headache, and myalgias are uncommon
    (D) appropriate initial therapy consists of antiviral drugs including acyclovir, famciclovir, or valacyclovir
    (E) recurrent outbreaks of these lesions occur in 60 to 90 percent of patients

274. A female patient reports a recent sexual contact with a partner who has just been treated for a suspected STD. During the examination, a urine test for pregnancy is found to be positive. Which of the following antibiotics is safe to prescribe before referring the patient to an obstetrician for prenatal care?

    (A) Acyclovir
    (B) Azithromycin
    (C) Cefixime
    (D) Metronidazole
    (E) All of the above

275. The diagnosis of toxic shock syndrome requires a temperature above 38.9°C (102°F), a systolic blood pressure (BP) below 90 mm Hg, an orthostatic decrease of systolic BP by 15 mm Hg or syncope, a rash with subsequent desquamation, and involvement of at least three organ systems. Which of the following systems is NOT considered in the diagnosis?

(A) Hematologic: thrombocytopenia < 100,000 platelets/μL

(B) Renal: increase in BUN and creatinine two times normal level; pyuria without evidence of infection

(C) CNS: disorientation without focal neurologic signs

(D) Respiratory: respiratory rate > 28 breaths per minute, evidence of bilateral alveolar infiltrates on chest x-ray

(E) Gastrointestinal: vomiting, profuse diarrhea

276. All of the following statements regarding TSS and toxic shock–like syndrome (TSLS) are TRUE EXCEPT

(A) the majority of cases of TSS are associated with menstruation

(B) *Staphylococcus aureus* and *Streptococcus pyogenes* are the most common organisms isolated from patients with TSS and TSLS

(C) TSST-1, an exotoxin implicated in the production of many TSS symptoms, has been isolated from 20 percent of randomly tested *S. aureus* isolates

(D) up to 60 percent of patients relapse if they are not treated with β-lactamase–stable antimicrobial drugs

(E) residual neurologic deficits, including memory deficits, decreased concentration, and diffuse electroencephalographic abnormalities, are seen in 50 percent of TSS survivors

277. An HIV-positive patient presents to the ED complaining of shortness of breath and nonproductive cough. Chest x-ray shows diffuse interstitial infiltrates, and O_2 saturation is 85 percent on room air. All of the following statements regarding this patient's probable diagnosis are TRUE EXCEPT

(A) *Pneumocystis carinii* pneumonia (PCP) is the most common opportunistic infection in AIDS patients

(B) pentamidine isothionate is an effective alternate therapy to TMP-SMX

(C) a normal chest x-ray rules out acute PCP infection

(D) 65 percent of patients relapse within 18 months

(E) oral steroid therapy should be started in patients with a Pao_2 < 70 mm Hg, or an alveolar–arterial gradient > 35

278. CNS disease occurs in 75 to 90 percent of patients with AIDS. Which of the following is the MOST common cause of opportunistic infection of the CNS in AIDS patients?

(A) Cryptococcal meningitis

(B) Bacterial meningitis

(C) HSV encephalitis

(D) Toxoplasmosis

(E) AIDS dementia

279. Up to 5 percent of ED visits for AIDS patients are related to complications of pharmacologic therapy. Which of the following medications is LEAST likely to be responsible for a rash in an HIV patient?

(A) Acyclovir

(B) TMP-SMX

(C) Clindamycin

(D) Ibuprofen

(E) Dapsone

280. All of the following statements regarding CMV retinitis are TRUE EXCEPT

(A) patients may present with photophobia, scotoma, eye redness, pain, or change in visual acuity

(B) treatment with ganciclovir (5 mg/kg) should be initiated

(C) patients may have funduscopic findings of CMV without ophthalmologic symptoms

(D) CMV retinitis occurs in 10 to 15 percent of AIDS patients

(E) funduscopic examination shows cotton-wool spots

281. A patient who fell down a cliff while backpacking is brought to the ED after a prolonged rescue 8 h after falling. The patient sustained multiple lacerations and abrasions that are covered by dirt and grass. The patient is a 45-year-old U.S. native who cannot remember the last time she received tetanus prophylaxis. Which of the following represents the BEST management?

(A) Adult tetanus toxoid (Td) 0.5 mL intramuscularly

(B) Human tetanus immune globulin (TIG) 250 U intramuscularly

(C) Td 0.5 mL intramuscularly and TIG 250 U intramuscularly in the opposite extremity

(D) No prophylaxis is necessary because the patient is a U.S. native who received primary immunization as a child

(E) Td 0.5 mL intramuscularly and TIG 250 U intramuscularly, followed by additional doses of Td at 1 month and 6 months

282. *Clostridium tetani* is the organism responsible for causing tetanus. All of the following statements regarding tetanus are TRUE EXCEPT

(A) tetanospasmin, an exotoxin produced by *C. tetani*, is responsible for the clinical manifestations of tetanus

(B) tetanospasmin is released into the CNS after *C. tetani* crosses the blood–brain barrier

(C) clinical manifestations of tetanus include generalized muscular rigidity, violent muscular contractions, and instability of the autonomic nervous system

(D) the most common presenting complaint of patients with generalized tetanus is pain and stiffness in the masseter muscle

(E) tetanospasmin prevents the release of GABA and glycine from presynaptic nerve terminals

283. Which of the following animals is NOT a potential carrier of rabies?

(A) Dogs
(B) Bats
(C) Skunks
(D) Squirrels
(E) Cows

284. A colleague seeks your advice regarding travel immunizations. He is leaving in 2 weeks to be part of a medical missionary team in remote areas of Africa and Southeast Asia and plans to take malaria prophylaxis. Which of the following statements is LEAST correct regarding rabies prophylaxis in this case?

(A) Preexposure prophylaxis is recommended because the areas being visited are known to be endemic

(B) Prophylaxis with HDCV 1 mL intramuscularly should be administered in three doses at days 0, 7, and 21 or 28

(C) Active immunity to rabies persists for at least 2 years in most vaccine recipients

(D) There is no need to check rabies antibody titers after immunization has been completed

(E) If an exposure occurs, immediate treatment consists of cleaning wounds with soap, debriding devitalized tissue, copious irrigation with sterile saline or water, and avoidance of suturing

285. A 40-year-old male who immigrated 6 months previously to the United States from Guatemala presents to the ED with complaints of fever, chills, malaise, and abdominal pain. He reports having had similar symptoms just before immigrating and received treatment with an unknown medicine from a Guatemalan clinic. A Giemsa-stained blood smear confirms the presence of malarial parasites. Which of the following regimens is recommended in adults for the treatment of uncomplicated malaria caused by *Plasmodium vivax*?

(A) Quinine sulfate 650 mg orally three times a day for 5 to 7 days

(B) Quinine sulfate 650 mg orally three times a day for 5 to 7 days, plus doxycycline 100 mg orally two times a day for 7 days

(C) Chloroquine phosphate 1-g load, followed by 500 mg in 6 h, and then 500 mg/day for 2 days

(D) Quinidine gluconate 10 mg/kg intravenous load and then 0.02 mg/kg/min infusion for 48 h plus doxycycline 100 mg intravenously every 12 h for 48 h

(E) Chloroquine phosphate 1-g load, followed by 500 mg in 6 h, and then 500 mg/day for 2 days, plus primaquine phosphate 26.3-mg load per day for 14 days upon completion of chloroquine therapy

286. A frequent traveler reports previously taking chloroquine for malaria prophylaxis while visiting India. The patient is now planning an extended trip to Sub-Saharan Africa and would like another supply of chloroquine. All of the following are TRUE regarding this patient's upcoming travel EXCEPT

(A) 300 mg chloroquine base orally every week is recommended, with continuation of prophylaxis for 4 weeks after the last exposure

(B) the patient should remain in well-screened areas between dusk and dawn, use mosquito nets, and wear long-sleeved clothing

(C) a pyrethrum-containing insect spray should be used in the evening and insect repellant containing DEET should be applied to exposed skin

(D) malaria can be contracted even if chemoprophylaxis is taken and personal protection recommendations are followed

(E) the patient should receive prophylaxis for chloroquine-resistant *P. falciparum* with mefloquine 228 mg base orally every week

287. Many cases of diarrhea are caused by consumption of contaminated food and water. Which of the following statements regarding food-borne illness is FALSE?

(A) Food-borne illness affects approximately 6 to 80 million Americans annually and causes 9,000 deaths each year

(B) The relative risk of food-borne infection with viruses, bacteria, or parasites ranges from 20 to 50 percent for all travelers depending on the geographic region visited

(C) Gastric pH, intestinal motility, and indigenous intestinal bacteria are physiologic mechanisms that can help prevent disease resulting from food-borne pathogens

(D) The most common pathogens causing food-borne illnesses are *Salmonella*, *Campylobacter*, *Shigella*, *Escherichia coli* O157, and the Norwalk viruses

(E) Viruses are the most common etiology of travelers' diarrhea

288. Which of the following laboratory studies or pieces of historical information is LEAST helpful when evaluating a patient for suspected bacterial diarrhea?

(A) A 3- to 4-day history of food and water exposure

(B) Information regarding frequent restaurant meals, consumption of raw foods and meats, overseas travel, exposure to day-care centers, and ingestion of stream or lake water

(C) Stool studies for fecal leukocytes

(D) Information regarding immunocompetence and recent use of antibiotics, antacids, H_2 blockers, and proton pump inhibitors

(E) A history of other contacts who have developed similar symptoms

289. Which of the following organisms is the major cause of most travelers' diarrhea?

(A) *E. coli*
(B) *Campylobacter*
(C) *Vibrio*
(D) *Giardia*
(E) *Shigella*

290. A 37-year-old male arrives at the ED at 9:00 A.M. complaining of diarrhea that began at 5:00 A.M. The patient felt fine the night before after eating dinner at 8:00 P.M. at a local seafood restaurant. His dinner companion reportedly also developed copious diarrhea the same morning and is going to meet the patient at the ED. Which of the following organisms is MOST likely responsible for the food-borne illness?

(A) *S. aureus*
(B) A Norwalk virus
(C) Enterotoxigenic *E. coli*
(D) *Vibrio parahaemolyticus*
(E) *Campylobacter*

291. Etiologic agents in tick-borne infections include bacterial, rickettsial, viral, and protozoal organisms. All of the following infections can be acquired from a tick bite EXCEPT

(A) Rocky Mountain spotted fever
(B) Q fever
(C) relapsing fever
(D) tularemia
(E) babesiosis

292. All of the following statements are TRUE regarding influenza EXCEPT

(A) influenza types A, B, and C may cause human infection
(B) migrating aquatic fowl are thought to be the natural animal reservoir for influenza type A
(C) antiviral therapy with amantidine and rimantidine is effective against influenza types A, B, and C
(D) annual influenza vaccination is recommended for healthcare workers
(E) influenza pneumonia carries a high mortality rate, and more than 90 percent of deaths occur in patients older than 70 years

293. Gas-forming soft tissue infections are life threatening and must be diagnosed early and treated aggressively. Which one of the following symptoms or findings is LEAST likely to be seen with these infections?

(A) Increasing symptoms over 7 to 10 days
(B) Pain out of proportion to physical findings
(C) Brawny edema with crepitance on palpation
(D) Bullae or malodorous serosanguinous discharge
(E) Low-grade fever, with tachycardia out of proportion to the fever

294. Which of the following patients is MOST likely to benefit from antibiotic therapy in addition to abscess incision and drainage?

(A) A previously healthy female with a Bartholin's gland abscess and no history suggesting a high risk for STD
(B) A healthy 25-year-old male with recurrence of a pilonidal abscess that first occurred 2 years previously
(C) A febrile 50-year-old female with NIDDM and recurrence of axillary hydradenitis suppurativa
(D) A 35-year-old male with a sebaceous gland cyst that has been present for 2 years and has now become infected
(E) An intravenous drug user without fever or tachycardia presenting with a 2-cm^2 deltoid abscess that developed 7 days after "skin popping"

295. The CDC publishes a list of reportable communicable diseases that is updated and revised routinely. A 20-year-old patient is found to have a sexually transmitted disease. Which of the following is NOT included on the CDC list of reportable diseases?

(A) Chancroid
(B) Gonorrhea
(C) HIV
(D) Syphilis
(E) Chlamydia

296. A patient presents to the ED with symptoms of Bell's palsy. Which of the following signs or symptoms are atypical and suggest a more worrisome diagnosis?

(A) Facial hemiparesis
(B) Taste disturbance
(C) Decreased blinking
(D) Sparing of the forehead muscles on the affected side
(E) Hearing increased on the affected side

297. All of the following statements are TRUE regarding CMV retinitis EXCEPT

(A) decreased vision or floaters in the visual field are typical complaints

(B) prompt treatment with gancyclovir or foscarnet can reverse visual deficits

(C) without treatment, CMV retinitis will progress to permanent blindness

(D) CMV retinitis occurs in more than 10 percent of AIDS patients

(E) in addition to retinitis, CMV can cause esophagitis, colitis, or adrenalitis

298. Universal precautions were recommended in 1987 by the CDC to protect healthcare workers from the potential hazards of exposure to blood and other body fluids. All of the following practices are part of the recommended universal precautions EXCEPT

(A) wear puncture-proof gloves when handling needles or sharp instruments with the potential for puncturing skin

(B) mask and eye protection are indicated if mucous membranes of the mouth, nose, and eyes may be exposed to drops of blood or other body fluids

(C) do not recap or bend needles

(D) use a bag-valve mask to prevent the need for mouth-to-mouth resuscitation

(E) healthcare workers with weeping dermatitis should avoid direct patient care until the condition resolves

299. The risk of tuberculosis (TB) among healthcare workers has increased, as has a resurgence of the disease. All of the following factors increase risk of TB transmission EXCEPT

(A) exposure to a highly contagious source case

(B) increased ventilatory rate of the healthcare worker

(C) increased air-exchange rate in the work environment

(D) working in an inner city environment

(E) increased duration of exposure to infected patients

INFECTIOUS DISEASE EMERGENCIES

ANSWERS

270. The answer is E. *(Chapter 137)* Although this patient's gram stain suggests gonococcal infection, there is a high incidence of concomitant chlamydial infection. Therefore, he should be treated for both gonorrhea and chlamydia. In addition, a serum test for syphilis and counseling regarding testing for human immunodeficiency virus (HIV) are warranted. This patient should also be educated about condom use and advised to have his sexual partners checked for sexually transmitted diseases (STDs). Metronidazole is not routinely administered unless trichomonas is seen on microscopic urinalysis.

271. The answer is B. *(Chapter 137)* All of the antibiotic regimens listed are recommended by the Centers for Disease Control and Prevention (CDC) guidelines as effective therapies for gonococcal infection except the single dose of azithromycin 2 g orally. The CDC guidelines suggest 2 g spectinomycin intramuscularly as an acceptable alternative therapy. Azithromycin 1 g orally as a single dose is effective against localized *chlamydial* infection such as cervicitis or urethritis or for postexposure prophylaxis but is insufficient to treat pelvic inflammatory disease.

272. The answer is B. *(Chapter 137)* There are three stages of syphilis. The primary stage usually occurs about 21 days after initial infection and is characterized by a painless chancre on the penis, vulva, or other area of sexual contact. These typical lesions usually resolve within 3 to 6 weeks. The second stage of syphilis occurs 3 to 6 weeks after the end of the primary stage. Stage II includes nonspecific symptoms (headache, sore throat, fever, malaise), diffuse lymphadenopathy, and rash. The rash is usually dull red and papular, first occurring on the trunk and flexor surfaces and then spreading to the palms and soles. The tertiary stage of syphilis may occur years after inital infection and is characterized by cardiovascular and nervous system involvement. Findings can include tabes dorsalis, acute meningitis, dementia, and thoracic aneurysm. HIV-positive patients may have an accelerated course.

273. The answer is C. *(Chapter 137)* This patient has acute herpes simplex infection, spread by direct contact with mucosal skin or with nonintact skin. Smears of the lesions may stain for intranuclear bodies, but direct culture of the lesions has a greater sensitivity. Most patients (60 to 90 percent) have at least one recurrent outbreak because the virus remains latent after initial infection. Appropriate therapy includes different regimens of acyclovir, famciclovir, or valacyclovir. Dysuria and systemic symptoms such as fever, headache, and myalgias are common, and some patients develop aseptic meningitis.

274. The answer is E. *(Chapter 137)* The patient's symptoms and examination findings would determine the treatment. All of the antibiotics listed, plus penicillin and ceftriaxone, are considered safe during pregnancy. If the safety of any treatment is in doubt, an obstetrician should be consulted.

275. The answer is D. *(Chapter 138)* The CDC formulated a case definition of toxic shock syndrome (TSS) in 1980. In addition to the findings of a fever, hypotension, and rash, at least three of the following organ systems must be involved—gastrointestinal: vomiting, profuse diarrhea; musculoskeletal: severe myalgias or twofold increase in CPK; renal: increase in blood urea nitrogen (BUN) and creatinine two times normal level, pyuria without evidence of infection; mucosal inflammation: vaginal, conjunctival, or pharyngeal hyperemia; hepatic involvement: hepatitis (twofold elevation of bilirubin, AST, ALT); hematologic: thrombocytopenia < 100,000 platelets/μL; central nervous system (CNS): disorientation without focal neurologic signs. Although not included in the case definition, involvement of the respiratory system, and development of adult respiratory distress syndrome (ARDS) and refractory hypotension are late manifestations of TSS that represent end-organ damage.

276. **The answer is A.** *(Chapter 138)*   TSS was initially a disease of young, healthy, menstruating women (50 percent of cases in 1986 and 1987). Changes in tampon composition and a heightened public and professional awareness of the risks of tampon use are credited for a change in epidemiology. At present, men comprise one-third of patients with TSS, and another 25 percent of cases have been associated with postpartum and *S. aureus* vaginal infections in nonmenstruating women. In addition, TSS has been associated with nasal packing (nasal tampons) and has been reported after influenza and influenza-like illnesses. *Staphylococcus aureus* and *S. pyogenes* are associated with TSS and TSLS, respectively. The TSST-1 exotoxin is a significant factor in the development of many TSS symptoms. Sequelae of TSS are numerous and include a high rate of neurologic deficits. Up to 60 percent of patients who do not receive β-lactamase–stable antibiotics have recurrence of the disease, usually within 2 months of the initial episode, but sometimes up to 1 year later. This second episode is usually less severe than the first, but deaths have resulted from recurrences of mild cases.

277. **The answer is C.** *(Chapter 139)*   PCP is the most common opportunistic infection in AIDS patients, and more than 80 percent of patients acquire PCP at some time during their illness. Common symptoms include nonproductive cough, shortness of breath, and exertional dyspnea. Chest x-ray findings often demonstrate bilateral alveolar infiltrates, but 5 to 10 percent of patients have a negative chest film. PCP is often the presumptive diagnosis in HIV-positive patients with unexplained hypoxia. Initial therapy for PCP is trimethoprim-sulfamethoxazole (TMP-SMX) orally or intravenously; pentamidine isothionate is an acceptable alternative. An ABG should be obtained and results used to determine the need for initiation of steroid therapy. Reinfection is common, and prophylactic therapy with TMP-SMX, inhaled pentamidine, or dapsone is recommended.

278. **The answer is D.** *(Chapter 139)*   Common etiologies of neurologic symptoms in AIDS patients include AIDS dementia, *Toxoplasma gondii*, and *Cryptococcus neoformans*. Of these, toxoplasmosis is most likely to cause focal encephalopathy. It may present with headache, fever, focal neurologic deficits, altered mental status, or seizures. Computed tomographic (CT) findings of ring-enhancing lesions are suggestive of toxoplasmosis; however, lymphoma, fungal infections, and cerebral tuberculosis may present with similar findings. Other infections such as HSV encephalitis, bacterial meningitis, brain abscess, cytomegalovirus (CMV) encephalitis, and neurosyphilis should be considered in the differential diagnosis of neurological symptoms in AIDS patients.

279. **The answer is A.** *(Chapter 139)*   Drug reactions are common among HIV patients, and all of the medications listed except acyclovir have been associated with rash. In addition to TMP-SMX, clindamycin, ibuprofen, and dapsone, isoniazid, and pentamidine have been shown to cause rash in HIV patients. Acyclovir has been associated with headache and gastrointestinal symptoms including nausea, vomiting, and diarrhea.

280. **The answer is E.** *(Chapter 139)*   All of the statements regarding CMV retinitis are true except E. Characteristic funduscopic findings of CMV retinitis are fluffy white retinal lesions, often perivascular. Cotton-wool spots are the most common eye finding in

AIDS patients and are thought to be secondary to microvascular lesions unrelated to CMV. These lesions often resolve spontaneously, and no specific therapy is indicated.

281. The answer is C. *(Chapter 140)* This patient should receive Td because she cannot remember the last time she received tetanus prophylaxis. In addition, she should receive TIG becayse the wounds are more than 6 h old and are contaminated with dirt. Tetanus prophylaxis in the ED is especially important in elderly Americans (>70 years of age), the majority of whom lack adequate immunity to tetanus. Intravenous drug users and immigrants are also at disproportionate risk of contracting tetanus.

282. The answer is B. *(Chapter 140)* Tetanospasmin, an exotoxin produced by *C. tetani*, is responsible for the clinical manifestations of tetanus. These manifestations include muscular rigidity, violent muscular contractions, and autonomic nervous system instability. The most common presenting complaint for patients with generalized tetanus is pain and stiffness in the masseter muscle. Tetanospasmin produces these effects by preventing release of γ-aminobutyric acid (GABA) and glycine from presynaptic terminals thus preventing the normal inhibitory control in the CNS. *Clostridium tetani* remains localized to the site of the injury. The exotoxin tetanospasmin reaches the CNS by retrograde intraneuronal transport from the peripheral nervous system.

283. The answer is D. *(Chapter 141)* In developing countries, the most common reservoir of rabies virus is the dog. However, in the United States, new human rabies cases are most commonly associated with exposure to wild carnivores. Rabid wildlife species recorded by the CDC in 1988 include skunks, racoons, bats, and foxes. Domestic species found to be rabid include cats, cows, dogs, and other livestock. Rodents (e.g., squirrels, chipmunks, hamsters, rats, and mice) and lagomorphs (e.g., rabbits and hares) are not rabies carriers.

284. The answer is D. *(Chapter 141)* Rabies prophylaxis should be considered for travelers to areas where rabies is endemic and for people who engage in wildlife trapping, animal handlers, and veterinarians. The regimen for prophylaxis consists of three doses of human diploid cell vaccine (HDCV) 1 mL intramuscularly at days 0, 7, and 21 or 28. In most vaccinated persons, immunity lasts for 2 years. Rabies antibody titers are usually not required after immunization has been completed but should be considered in anyone who is immunocompromised or is taking immunosuppressive drugs. In this case, the patient may be taking chloroquine simultaneously for malaria prophylaxis, and antibody titers may be warranted. Postvaccination titers should be checked 2 to 4 weeks after immunization has been completed. For any exposure that occurs, immediate treatment consists of thoroughly cleaning the wounds with soap, removing devitalized tissue, copious irrigation with sterile saline or water, and avoidance of suturing. Following these postexposure recommendations reduces the subsequent incidence of rabies by about 90 percent.

285. The answer is E. *(Chapter 142)* In this case, the infecting organism is probably *P. vivax* because of the geographic location of the patient's exposure. It is more likely that the patient is suffering a relapse than a reexposure. Relapses may occur in patients with *P. vivax* or *P. ovale* because chloroquine therapy does not reach exoerythrocytic parasites that remain dormant in the liver. The recommended therapy for uncomplicated, non–chloroquine-resistant *P. vivax* is chloroquine phosphate 1-g load, 500 mg in 6 h, and then 500 mg/day for 2 days, plus primaquine phosphate 26.3-mg load (15-mg base) per day for 14 days upon completion of chloroquine therapy. Unless primaquine therapy follows chloroquine therapy, relapses of malaria are common. Relapses of malaria also occur in patients who have previously received "successful" therapy.

286. The answer is A. *(Chapter 142)* The CDC reports that between 1990 and 1994 more than half of all cases of malaria among U.S. citizens were due to *P. falciparum* and were acquired from travels in Sub-Saharan Africa. There have also been reports of widespread chloroquine-resistant *P. falciparum* throughout this area. The appropriate chemoprophylaxis in this case would be mefloquine rather than chloroquine. In addition, travelers should use mosquito netting, wear long-sleeved clothing, stay in well-screened areas between dusk and dawn, and use pyrethrum-containing insect sprays. Spray can be applied to clothes for additional protection, and an insect repellant containing *N,N*-diethylmetatoluamide (DEET) should be applied to exposed skin. Even with appropriate chemoprophylaxis and personal protection, it is possible to contract malaria.

287. **The answer is E.** *(Chapter 144)* The incidence of food-borne illness is staggering, and the increasing availability of imported fruits and vegetables and an increase in international travel has facilitated the transmission of these diseases across continents. Exact prevalence is difficult to determine because most infections are undiagnosed and unreported. The use of antacids, H_2 blockers, antibiotics affecting indigenous intestinal bacteria, and antiperistaltic agents can all increase susceptibility to developing a food-borne illness. Viral infections are the most common overall cause of diarrheal disease, but travelers' diarrhea is most likely of bacterial etiology.

288. **The answer is C.** *(Chapter 144)* Information regarding ill contacts, recent food and water exposure, and host susceptibility are important factors in making a diagnosis of food-borne illness. Most infectious diarrhea is self-limiting, and routine studies for ova and parasites and stool cultures are not cost effective. If symptoms persist for more than 3 or 4 days, especially when accompanied by dehydration or fever, laboratory studies may be indicated. Fecal leukocytes in stool samples suggest a bacterial pathogen, but the absence of fecal leukocytes does not exclude a bacterial etiology; therefore, the test has limited diagnostic efficacy.

289. **The answer is A.** *(Chapter 144)* Enterotoxigenic *E. coli* is the major cause of travelers' diarrhea. Other strains associated with travel include enterohemorrhagic and enteroinvasive *E. coli*. All of the organisms listed are also travel-related pathogens, mostly seen after international travel by U.S. citizens. Additional etiologies of travelers' diarrhea include *Salmonella*, *Brucella*, *Cryptosporidium*, and hepatitis A.

290. **The answer is D.** *(Chapter 144)* The patient's symptoms developed 9 h after the ingestion of the suspected contaminated food. Of the organisms listed, only *V. parahaemolyticus* has an incubation period of 6 to 24 h. *Staphylococcus aureus* and Norwalk viruses usually produce symptoms 1 to 6 h after exposure. Enterotoxigenic *E. coli* produces symptoms 24 to 48 h after exposure, and *Campylobacter* produces symptoms 2 to 6 days after ingestion of contaminated food. *Vibrio* poisoning is commonly associated with ingestion of seafood.

291. **The answer is B.** *(Chapter 145)* All of the diseases listed except Q fever may be contracted by a tick bite. Rocky Mountain spotted fever is caused by a rickettsial organism, *Rickettsia rickettsia*. Relapsing fever is caused by a spirochete, *Borrelia burgdorferi*. Tularemia is caused by a gram-negative nonmotile coccobacillus, *Francisella tularemia*. The protozoan parasites, *Babesia microti* and *B. equi*, cause babesiosis. Q fever is unique in that it is the only rickettsial infection acquired by aerosol inhalation rather than by an arthropod vector. Q fever is common among domesticated farm animals in the United States and is shed in urine, feces, and afterbirth. The rickettsial organism responsible for causing Q fever is *Coxiella burnetti*.

292. **The answer is C.** *(Chapter 145)* Most viral zoonotic pneumonias are caused by influenza. Influenza types A, B, and C infect humans, but only influenza type A is transmitted between vertebrate animals and humans. In addition to migrating waterfowl, horses and marine mammals can serve as reservoirs. There is also evidence for transmission of influenza virus between specific species, such as humans and pigs. Pandemics of human influenza are believed to occur as a combination of antigenic drift of viral surface proteins (hemagglutinin and neuraminidase) and a zoonotic reservoir for the virus. Influenza pneumonia carries a high mortality rate, especially in patients older than 70 years. Antiviral therapy with amantadine and rimantadine is effective against influenza A but not against types B or C. Annual influenza vaccination is recommended for healthcare workers.

293. **The answer is A.** *(Chapter 146)* Gas-forming soft tissue infections are rapidly progressive. The incubation period is short, with symptoms occurring fewer than 3 days after inoculation. Patients frequently describe pain out of proportion to physical findings and a sensation of "heaviness" of the affected part. On examination, the skin is often bronze-colored with brawny edema and crepitance. Bullae and a malodorous serosanguinous discharge may be seen. Patients are often irritable or confused and have low-grade fevers with tachycardia out of proportion to the fever. Common laboratory findings include leukocytosis, anemia, metabolic acidosis, thrombocytopenia, coagulopathy, myoglobinemia, and myoglobinuria and abnormalities of kidney or liver function tests. Radiologic studies may demonstrate gas within soft tissue planes and within the peritoneal or retroperitoneal spaces.

294. **The answer is C.** *(Chapter 146)* Cutaneous abscesses represent 1 to 2 percent of all presenting complaints to EDs. Most patients can be treated with incision and drainage of the abscess and discharged from the ED with follow-up in 2 to 3 days. Antibiotic use is controversial. The risk of systemic infection after local incision and drainage appears to be low. In patients with diabetes, alcoholism, or other underlying immunocompromised states, the threshold for antibiotic use should be lower. In addition, patients with signs of systemic disease such as fever, chills, or cellulitis extending beyond the abscess borders should be strongly considered for antibiotic therapy.

295. **The answer is C.** *(Chapter 147)* All of the STDs listed except HIV are reportable communicable diseases according to the CDC guidelines. HIV is reportable in the pediatric population (< 13 years old). In patients older than 13 years, HIV disease is not reportable until the disease has progressed to AIDS. The current CDC definition of AIDS requires an HIV-infected adult to have: (1) a CD4 T lymphocyte count of less than 200, (2) a CD4 T lymphocyte count less than 14 percent of total lymphocytes, or (3) any of the following: pulmonary tuberculosis, recurrent pneumonia, invasive cervical cancer, or 23 other clinical conditions that are listed on the World Wide Web at www.cdc.gov/epo/mmwr/mmwr.html.

296. **The answer is D.** *(Chapter 150)* Herpes simplex virus 1 is a frequent cause of cranial nerve (CN) VII (Bell's) palsy. All of the signs or symptoms described can be found with a simple peripheral CN VII palsy, except sparing of the forehead musculature on the affected side. Central CN VII lesions spare the forehead musculature because of cross-innervation from the opposite side. However, a peripheral lesion should cause the patient to be unable to wrinkle the brow on the ipsilateral side. If the forehead is spared, additional investigations such as head CT or magnetic resonance imaging are warranted. The differential diagnosis of Bell's palsy includes tumor, stroke, Guillain-Barré syndrome, Lyme disease, and Ramsay Hunt syndrome. In addition, if a Bell's palsy is found with an otitis media, mastoiditis, or parotitis, an ENT specialist should be consulted.

297. **The answer is B.** *(Chapter 150)* CMV is a common herpes virus that is present in 40 to 100 percent of adults, depending on geographic location, socioeconomic status, attendance at day care, and sexual behavior. Symptomatic CMV infections usually occur in the advanced stages of HIV disease and can cause significant morbidity. CMV retinitis occurs in more than 10 percent of AIDS patients and may be treated acutely with gancyclovir for 2 to 3 weeks, followed by lifetime suppressive therapy. The natural course of CMV retinitis involves progression to blindness, but the disease process may be slowed with the use of gancyclovir. Gancyclovir cannot cure patients of their CMV, and it does not reverse loss of sight that has already occurred. In addition to retinitis, CMV can cause esophagitis, colitis, or adrenalitis in HIV patients.

298. The answer is A. *(Chapter 148)*   The CDC instituted six basic universal precautions, including all of the listed recommendations, except the recommendation regarding puncture-proof gloves. Gloves should be worn routinely when contact with blood or other body fluids is anticipated. However, to date, no acceptable puncture-proof glove is available. Needles should never be recapped, and they should be disposed of in special "sharps" containers. Pregnant healthcare workers should be aware of the risk of perinatal HIV transmission.

299. The answer is C. *(Chapter 148)*   Certain groups of healthcare workers are at greater risk for contracting TB. Factors to consider include contact with a large number of infected patients, exposure to highly infectious patients, increased ventilation rate of the worker, the duration of exposure, and air-exchange rates in the environment. An increased air-exchange rate in the environment allows for greater filtration of air and a reduction in the number of potentially infective particles in the environment. Healthcare workers in the inner city are at greatest risk for contracting TB. OSHA regulations require healthcare workers and visitors who enter rooms of known or suspected TB patients to wear high-efficiency particulate air masks. All healthcare workers are advised to participate in TB screening and prophylaxis programs.

METABOLIC, ENDOCRINOLOGIC, AND RHEUMATOLOGIC EMERGENCIES

QUESTIONS

DIRECTIONS: Each question below contains five suggested responses. Choose the **one best** response to each question.

Questions 300–301

300. A patient presents to the ED and has the following laboratory values: sodium 139 mEq/L, potassium 4.1 mEq/L, chloride 112 mEq/L, bicarbonate 15 mEq/L, blood urea nitrogen (BUN) 22, creatinine 1.5, and glucose 180. All of the following could be the etiology of these laboratory findings EXCEPT

(A) salicylates
(B) renal tubular acidosis, type II
(C) acute diarrhea
(D) ureterosigmoidostomy
(E) pancreatic fistula

301. What is the calculated osmolarity for the patient in question 300?

(A) 157 mOsm/L
(B) 274 mOsm/L
(C) 296 mOsm/L
(D) 310 mOsm/L
(E) 347 mOsm/L

302. Syndrome of inappropriate antidiuretic hormone (SIADH) secretion can be caused by each of the following EXCEPT

(A) meningitis
(B) pneumonia
(C) hyperthryoidism
(D) thiazide diuretics
(E) monoamine oxidase inhibitors

303. A patient is sent to the ED from his doctor's office because of hypocalcemia. One would expect all of the following EXCEPT

(A) Chvostek's sign
(B) muscle spasms
(C) prolonged QT interval
(D) Tinel's sign
(E) weakness

304. A patient presents to the ED complaining of sudden onset of shortness of breath 1 day after a 5-h plane ride. Arterial blood gas on room air at sea level is: pH = 7.32, Pao_2 = 74 mm Hg, PCO_2 = 30 mm Hg. What is the alveolar-arterial (A-a) gradient for this patient?

(A) 20 mm Hg
(B) 30 mm Hg
(C) 40 mm Hg
(D) 50 mm Hg
(E) 60 mm Hg

305. A young male presents to the ED unable to give a history. As part of the work-up, you find an anion gap (AG) of 38. All of the following are possible etiologies of this patient's problem EXCEPT

(A) lactic acidosis
(B) ethylene glycol
(C) hyperglycemic hyperosmolar state
(D) renal failure
(E) isopropanol

306. All of the following statements are true of hyperkalemia EXCEPT

(A) leukocytosis may cause a pseudohyperkalemia
(B) calcium chloride should be given for severe cases of hyperkalemia
(C) kayexalate will not work for patients who have had a colon resection
(D) inhaled albuterol can be used to treat hyperkalemia
(E) the effects of hyperkalemia are decreased in patients with hyperglycemia

307. Which of the following statements regarding hypoglycemia is FALSE?

(A) Counterregulatory hormones are released in a hypoglycemic state

(B) Hypoglycemia causes both autonomic and neuroglycopenic symptoms

(C) Hypoglycemic patients commonly present with altered levels of consciousness, lethargy, confusion, or agitation

(D) Hypoglycemia is diagnosed when the blood glucose is less than 60 mg/dL

(E) Glucagon is ineffective in the treatment of alcohol-induced hypoglycemia

308. All of the following are important in quickly mediating and correcting states of hypoglycemia EXCEPT

(A) glucagon

(B) epinephrine

(C) glucocorticoid

(D) decrease in insulin secretion

(E) glycogenolysis

309. What is the MOST common cause of hypoglycemia in patients presenting to the ED?

(A) First time presentation of diabetes

(B) Alcohol related

(C) Oral hypoglycemics

(D) Insulinoma

(E) Liver failure

310. Which scenario is MOST typical of alcoholic ketoacidosis?

	Glucose	Alcohol	Ketones	AG
(A)	Normal	High	Large	Present
(B)	High	Low	Large	Present
(C)	High	High	Small	Absent
(D)	Mild elevation	Low	Large	Present
(E)	Mild elevation	High	Small	Absent

311. Which of the following statements about alcoholic ketoacidosis (AKA) is FALSE?

(A) Therapy includes intravenous administration of glucose and saline solutions

(B) As AKA is treated, the nipride test becomes more positive

(C) The development of Wernicke's encephalopathy can be prevented by administration of thiamine before glucose infusion

(D) Most patients fully recover

(E) AKA occurs only in chronic alcoholics

312. All of the following statements about hypothyroidism are TRUE EXCEPT

(A) prevalence is greater in women than in men

(B) amiodarone and lithium may mask the presentation secondary to elevation of thyroid hormone levels

(C) in secondary hypothyroidism, thyroid-stimulating hormone (TSH) levels are usually low

(D) although hypothyroidism is common in those older than 60 years, a paucity of symptoms may make the diagnosis difficult

(E) postablation hypothyroidism is a cause of primary hypothyroidism

313. All the following abnormalities are common in a patient with myxedema EXCEPT

(A) respiratory: hypoventilation, hypoxia

(B) central nervous system: confusion, lethargy, coma

(C) electrolyte: hypernatremia, water retention

(D) cardiovascular: bradycardia

(E) thermoregulatory: hypothermia

314. All of the following pathways occur as diabetic ketoacidosis develops EXCEPT

(A) hyperglycemia → glycosuria → dehydration and loss of electrolytes

(B) hyperglycemia → cell dehydration → altered level of consciousness

(C) insulin and glucagon deficiency → increased hepatic gluconeogenesis

(D) lipolysis → ketosis → acidosis

(E) muscle breakdown → azotemia → loss of sodium

315. Which of the following statements is TRUE regarding administration of sodium bicarbonate solution during the management of diabetic ketoacidosis (DKA)?

(A) It prevents paradoxical spinal fluid acidosis and cerebral edema

(B) It shifts potassium ions extracellularly and corrects the hypokalemia

(C) It shifts the oxyhemoglobin dissociation curve to the right, facilitating off-loading of oxygen at the tissue level

(D) Complications include rebound alkalosis and sodium overload

(E) It is recommended in all DKA patients with severely altered levels of consciousness

316. All of the following are appropriate treatments for DKA EXCEPT

(A) administering 3 to 5 L normal saline in the first 4 to 6 h

(B) replacing the 3 to 5 mEq KCl/kg deficit gradually over the first 2 to 3 days

(C) infusing insulin at 0.1 U/kg/h after the initial bolus is given

(D) stopping insulin administration when glucose levels fall to 250 mg/dL

(E) administering phosphate if levels fall below 1.0 mg/dL

317. Which of the following statements concerning hyperosmolar hyperglycemic nonketotic syndrome (HHNS) is TRUE?

(A) The mortality rate of HHNS is less than that of DKA

(B) HHNS and DKA are easily distinguishable

(C) A majority of HHNS patients present with coma

(D) Metabolic acidosis excludes the diagnosis

(E) Seizures occur in up to 15 percent of patients with HHNS

318. Precipitating factors for HHNS include all of the following EXCEPT

(A) infections

(B) extensive burns

(C) thiazide diuretics

(D) ingestion of large quantities of sugar-containing fluids

(E) salicylic acid

319. Which of the following statements regarding lactic acidosis is FALSE?

(A) It is an uncommon cause of metabolic acidosis

(B) The source of elevated lactic acid comes from the conversion of pyruvate to lactate

(C) In anoxic states, the cellular lack of NAD prevents mitochondrial reduction of lactate to pyruvate

(D) Lactic acidosis caused by tissue hypoxia is classified as type A lactic acidosis

(E) Liver and kidney gluconeogenesis contribute significantly to lactate utilization

320. An ill-appearing 48-year-old European female presents to the ED with nonspecific complaints. Laboratory tests show an elevated AG, lactate level of 5.0, pH 7.34, and a normal glucose level. Detailed history reveals that she is taking oral phenformin. All of the following apply to this patient's lactic acidosis EXCEPT

(A) the patient most likely has type B lactic acidosis

(B) sodium bicarbonate should be administered

(C) myocardial contractility and hypotension may occur at pH levels below 7.1

(D) phenformin has been withdrawn from the U.S. market

(E) ethanol use can cause a similar presentation

321. Which of the following statements regarding hyperthyroidism is FALSE?

(A) Free T_3 is more biologically active than T_4 but has a shorter half-life

(B) Hyperthyroidism during pregnancy is almost always due to Graves' disease

(C) Lithium, iodine, and amiodarone have all been associated with hyperthyroidism

(D) Normal T_4 levels eliminate the possibility of hyperthyroidism

(E) Mortality rates from thyroid storm range from 20 to 50 percent

322. Assuming no allergies, which of the following is TRUE for all patients with thyroid storm?

(A) Give aspirin to control fever

(B) Administer propranolol to block the adrenergic drive

(C) Give propylthiouracil (PTU) 1 h before iodide therapy

(D) Draw free T_4/TSH levels before and 1 h after administering antithyroxine

(E) Avoid steroids because these increase conversion of T_4 to T_3

323. Which of the following is TRUE regarding hormones produced in the adrenal glands?

(A) Corticotropin-releasing factor emanates from the pituitary and stimulates cortisol release

(B) Cortisol is a potent hormone that increases glucose uptake into cells

(C) Aldosterone is an important mineralocorticoid that increases sodium resorption and potassium excretion

(D) Adrenally produced androgens are an important source of androgens in men

(E) Adrenal insufficiency occurs primarily because of decreased epinephrine and norepinephrine production in the medulla

324. An 18-year-old, ill-appearing female presents to the ED with low blood pressure. She has a 1 day history of headache and fever. Examination is significant for petechial skin lesions. Waterhouse-Friderichsen syndrome is suspected. All of the following statements are TRUE EXCEPT

(A) bilateral adrenal gland hemorrhage frequently occurs with this disorder
(B) the bacterial organism implicated in this severe infection is *Neisseria meningitidis*
(C) although controversial, administration of glucocorticoids is indicated in most cases
(D) abdominal CT is not sensitive in determining adrenal hemorrhages
(E) pregnancy is a risk factor for developing adrenal hemorrhage

325. A 48-year-old female with a history of sarcoidosis comes to the ED with a chief complaint of syncope. She admits to anorexia, nausea, vomiting, and abdominal pain. She stopped going to work because she is too tired. Physical examination is significant for hyperpigmented lesions and alopecia. Initial laboratory findings show a glucose level of 50 mg/dL and a potassium level of 5.4 mEq/L. What is the MOST likely diagnosis?

(A) Conn's syndrome
(B) Nephrogenic diabetes insipidus
(C) Hyperthyroidism
(D) Adrenal insufficiency
(E) Depression

326. A 24-year-old male comes to the ED in adrenal crisis. His wife reports that he has been feeling poorly for about 48 h. He is mumbling incoherently, blood pressure is 80/60, and temperature is 103°F. Which of the following actions is LEAST likely to benefit this patient initially?

(A) Starting mineralocorticoid therapy
(B) Infusing isotonic saline
(C) Administering dextrose
(D) Administering 100 to 200 mg hydrocortisone
(E) Administering appropriate intravenous antibiotics

327. Each of the following cardiac conditions is associated with systemic lupus erythematosus (SLE) EXCEPT

(A) pericarditis
(B) aortic stenosis
(C) angina
(D) costochondritis
(E) myocarditis

328. A 10-year-old female comes to the ED with bilateral knee and ankle joint pain and subcutaneous nodules over the extensor surfaces. Which of the following additional criteria is needed to confirm the diagnosis of acute rheumatic fever (ARF)?

(A) Fever
(B) Arthralgia
(C) Petechial rash
(D) Evidence of preceding streptococcal infection
(E) Chorea

329. A 58-year-old female presents to the ED with headache, tender temples, and flashes of blindness consistent with temporal arteritis. Which of the following actions is MOST appropriate?

(A) Consulting surgery for an immediate temporal artery biopsy
(B) Confirming the diagnosis with an elevated erythrocyte sedimentation rate and then consulting surgery
(C) Referring the patient back to her primary medical doctor (PMD) in the morning for extensive rheumatologic evaluation
(D) Initiating high doses of indomethacin
(E) Initiating prednisone therapy

330. A 56-year-old male with no medical history presents to the ED with a 1 to 2 day history of a painful elbow. He denies trauma. Examination demonstrates a warm, tender, erythematous joint. Range of motion is limited secondary to pain. All of the following are TRUE EXCEPT

(A) a diagnostic arthrocentesis should be performed
(B) uric acid crystals may be seen upon examination of joint fluid with a polarizing microscope
(C) serum urate levels are often normal in gout patients
(D) administration of intravenous colchicine is the first line of treatment for this patient
(E) during an acute flare, other medications used to prevent recurrences of gouty arthritis should not be adjusted

331. A 21-year-old male complains of new-onset left knee pain without antecedent trauma. He last had sex 1 week before and does not use condoms. Which of the following statements is TRUE?

(A) Cultures for gonorrhea should be obtained from the oropharynx, urethra, and rectum
(B) Synovial fluid from joints infected with gonoccocus often does not show the organism
(C) Intravenous antibiotics should be considered when gonorrhea infection is present in weight-bearing joints
(D) In some patients with gonorrhea, vesiculopustular lesions are found on the fingers
(E) All of the above

332. A 33-year-old intravenous drug user presents to the ED with complaints of fever and arthralgias. On visual inspection, there is no obvious swelling of the extremities. Which of the following joints are at greatest risk for infection in this patient?

(A) Atlanto-axial-occipital joint
(B) Metacarpal and interphalangeal joints
(C) Sternoclavicular, sacroiliac, and intervertebral joints
(D) Elbow and shoulder joints
(E) None of the above; all joints are equally affected

333. All of the following support the diagnosis of a ruptured Baker's cyst rather than a deep venous thrombosis (DVT) EXCEPT

(A) swelling that spares the foot
(B) a "crescent sign"
(C) rapid diminution of popliteal fullness
(D) sudden onset calf pain and swelling
(E) arthrogram showing no thrombus

334. Which one of the following is the causative agent in Lyme disease?

(A) *Borrelia burgdorferi*
(B) *Ehrlichia chaffeensis*
(C) Isolated neurotoxin from a tick
(D) *Rickettsia rickettsii*
(E) *Babesia* species

335. All of the following are consistent with a diagnosis of Kawasaki's syndrome EXCEPT

(A) 80 percent of cases occur in patients younger than 4 years
(B) conjunctivitis is common
(C) cervical lymphadenopathy is present in the majority of children
(D) sterile pyuria is an associated feature
(E) only 15 percent of patients treated with intravenous immunoglobulin within the first 10 days of illness develop coronary artery aneurysms

336. All of the following are criteria for admitting patients with Henöch-Schonlein purpura (HSP) EXCEPT

(A) age younger than 2 years
(B) renal function monitoring
(C) rehydration for recurrent emesis
(D) lack of PMD
(E) control of abdominal pain

METABOLIC, ENDOCRINOLOGIC, AND RHEUMATOLOGIC EMERGENCIES

ANSWERS

300–301. **The answers are A and C, respectively.** *(Chapters 21, 23)* The anion gap (AG) is the difference between the measured sodium level and the sum of the measured chloride and CO_2 levels. Normal AG $= 12 \pm 4$. The etiologies of this patient's normal AG (hyperchloremic) metabolic acidosis can be remembered by a helpful mnemonic, *HARDUP*: H for hypoaldosteronism (Addison's disease), A for acetazolamide, R for renal tubular acidosis, D for diarrhea, U for ureterosigmoidostomy, and P for pancreatic fistula. Salicylate toxicity causes an elevated AG with a normal osmolar gap. Serum osmolarity is measured directly by determining the freezing point of the serum. It is calculated from the sodium, glucose, and BUN values with the following equation:

$$\text{osmolarity} = 2(\text{Na}) + \text{glucose}/18 + \text{BUN}/2.8.$$

The normal serum osmolarity is 275 to 296 mOsm/L. In this case, the calculated serum osmolarity is 296 mOsm/L. A difference between the measured and calculated osmolarity (osmolol gap) of more than 10 mOsm/L indicates the presence of osmotically active substances (such as alcohols) in the blood.

302. **The answer is C.** *(Chapter 23)* The diagnosis of SIADH is primarily one of exclusion that should be made in the absence of hypovolemia, hypervolemia, renal failure, and drugs that impair water excretion. The causes of this syndrome are diverse, ranging from central nervous system disorders and tumors (lung cancer, lymphoma, thymoma) to pulmonary and endocrine disorders, including glucocorticoid insufficiency and hypothyroidism. There are miscellaneous causes such as porphyria, pain, and nausea. Opiates, chlorpropamide, nonsteroidal antiinflammatory medications, cyclophosphamide, phenothiazines, mono-amine oxidase inhibitors, tricyclic antidepressants, and thiazide diuretics are among the drugs that have been implicated in this syndrome.

303. **The answer is D.** *(Chapter 23)* The severity of signs and symptoms of hypocalcemia depends greatly on the rapidity of the fall of the calcium. Hypocalcemia is uncommon in the ambulatory setting unless the patient recently had surgery and is hypoparathyroid or has chronic renal disease. Symptoms of hypocalcemia include weakness, fatigue, perioral paresthesias, muscle spasms, and impaired memory. Hypocalcemia should be considered in refractory heart failure. Chvostek's and Trousseau's signs are evidence of hypocalcemia. A positive Tinel's sign signals carpal tunnel syndrome.

304. **The answer is C.** *(Chapter 22)* The A-a oxygen gradient measures the extent to which lung function is impaired. The A-a gradient in a healthy individual is less than 15 mm Hg. The formula to calculate the alveolar oxygen level at room air is: $150 - (\text{arterial } CO_2 \times 1.2)$. The gradient is the difference between this number and the Pa_{O_2}. In this case, 114 mm Hg $-$ 74 mm Hg $=$ 40 mm Hg.

305. **The answer is E.** *(Chapter 21)* Isopropanol, also known as isopropyl alcohol, is commonly found in rubbing alcohol. The clinical features of isopropanol intoxication are similar to those of ethanol intoxication. Laboratory studies of patients who have ingested this alcohol show a normal or minimal AG, with an elevated osmolar gap. Patients with an AG greater than 35 usually have ethylene glycol or methanol intoxication, hyperglycemic hyperosmolar coma, or lactic acidosis. *MUDPILES* is the mnemonic for the etiologies of an AG acidosis: M for methanol, U for uremia, D for diabetic ketoacidosis, P for paraldehyde, I for iron/isoniazid, L for lactic acidosis, E for ethanol and ethylene glycol, and S for salicylates.

306. The answer is E. *(Chapter 23)* Hemolysis, leukocytosis, and thrombocytosis all can produce a pseudohyperkalemia. Effects of hyperkalemia are more pronounced in patients with concomitant hyponatremia and hypocalcemia. There are many different ways to treat hyperkalemia. Kayexalate (sodium polystyrene sulfonate) is an ion-exchange resin that works in the distal colon to extract potassium. High-dose inhaled albuterol is a useful temporizing measure to move potassium into the intracelluar space. Glucose with insulin can also cause a temporary shift of potassium into the intracellular space. Sodium bicarbonate causes an alkalosis that tends to reduce serum potassium levels. Calcium (preferably CaCl because of the higher concentration of calcium) stabilizes the cell membrane. Dialysis should be used to rapidly remove potassium when the hyperkalemia is severe.

307. The answer is D. *(Chapters 23, 202)* The serum glucose level that causes hypoglycemic symptoms is variable. Levels of 35 mg/dL and lower are present in asymptomatic individuals, and levels in the "normal" range can cause symptoms of hypoglycemia that resolve with glucose administration. Patients with hypoglycemia experience both neuroglycopenic and autonomic symptoms. Neuroglycopenic symptoms result from a direct effect on the brain and manifest as dizziness, confusion, tiredness, difficulty speaking, and headache. Autonomic or sympathomimetic symptoms are due to release of the counterregulatory hormone epinephrine and include diaphoresis, anxiety, trembling, and nausea. Glucagon is ineffective in alcoholics and the elderly because they have low glycogen stores.

308. The answer is C. *(Chapters 23, 202)* The counterregulatory hormones glucagon and epinephrine are released in response to hypoglycemia. Within minutes, glycogenolysis is activated and glucose is released into the bloodstream. Simultaneous to this process, there is a notable decrease in insulin secretion. Glucocorticoid and growth hormone are slower-acting mediators.

309. The answer is B. *(Chapters 23, 202)* Both alcohol use and diabetes are common causes of hypoglycemia. The established diabetic patient who eats inadequately, has inappropriate medication dosing, is on a multiple-drug regimen, or has a complicating medical problem may present with hypoglycemia. New-onset diabetes presents with hyperglycemia. Insulinomas, overdose of oral hypoglycemics, and liver failure are less frequent causes of low blood sugar.

310. The answer is D. *(Chapter 204)* The laboratory presentation of alcoholic ketoacidosis is variable but tends to follow the pattern described in answer D. Glucose levels are mildly elevated. The alcohol level is uncharacteristically low given the patient's history of regular alcohol consumption. Ketones are present in large numbers and cause an elevated AG. The three ketones produced are β-hydroxybutyrate, acetoacetate, and acetone. Acetone is nonacidotic and rapidly excreted in the urine.

311. The answer is E. *(Chapter 204)* Although AKA classically presents in chronic alcoholics, it can also occur in first-time drinkers who consume insufficient food. Standard therapy of AKA consists of administration of glucose, thiamine, and saline solutions. This regimen restores volume, replenishes glucose, and prevents Wernicke's encephalopathy from developing. As acetoacetate increases and β-hydroxybutyrate decreases, the nipride test becomes more positive. Thus, as the patient's clinical condition improves, laboratory values may transiently worsen. Most patients without co-morbid conditions recover fully from AKA.

312. **The answer is B.** *(Chapter 207)* Hypothyroidism has a higher prevalence in women and is especially common in individuals older than 60 years. A high suspicion must be maintained in elderly patients because there is often a paucity of classic signs and symptoms. Autoimmune disorders, idiopathic causes, and postablation of thyroid tissue are common etiologies. In primary hypothyroidism, the TSH levels are high; in secondary hypothyroidism, the TSH levels are low. Amiodarone and lithium may induce hypothyroidism by increasing iodine levels, thereby inhibiting thyroxine production.

313. **The answer is C.** *(Chapter 207)* The rare patient who develops myxedema because of prolonged and severe hypothyroidism exhibits all of the listed abnormalities except hypernatremia. The hypothyroid patient typically becomes overloaded with water, leading to dilutional hyponatremia. The etiology of this hyponatremia is not clearly understood. The patient in a myxedematous state is usually hypothermic, lethargic, hypoventilating, and bradycardic.

314. **The answer is C.** *(Chapter 203)* Diabetic ketoacidosis occurs when inadequate insulin is secreted from pancreatic cells. In response, glucagon levels soar. The elevated glucagon levels result in gluconeogenesis and glycogenolysis. This hyperglycemic state produces an osmotic diuresis, leading to cell dehydration, electrolyte abnormalities, and an altered level of consciousness. The catabolic processes of lipolysis and muscle breakdown are also activated.

315. **The answer is D.** *(Chapter 203)* Administration of sodium bicarbonate is controversial. It may cause paradoxical spinal fluid acidosis, adversely affecting brain function. In addition, it shifts potassium ions intracellularly and worsens hypokalemia. The acidosis in diabetic states is protective and shifts the oxyhemoglobin curve to the right. Administering bicarbonate solutions may shift the curve back to the left.

316. **The answer is D.** *(Chapter 203)* Patients with DKA have an average water deficit of 5 to 10 L secondary to the osmotic diuresis that occurs with high serum glucose levels. Normal saline administration prevents a rapid fall in osmolality that could lead to excessive transfer of water into the central nervous system. Although the initial serum potassium level is elevated, repletion of potassium is necessary to restore low intracellular levels. To prevent hypoglycemia, dextrose should be added to intravenous fluids when the serum glucose falls to a level between 250 and 300 mg/dL. Even with this level of glucose, continued insulin is needed to resolve the acidosis and ketonemia. Phosphate levels only become critical when below 1.0 mg/dL.

317. **The answer is E.** *(Chapter 205)* HHNS occurs primarily in diabetics, although most cases are undiagnosed at the time of presentation. The mortality of HHNS is three to seven times greater than that for DKA. HHNS is characterized by severe dehydration (8–12 L deficit), hyperglycemia (greater than in DKA), and hyperosmolality. In patients with HHNS, high levels of glucose occur without the ketone body formation seen in DKA. However, metabolic acidosis may occur in HHNS from other causes (e.g., excessive lactic acid levels or uremia). Neurologic signs can be prominent in HHNS, with about 15 percent of patients manifesting seizures. Although HHNS is frequently referred to as hyperosmolar nonketotic coma, coma occurs in fewer than 10 percent of such patients. HHNS and DKA can be difficult to distinguish clinically.

318. **The answer is E.** *(Chapter 205)* Any comorbid disease process can precipitate HHNS in a diabetic patient. In the nondiabetic population, HHNS can occur after dehydration from heat strokes, burns, or dialysis. Drugs, especially diuretics or those that mediate insulin, are common precipitating factors. Ingestion of enormous amounts of sugar-containing fluids is an unusual cause. Aspirin has not been implicated.

319. **The answer is A.** *(Chapter 21)* Lactic acidosis is the most common cause of metabolic acidosis. Lactate is produced in the anaerobic glycolysis pathway. Normally, phys-

iologic levels of lactate are cleared through gluconeogenesis in the kidney and liver. When this system is overwhelmed and NAD is lacking, lactate levels rise. This commonly occurs in hypoxic or hypovolemic states and is referred to as type A lactic acidosis.

320. **The answer is B.** *(Chapter 184)* This patient suffers from phenformin-induced lactic acidosis. Phenformin is an oral hypoglycemic agent used in Europe that is no longer used in the United States. Other drugs such as alcohol, methanol, and antiretrovirals are also associated with type B lactic acidosis. The clinical findings of lactic acidosis are nonspecific. At a pH of 7.1 or lower, depressed cardiac function and hypotension may develop. Administration of sodium bicarbonate solution is controversial. Current recommendations suggest withholding alkali therapy if the pH is above 7.1.

321. **The answer is D.** *(Chapter 206)* Although most cases of hyperthyroidism are characterized by low levels of free thyroxine (T_4), levels are normal in some thyrotoxic patients. T_4 is the predominant circulating thyroid hormone. By cleaving an iodine molecule, triiodothyronine (T_3) is produced. T_3 is more biologically active than T_4, but its half-life is only 1 day. Graves' disease is by far the most common cause of hyperthyroidism, even in pregnancy. In addition to lithium, iodine, and amiodarone, a patient's own thyroid medication can induce a hyperthyroid state. Despite treatment, mortality rates of thyroid storm are high, ranging from 20 to 50 percent.

322. **The answer is C.** *(Chapter 206)* Aspirin use is contraindicated in the setting of thyroid storm because salicylates increase free T_3 and T_4 levels by displacing the molecules from their carrier thyronine-binding globulin hormone. Free T_4 and TSH levels should be drawn before, not after, therapy. β Blockers such as propranolol are contraindicated in patients with bronchospastic disease or heart block. A selective β_1 blocker (e.g., esmolol) can be used in this setting. Administration of PTU before iodide prevents the incorporation of iodide into the new thyroxine hormone. Steroid use is associated with increased survival, especially in cases with the potential for adrenal insufficiency.

323. **The answer is C.** *(Chapter 208)* Adrenal insufficiency is a deficiency produced by inadequate hormone production from the adrenal cortex, not the medulla. Adrenal medulla deficiency does not result in clinical disease. The following hormones are released from the adrenal gland: (a) aldosterone: increases sodium resorption and potassium excretion; (b) cortisol: maintains adequate glucose levels by decreasing glucose uptake and facilitating gluconeogenesis; and (c) androgens: important for certain sexual characteristics. Cortisol is released in response to pituitary release of adrenocorticotropic hormone (ACTH). ACTH is stimulated by corticotropin-releasing factor from the hypothalamus. The male gonads are the most important source of androgens; adrenal production is trivial by comparison.

324. **The answer is D.** *(Chapter 208)* The Waterhouse-Friderichsen syndrome is a life-threatening disorder resulting from overwhelming septicemia due to infection with *N. meningitidis*. Only about 10 percent of meningococcemia cases result in this syndrome. Bilateral adrenal hemorrhage is common. Computed tomography (CT) and ultrasound are both helpful in making the diagnosis. Although steroids are controversial, they are usually administered before antibiotic therapy. Risk factors for adrenal hemorrhage include stress, trauma, anticoagulants, pregnancy, surgery, and burns.

325. **The answer is D.** *(Chapter 208)* Adrenal insufficiency manifests insidiously. The findings in this patient are explained by deficiencies in androgens, corticosteroids, and mineralocorticoids. Hyperpigmented lesions represent lack of suppression of ACTH and melanocyte-stimulating hormone. Conn's syndrome results from overproduction of adrenal hormones. Isolated nephrogenic diabetes insipidus would not produce low glucose and elevated potassium. Hyperthyroidism has a vastly different clinical presentation, and glucose levels are often elevated. Depression alone would not account for the hyperpigmented skin or the electrolyte changes.

326. **The answer is A.** *(Chapter 208)*   This patient's initial stabilization should include all of these measures except beginning mineralocorticoid therapy. Hydrocortisone replenishes the patient's inadequate steroid levels and provides some mineralocorticoid effect. Therefore, early administration of mineralocorticoids is not necessary. Correction of hypoglycemia and hypotension are essential. Early antibiotic administration is important to prevent potentially fatal infections leading to adrenal crisis.

327. **The answer is B.** *(Chapter 276)*   Both pericarditis and myocarditis are common clinical manifestations in SLE patients. Although pericarditis may be accompanied by effusion, it rarely progresses to pericardial tamponade. Chronic steroid therapy may lead to premature atherosclerotic disease. Therefore, angina and myocardial infarctions should be considered. Costochondritis is a component of lupus arthritis. Aortic stenosis may be seen in association with ankylosing spondylitis, but not with SLE.

328. **The answer is D.** *(Chapter 132)*   This patient has two major Jones' criteria for ARF. To make the diagnosis, evidence of streptococcal antibodies is needed. Major Jones' criteria include carditis, polyarthritis, erythema marginatum, chorea, and subcutaneous nodules. Fever, arthralgia, and previous rheumatic fever are minor criteria. Evidence of antecedent streptococcal infection plus either two major or one major and two minor criteria are necessary to diagnose ARF.

329. **The answer is E.** *(Chapter 219)*   Temporal arteritis can cause sudden and permanent loss of vision. This sudden loss of vision is due to narrowing of the ophthalmic or posterior ciliary arteries. Permanent visual loss occurs in approximately 10 percent of these patients. Although a surgical biopsy of the artery is recommended, antiinflammatory treatment with steroids can save sight and should be initiated in the ED based on clinical suspicion alone.

330. **The answer is D.** *(Chapter 278)*   A first-time painful, swollen joint must be tapped to rule out septic arthritis. The synovial fluid of a gouty joint appears like egg-drop soup, with urate crystals and white blood cells visualized under the microscope. Serum urate may be normal during an acute gouty attack. If a patient is taking chronic suppressive therapy, it should be continued to avoid exacerbating crystal precipitation. Initial therapy for the acute attack consists of indomethacin or oral colchicine. Intravenous colchicine should be used with caution if at all because of serious side effects that include bone marrow suppression, neuropathy, myopathy, and death.

331. **The answer is E.** *(Chapter 278)*   A high index of suspicion must be maintained to diagnose gonococcal arthritis. Urethral or vaginal discharge is not uniformly present. A thorough history and examination should be performed in any sexually active patient complaining of joint pain without antecedent trauma. Because synovial fluid rarely shows the organism, in suspected gonococcal arthritis, cultures obtained from the urethra, cervix, rectum, mouth, and blood may be needed to confirm the diagnosis.

332. **The answer is C.** *(Chapter 278)*   A thorough examination of all joints should be performed in intravenous drug users with fever and arthralgias. Joints that have a predisposition for infection and are often overlooked include the sternoclavicular, sacroiliac, and intervertebral. If these joints are tender to palpation, additional work-up with bone scan or joint aspiration is indicated.

333. **The answer is D.** *(Chapter 55)*   Baker's cysts occur when fluid from a chronic inflammatory arthritis dissects into potential space in the popliteal region. When this collection of fluid ruptures, it can produce pain very similar to that of a DVT. Classically, swelling that spares the foot, a bluish discoloration around the ankle ("crescent sign"), and a sudden decrease in popliteal fullness all support the diagnosis of a ruptured Baker's cyst. The gold standard test is the arthrogram or duplex Doppler scan. The rapidity of pain onset when a Baker's cyst ruptures does not help differentiate it from DVT.

334. **The answer is A.** *(Chapter 145)* All of the agents are transmitted through ticks. Ticks should be carefully removed from patients by grasping the head with forceps and applying gentle pressure. *Ehrlichia chaffeensis* causes ehrlichiosis, isolated neurotoxin causes tick paralysis, *R. rickettsii* causes Rocky Mountain spotted fever, and *Babesia* species causes babesiosis. Lyme disease is the most frequently transmitted vector-borne infection in the United States. The three stages of this disease culminate in a prolonged and chronic arthritis.

335. **The answer is E.** *(Chapters 131, 132)* Kawasaki's syndrome is a generalized vasculitis of small and medium-sized arteries. The classic presentation includes fever, conjunctivitis, lip and oral mucosal changes, strawberry tongue, extremity edema or erythema, polymorphous rash, and cervical lymphadenopathy. Associated features affect the cardiovascular, central nervous, hematologic, genitourinary, pulmonary, and gastrointestinal systems. Urethritis with a sterile pyuria can be seen. Coronary artery aneurysms develop in about 20 percent of patients who receive no intravenous immunoglobulin therapy but in only 3 to 4 percent of those who are treated within the first 10 days of illness.

336. **The answer is A.** *(Chapter 132)* Patients with suspected HSP should be admitted to the hospital for monitoring of renal function, rehydration, severe abdominal pain, lack of a PMD who is available for close follow-up, or when the diagnosis is in doubt. There is no specific age requirement for admission.

NEUROLOGIC AND PSYCHIATRIC EMERGENCIES

QUESTIONS

DIRECTIONS: Each question below contains five suggested responses. Choose the **one best** response to each question.

337. A 20-year-old female undergraduate student presents complaining of a gradual onset of right-sided headache. The headache is accompanied by nausea and photophobia and prevents her from studying for exams. Which of the following is LEAST likely to be associated with her headache?

(A) Aura
(B) Birth control pills
(C) Family history of similar headaches
(D) Menstruation
(E) Unilateral tearing with conjunctival injection

338. A 60-year-old male presents complaining of a typical spring headache, 2 months after a femoral-popliteal bypass. He states that the pain is excruciating, began over the left eye, and is causing the eye to tear and throb. Which abortive therapy is the LEAST appropriate?

(A) Ergotamine
(B) Ketorolac
(C) Prochlorperazine
(D) Oxygen inhalation
(E) Intranasal lidocaine

339. Temporal arteritis is a vasculitis that affects women more frequently than men. Which one of the following is NOT usually associated with temporal arteritis?

(A) Age > 50 years
(B) ESR > 50
(C) Ischemic papillitis
(D) Tender, pulsatile temporal artery
(E) Polymyalgia

340. Amaurosis fugax is caused by occlusion of which one of the following arteries?

(A) Anterior cerebral artery
(B) Basilar artery
(C) Carotid artery
(D) Posterior cerebral artery
(E) Vertebral artery

341. A 58-year-old female is brought to the ED by her family. They state that her words do not make sense, the right side of her face is drooping, and she is weak on the right side. On examination you note that the patient is awake and alert, has an expressive aphasia, right-sided facial droop, three-fifths right arm strength, four-fifths right leg strength, and decreased sensation to pin-prick on the right side. Which stroke syndrome is MOST likely?

(A) Anterior cerebral artery infarct
(B) Basilar artery occlusion
(C) Middle cerebral artery infarct
(D) Lacunar infarct
(E) Intracerebral hemorrhage

342. A 62-year-old female with a history of TIA affecting the right side complains of 8 h of a dense right-sided paralysis and dysarthria. No previous studies have been completed. What is the MOST appropriate disposition?

(A) Admit to the medical ward
(B) Admit to the rehabilitation ward
(C) Discharge to home and arrange follow-up with the primary care physician
(D) Transfer the patient to a skilled nursing facility
(E) Conduct a stroke work-up in the ED and then discharge to home

343. A 25-year-old male is brought to the ED by his sister who states that he started vomiting that morning after complaining of a severe headache. On examination, he is drowsy but arousable with mild nuchal rigidity and no focal neurologic deficit. Which of the following is LEAST likely to be needed for his work-up and treatment?

(A) CT of the head
(B) Blood glucose determination
(C) Antiemetic
(D) Lumbar puncture
(E) Nimodipine

344. Which of the following MOST likely represents vertigo of peripheral origin?

(A) Ataxia
(B) Diplopia
(C) Dysphagia
(D) Facial numbness
(E) Unilateral hearing loss

345. A 26-year-old female is brought to the ED after three successive witnessed grand mal seizures without recovery of consciousness. Upon arrival, she is obtunded with no spontaneous eye opening and withdraws to pain only. Initial ED management could include all of the following EXCEPT

(A) endotracheal intubation
(B) barbiturate coma
(C) phenytoin infusion
(D) determination of blood glucose
(E) gastric lavage

346. A 37-year-old male intravenous drug user (IVDU) presents with the complaint of several days of general malaise, difficulty swallowing, occasional double vision, and subjective fever. On examination, the patient is noted to have grossly intact cranial nerves II to XII, a distended bladder, and a temperature of 99.1°F. What is the MOST appropriate next step?

(A) Admit to the ED observation unit
(B) Admit to the floor for observation
(C) Admit to the ICU
(D) Discharge to home with reassurance
(E) Discharge to home with follow-up in several days

347. Which of the following is LEAST consistent with Guillain-Barré syndrome?

(A) Ascending paralysis
(B) Preceded by exposure to toxins
(C) Sensory involvement
(D) Intact reflexes
(E) Resolution of symptoms in months

348. Parkinson's disease is characterized by all of the following EXCEPT

(A) akinesia or bradykinesia
(B) cogwheel rigidity
(C) intention tremor
(D) Lewy bodies
(E) impairment in posture and equilibrium

349. A 35-year-old female with a history of newly diagnosed myasthenia gravis presents to the ED with profound generalized muscle weakness for 2 days without a known precipitant. A test dose of 2 mg intravenous edrophonium results in visible muscle fasciculations and slowing of the patient's respiratory rate and depth. Which of the following actions is INAPPROPRIATE?

(A) Administering neostigmine
(B) Preparing for intubation
(C) Consulting a neurologist
(D) Establishing aspiration precautions
(E) Admission to the ICU

350. All of the following are consistent with multiple sclerosis (MS) EXCEPT

(A) multiple discrete lesions of the white matter
(B) increase of immunoglobulin in the CSF
(C) worsening spasticity with urinary tract infection
(D) diminution of symptoms with fever
(E) optic neuritis as first symptom

351. Which of the following seizure patients requires electroencephalographic (EEG) monitoring for optimal treatment?

(A) 35-year-old status post a witnessed tonic–clonic seizure with resolution of the postictal period in 10 min
(B) 40-year-old alcoholic status post two witnessed seizures in the ED, with lucid periods after each seizure
(C) 20-year-old status post first seizure
(D) 28-year-old with status epilepticus controlled with fosphenytoin
(E) 30-year-old with refractory status epilepticus requiring vecuronium

352. Which of the following is FALSE regarding myasthenia gravis?

(A) The clinical hallmark is nonfatigable muscle weakness
(B) Myasthenia gravis is often associated with other autoimmune diseases
(C) Confirmation of myasthenia is possible with the edrophonium test
(D) Overmedication can produce a clinical picture that mimicks myasthenic crisis
(E) Thymectomy is advocated for most myasthenic patients

353. A 7-year-old male presents to the ED 6 months status post revision of a CSF shunt. He complains of a persistent headache for 1 week, occasional nausea, and vomiting three to four times that day. Evaluation for shunt infection should include all of the following EXCEPT

(A) CT of the head
(B) shunt survey (plain films of the skull, chest, and abdomen)
(C) compression of the reservoir
(D) neurosurgical consult
(E) lumbar tap

354. Which of the following statements regarding bacterial meningitis is FALSE?

(A) Some bacteria are able to spread directly into the CNS, whereas others depend on hematogenous seeding
(B) Brudzinski's sign is not pathognomonic for meningitis
(C) Dexamethasone can be given to adult patients suspected of having meningitis
(D) Oral antibiotics change the clinical course
(E) Patients should receive prophylactic phenytoin to prevent seizures

355. Which of the following reflex findings would be pathologic in an adult?

(A) Bilateral patellar hyperreflexia
(B) Bilateral patellar hyporeflexia
(C) Bilateral snout reflexes
(D) Bilateral plantar reflexes
(E) Superficial anal reflex

356. Which of the following distinguishes delirium from dementia?

(A) Global cognitive impairment
(B) Periods of acute worsening of symptoms
(C) Clouded sensorium
(D) Reversibility
(E) Gradual onset of symptoms

357. Which of the following personality disorders is seen in a disproportionate number of ED patients?

(A) Antisocial
(B) Borderline
(C) Obsessive-compulsive
(D) Dependent
(E) Paranoid

358. Which of the following must be monitored in a schizophrenic patient controlled with clozapine?

(A) Liver function tests
(B) Amylase
(C) Glucose
(D) CBC
(E) Urinalysis

359. A 28-year-old female overdosed on her father's lithium. She presents with complaints of nausea, vomiting, and blurred vision. Initial lithium level is 2 mEq/L. Which of the following would NOT be appropriate ED management?

(A) Intravenous hydration
(B) Correction of electrolyte imbalance
(C) Urine pregnancy test
(D) Discharge to an inpatient psychiatric facility if asymptomatic after a 4-h observation period
(E) Alkalinization of the urine

360. A 25-year-old male is brought to the ED by ambulance on a psychiatric hold after wandering in a residential area looking for the source of the evil voices that he states are controlling his thoughts. Upon arrival, he is screaming and wildly agitated. Which of the following represents an appropriate initial dose of intramuscular haloperidol for this patient?

(A) 0.05 mg
(B) 0.5 mg
(C) 5.0 mg
(D) 50 mg
(E) 500 mg

361. Which of the following is more consistent with bulimia than with anorexia nervosa?

(A) Hypoglycemia
(B) Tachydysrhythmia
(C) Stress fracture
(D) Dysphagia
(E) Cathartic colon

362. Which of the following is LEAST consistent with a panic attack?

(A) Hallucinations
(B) Palpitations
(C) Chest tightness
(D) Dizziness
(E) Dyspnea

363. A 13-year-old female presents with the complaint that she cannot move her right leg. There are no other associated symptoms and no history of trauma, headache, or prior medical problems. The symptom began on the day she was to meet her father for the first time. Which of the following would be LEAST helpful in the management of this patient?

(A) Perform a Hoover test
(B) Tell her that nothing is wrong
(C) Hypnosis
(D) Tell her that she can talk with her father on the telephone rather than in person
(E) Reassure the patient that she will walk again

364. All of the following are symptoms of physician burnout EXCEPT

(A) illicit drug use
(B) chronic fatigue
(C) excessive irritability
(D) feelings of helplessness
(E) negative attitudes toward work

365. Which of the following is MOST impaired by REM sleep deprivation?

(A) Physical recuperation
(B) Intellectual tasks
(C) Psychological well being
(D) Social life
(E) Manual tasks

366. All of the following characteristics are associated with an increased suicide risk EXCEPT

(A) psychosis
(B) unemployment
(C) chronic illness
(D) first attempt
(E) readily available lethal weapon

367. Which of the following relations is LEAST likely to exist?

(A) Crime and substance abuse
(B) Trauma and alcohol abuse
(C) Mental illness and suicide gestures
(D) Cocaine and sexually transmitted diseases
(E) Intravenous drug use and long life expectancy

NEUROLOGIC AND PSYCHIATRIC EMERGENCIES

ANSWERS

337. **The answer is E.** *(Chapter 219)* The headache described is typical of a migraine. Migraine headaches can occur with or without an aura or prodrome. They can be provoked by changes in the body's internal milieu, environmental factors, certain foods, medications, and alcohols. There is usually a positive family history. Occasionally, patients have neurologic symptoms. Unilateral nasal congestion, tearing, and conjunctival injection are signs and symptoms seen with cluster headaches that predominantly affect men.

338. **The answer is A.** *(Chapter 219)* In general, abortive therapy for cluster headaches is similar to treatment for migraines. Treatment includes ergotamines, phenothiazines, serotonin agonists, nonsteroidal antiinflammatory drugs, and opiates. In addition, oxygen inhalation of 5 to 8 L/min for 10 min at symptom onset and instillation of 4 percent intranasal lidocaine into the ipsilateral nostril are useful modalities. Ergotamine is contraindicated in patients such as this one who have peripheral vascular disease. It should also be avoided in patients with focal neurologic signs, hypertension, coronary artery disease, and in those who are pregnant.

339. **The answer is D.** *(Chapter 219)* Temporal arteritis affects people older than age 50 years and is usually unilateral. Systemic signs and symptoms are generally present. They include fever, malaise, weight loss, anorexia, visual deficits, and polymyalgia. On examination, the temporal artery is tender and pulseless. The most common sequela is blindness, secondary to ischemic papillitis. If the diagnosis is strongly suspected, prednisone should be initiated in the ED to prevent the progression of blindness.

340. **The answer is C.** *(Chapter 220)* Amaurosis fugax is an ocular transient ischemic attack (TIA) involving the anterior circulation of the brain that is characterized by sudden onset of painless monocular blindness. The basilar, posterior cerebral, and vertebral arteries belong to the posterior circulation. The anterior cerebral artery is distal to the ophthalmic artery. The ophthalmic artery supplies the optic nerve and the retina and is the first branch off the internal carotid artery. Therefore, of the listed choices, the symptom can only be attributed to the carotid artery.

341. **The answer is C.** *(Chapter 220)* Patients with hemorrhagic stroke syndromes generally have decreased mentation. Anterior cerebral artery infarcts cause leg weakness more than arm weakness. Basilar artery occlusion causes the "locked-in" syndrome. Lacunar infarcts lead to pure motor or sensory deficits. Middle cerebral artery infarcts cause contralateral sensory deficit and motor weakness, with the arm and face weaker than the leg. When the dominant hemisphere is involved, patients often have a receptive or expressive aphasia.

342. **The answer is A.** *(Chapter 220)* All patients with new strokes should be admitted to the hospital for evaluation, education, and early rehabilitation. No newly diagnosed patient should go directly to rehabilitation or a nursing home. Only those patients with a previous history of an anterior circulation stroke who have been previously studied and present with a minor, completed, recurrent stroke or TIA and have a reliable support system may be discharged home. In this situation, primary care follow-up must be arranged

after the appropriate ED work-up. If this patient had presented earlier, she could have been a candidate for thrombolytic therapy.

343. **The answer is D.** *(Chapter 219)* Because of the patient's altered mental status, hypoglycemia should be ruled out. Otherwise his presentation is typical for a subarachnoid hemorrhage (SAH), with sudden onset of a severe, constant headache accompanied by nausea and vomiting. An emergent noncontrast computed tomography (CT) of the head is needed to confirm and localize the bleed. Up to 95 percent of all SAHs are identified by CT. A lumbar puncture is performed only if the CT does not locate the bleed. Nausea and vomiting should be treated with antiemetics to prevent elevation of intracranial pressure. Nimodipine treatment should be considered to reduce the incidence and severity of vasospasm that can lead to cerebral ischemia.

344. **The answer is E.** *(Chapter 223)* Peripheral vertigo is caused by disease processes affecting structures peripheral to the brain stem. The eighth cranial nerve and vestibular apparatus are both peripheral. Central lesions produce cerebellar signs and symptoms such as ataxia, diplopia, dysphagia, and facial numbness.

345. **The answer is B.** *(Chapter 224)* Initial management of status epilepticus includes stabilization of airway, breathing, and circulation; search for correctable precipitants such as hypoglycemia and toxic ingestion; and administration of appropriate anticonvulsant drugs. A barbiturate coma should be initiated only when status epilepticus is refractory to the standard regimen of benzodiazepines, phenytoin, and phenobarbital.

346. **The answer is C.** *(Chapter 225)* This clinical scenario is classic for botulism. An IVDU is at risk for wound botulism because of the possibility of injecting botulinum spores as a contaminant of the drugs. The botulism toxin is preformed and exerts its effect at the myoneural junction by preventing the release of acetylcholine. In addition to wound botulism, food-borne and infantile forms exist. Diagnosis depends on epidemiologic, clinical, and electrophysiologic findings and may be confirmed by finding the toxin or organism in food, stool, or the wound. Precipitous respiratory failure is possible; therefore, the patient should be admitted to the ICU and intubated as necessary.

347. **The answer is D.** *(Chapter 225)* Guillain-Barré syndrome may occur after contracting an infectious disease, a collagen vascular disease exacerbation, or an exposure to toxins. In general, the lower extremities are involved first and are affected more severely than the upper extremities. The bulbar musculature may also be involved. Reflexes are affected early, and lack of deep tendon reflexes is a hallmark finding. Recovery may take months to years but is usually complete.

348. **The answer is C.** *(Chapter 226)* Parkinson's disease is the most common of the chronic neurodegenerative diseases. The four hallmark neurologic signs include cogwheel rigidity, akinesia or bradykinesia, impairment in posture and equilibrium, and a resting tremor that becomes less prominent with purposeful movement. Other possible signs and symptoms include facial and postural changes, voice and speech abnormalities, depression, and muscle fatigue. Lewy bodies are cytoplasmic inclusions that represent the characteristic cellular changes seen with Parkinson's disease.

349. **The answer is A.** *(Chapter 226)* Patients with myasthenia gravis are treated with cholinesterase inhibitors that can produce signs and symptoms of cholinergic excess. Cholinergic crisis can be differentiated from myasthenic crisis by the Tensilon test. A test dose of edrophonium is administered to determine whether muscle weakness improves (indicating myasthenic crisis) or worsens (indicating cholinergic crisis). Once cholinergic crisis is diagnosed, administration of additional cholinesterase inhibitors such as neostigmine is contraindicated. The physician should be prepared to manage the airway, excessive secretions, bronchospasm, and impaired swallowing.

350. The answer is D. *(Chapter 229)* MS is a demyelinating disease characterized by focal, patchy destruction of myelin sheaths in the central nervous system (CNS). It manifests as recurrent attacks of a focal neurologic disease. Ten to 30 percent of patients in the United States initially present with optic neuritis. Diagnosis is established clinically and is supported by discrete white matter lesions on magnetic resonance imaging, conduction defects with evoked potentials, and increased immunoglobin in the cerebrospinal fluid (CSF). Urologic dysfunction causes significant morbidity and mortality. Urinary tract infections may aggravate symptoms such as lower extremity weakness or spasticity. Small increases in the body temperature of MS patients can worsen existing signs and symptoms and produce additional neurologic manifestations. Therefore, it is important to lower the temperature in a febrile MS patient.

351. The answer is E. *(Chapter 224)* It would be interesting to obtain an EEG after each clinically apparent seizure to demonstrate postictal slowing, indicating a true seizure. However, it is not necessary for immediate clinical management. When patients require paralytic agents, however, clinical assessment of seizure activity becomes impossible, and EEG monitoring is necessary to assess the effectiveness of anticonvulsant therapy.

352. The answer is A. *(Chapter 226)* All of the listed items are true except for nonfatigable weakness. In myasthenia gravis, neuromuscular transmission at the myoneural junction is dysfunctional secondary to antibody-mediated depletion of acetylcholine receptors. With repetitive activation of the motor nerve terminal, the affected muscle fiber becomes refractory to additional nerve impulses. This is manifested clinically as fatigable weakness.

353. The answer is E. *(Chapter 228)* All of the listed items are appropriate for evaluation of shunt infection except lumbar puncture because it often misses CSF shunt infections. A shunt tap rather than a lumbar tap should be performed by a neurosurgeon. All CSF fluid obtained from the shunt tap should be cultured, even if the analysis is normal. One-fifth of all taps will ultimately be positive for infection.

354. The answer is E. *(Chapter 227)* Hematogenous spread usually occurs with encapsulated organisms that can survive dissemination through the bloodstream and trigger inflammatory cascades in the host. Organisms reaching the CNS from direct spread are less virulent and are associated with selected patient groups such as those with immunodeficiency, trauma, neurosurgery, CSF shunts, or infected parameningeal structures. Brudzinski's sign indicates meningeal irritation but can be secondary to many processes. Dexamethasone has been shown to reduce morbidity in children with bacterial meningitis when given before or at the time of the first antibiotic. It is recommended in all children and considered in adults who have a heavy burden of organisms and a reduced level of consciousness. Antibiotics administered by any route can influence the clinical course of meningitis. Seizure is a potential complication of meningitis, occurring in about 25 percent of adults. Phenytoin may be used to treat seizures but is not recommended for prophylaxis.

355. The answer is C. *(Chapter 218)* Regressive pathologic reflexes include Babinski's reflex and snout, root, and grasp reflexes. They all indicate lack of inhibition from higher cortical centers. Asymmetry of deep tendon reflexes is a significant finding, but the finding of a symmetrical increase or decrease in patellar reflexes without other neurologic findings is usually normal. The superficial anal reflex is a normal contraction of the external anal sphincter when the skin or mucosa of the perianal region is stroked. A normal plantar reflex involves plantar flexion of the toes or entire foot after the sole is scratched near its lateral aspect, from the heel toward the toes.

356. The answer is C. *(Chapters 221, 280)* The two features that distinguish delirium from dementia are (1) acute onset with rapid deterioration of function and (2) clouding of consciousness. Delirium and dementia share cognitive impairment, periods of acute worsening, and reversibility. Medical illnesses such as urinary tract infection and hepatic encephalopathy are common precipitants of worsening dementia and new-onset delirium, especially in elderly patients.

357. **The answer is A.** *(Chapter 280)*   Patients with antisocial personality disorder show a pattern of maladaptive behavior. This can manifest as criminal behavior, fighting, lying, abuse and neglect of dependents, and recklessness. ED management is challenging. It is important to minimize anger toward such patients and to set firm limits on their behavior.

358. **The answer is D.** *(Chapter 282)*   Clozapine is an atypical antipsychotic drug used for patients with schizophrenia unresponsive to standard agents or for patients with severe extrapyramidal symptoms. Although clozapine induces less bradykinesia than most other neuroleptics, it tends to cause more sedation. Because it can cause agranulocytosis, a complete blood count (CBC) should be monitored weekly for the first 6 months of use and then every 2 weeks thereafter.

359. **The answer is D.** *(Chapter 282)*   Symptoms of acute lithium overdose may not be fully apparent for up to 48 h, so it would not be appropriate to discharge this patient to a psychiatric facility. She should be admitted to a medical facility and monitored for progression of symptoms. These include ataxia, hyperreflexia, incoordination, confusion, and seizures. All of the other listed measures are appropriate components of ED management.

360. **The answer is C.** *(Chapter 282)*   This patient is exhibiting signs and symptoms of acute psychosis and should be given an antipsychotic agent for his safety and the safety of the staff. Low-potency neuroleptics such as chlorpromazine (Thorazine) should be avoided because of the risk of hypotension. An appropriate dose of haloperidol is 5 to 10 mg intramuscularly, and this can be co-administered with lorazepam 1 to 2 mg intramuscularly for increased sedation.

361. **The answer is D.** *(Chapter 283)*   Eating disorders produce a number of physiologic and clinical changes. Bulimic patients often have dental problems secondary to recurrent gastric acid regurgitation and vigorous brushing. They can also induce dysphagia, hematemesis, and esophageal rupture with their excessive purging. Cathartic colon is seen in laxative abusers and occurs when the colon is no longer capable of propelling a fecal stream without large doses of laxatives. The other clinical manifestations—tachydysrhythmias, hypoglycemia, and stress fractures—are more consistent with anorexia nervosa than with bulimia.

362. **The answer is A.** *(Chapter 284)*   Panic attacks usually manifest with autonomic symptoms such as palpitations, chest tightness, dizziness, dyspnea, and diaphoresis. Attacks are associated with extreme anxiety and can mimic life-threatening medical conditions such as myocardial infarction. Psychotic features are not typical, and their presence requires screening for organic causes of the symptoms, in particular illicit drug use.

363. **The answer is B.** *(Chapter 285)*   Management of conversion reactions includes ruling out organic pathology, reassurance, removing precipitating factors, and psychiatric referral. In refractory cases, hypnosis or amobarbital (Amytal) interview may be required. Patients should not be confronted because they are unaware that the symptoms have no organic cause. The Hoover test is useful to distinguish pseudoparalysis from paralysis. The examiner holds the heels of the patient and asks the patient to lift the unaffected leg. With pseudoparalysis, the affected leg will push downward.

364. **The answer is A.** *(Chapter 288)*   Burnout is a state of physical, emotional, and mental exhaustion. It is manifested by negative attitudes toward self, work, life, and others; irritability toward others; anger and frustration; feelings of helplessness, isolation, and hopelessness; and chronic fatigue. It is thought to be a precursor to more severe forms of impairment that are manifested by alcohol use, drug use, and suicidal ideation.

365.   The answer is C.   *(Chapter 288)*   Rapid eye movement (REM) sleep is the period of time when the brain is on, but the body is off. It occurs toward the end of a normal 7- to 8-h nocturnal sleep period. It is thought to be vital for psychological well-being because patients deprived of REM sleep complain of irritability and moodiness. Physical recuperation occurs during delta sleep. Intellectual tasks, social life, and manual tasks are deleteriously affected by sleep deprivation but are not influenced by any specific phase of the sleep cycle.

366.   The answer is D.   *(Chapter 281)*   Multiple attempts, rather than the first attempt, are associated with a high risk for successful suicide. Psychosis, unemployment, chronic illness, and easy access to a lethal weapon are all risk factors for suicide. Other characteristics that make a patient a high suicide risk include male sex, planned event, and performance of the attempt in an area of unlikely rescue.

367.   The answer is E.   *(Chapter 287)*   Illicit substance users are 18 times more likely to be involved in criminal activities. Elevated serum alcohol levels are found in at least 35 percent of trauma patients. Mental health patients have an increased frequency of suicidal ideation and gestures. Women commonly turn to prostitution to support their drug habits. Intravenous drug users have an increased risk of intentional and accidental overdose, infection, and blood-borne diseases, thereby decreasing their normal life expectancy. Crime, substance abuse, trauma, and medical problems are all interrelated and underscore the need for physicians to be proactive in health education and legislative activities.

OBSTETRIC AND GYNECOLOGIC EMERGENCIES

QUESTIONS

DIRECTIONS: Each question below contains five suggested responses. Choose the **one best** response to each question.

368. All of the following are TRUE of spontaneous abortion (SAB) EXCEPT

(A) more than 50 percent of the abortuses have chromosomal abnormalities

(B) most SABs occur before 8 or 9 weeks of gestation

(C) maternal factors such as uterine adhesions and pelvic structural abnormalities may lead to SABs

(D) the incidence of SAB climbs with increasing maternal age

(E) the pain associated with SAB usually occurs after the bleeding has commenced

Questions 369–370.

369. A 25-year-old female presents to the ED with right lower quadrant pain. Her last normal menstrual period was 26 days ago. She is expecting her menses to begin any day. What is the first study you should order on this patient?

(A) Urinalysis

(B) Complete blood count (CBC)

(C) Quantitative βhCG

(D) Qualitative βhCG

(E) Ultrasound

370. With respect to the patient in question 369, which of the following is the LEAST likely etiology of the pain?

(A) Ectopic pregnancy

(B) Mittelschmerz

(C) Ovarian torsion

(D) Endometriosis

(E) Appendicitis

371. A 30-year-old pregnant female presents to the ED complaining of vaginal bleeding. All of the following statements are true concerning this patient EXCEPT

(A) most patients with bleeding in early pregnancy have normal pregnancy outcomes

(B) urinary tract infection can precipitate spontaneous abortion

(C) lack of adnexal mass on bedside ultrasound makes ectopic unlikely

(D) she should have her Rh status checked

(E) the quantitative βhCG level should be monitored

372. All of the following are true of intraperitoneal blood and culdocentesis EXCEPT

(A) the test is positive when clotting blood is aspirated

(B) cervical motion tenderness may be present in a patient with intraperitoneal blood

(C) a ruptured corpus luteum cyst can produce a positive test

(D) culdocentesis is positive in the majority of ectopic pregnancies, ruptured and unruptured

(E) aspiration of clear fluid denotes a negative test

373. All of the following are risk factors for pelvic inflammatory disease (PID) EXCEPT

(A) multiple sexual partners

(B) adolescence

(C) history of gonococcal salpingitis

(D) use of intrauterine (IUD) contraceptive device

(E) low socioeconomic status

374. All of the following regimens are recommended for the treatment of acute PID EXCEPT

(A) ceftriaxone 125 mg intramuscularly plus doxycycline 100 mg orally twice a day for 10 to 14 days

(B) cefoxitin 2 g intravenously every 6 h plus doxycycline 100 mg intravenously twice a day or orally for 10 to 14 days

(C) cefoxitin 2 g intramuscularly plus probenecid 1 g orally and ofloxacin 400 mg orally twice a day for 14 days

(D) clindamycin 900 mg intravenously every 8 h plus gentamycin loading dose of 2 mg/kg intravenously followed by a maintenance dose of 1.5 mg/kg every 8 h

(E) cefotetan 2 g intravenously every 12 h plus doxycycline 100 mg intravenously twice a day or orally for 10 to 14 days

375. All of the following are TRUE concerning vulvovaginitis EXCEPT

(A) bacterial vaginosis is the most common etiology

(B) alkaline cervical secretions predispose a woman to infection

(C) older women usually do not have symptoms until the vulvovaginitis is advanced

(D) pinworms (*Enterobius vermicularis*) can cause vaginal irritation

(E) the classic "strawberry cervix" is commonly seen in patients with *Trichomonas vaginalis*

376. All of the following physiologic changes take place during normal pregnancy EXCEPT

(A) respiratory rate is increased

(B) blood volume increases

(C) systolic blood pressure decreases

(D) serum blood urea nitrogen (BUN) decreases

(E) leukocyte count increases

377. All of the following statements concerning drugs in pregnancy are TRUE EXCEPT

(A) with the exception of large molecules, virtually all drugs cross the placenta

(B) category A drugs are safe during the first trimester of pregnancy

(C) diuretics are not generally recommended in pregnancy

(D) erythromycin estolate can be safely prescribed in pregnancy

(E) cephalosporins can be used at any time during pregnancy

378. The MOST important factor in determining fetal risk from diagnostic imaging is the amount of ionizing radiation produced by the test. Rank the following radiation exposures from lowest to highest dose of radiation.

1. Head computed tomography (CT)
2. Posteroanterior and lateral chest x-ray
3. Lumbrosacral spine series (three films)
4. Abdominal CT
5. Intravenous pyelogram (IVP)

(A) 2, 3, 1, 4, 5

(B) 2, 1, 3, 5, 4

(C) 3, 2, 1, 5, 4

(D) 1, 4, 2, 3, 5

(E) 2, 1, 5, 3, 4

379. A woman in the third trimester of pregnancy presents to the ED complaining of abdominal pain without vaginal bleeding. Vital signs are remarkable for a systolic blood pressure of 160, heart rate of 105, and a respiratory rate of 18. Which one of the following statements is TRUE concerning this patient?

(A) A normal ultrasound excludes the diagnosis of placental abruption

(B) Lack of vaginal bleeding excludes the diagnosis of placental abruption

(C) A pelvic examination should be avoided

(D) A CBC, electrolytes, and renal and liver function tests (LFTs) should be obtained

(E) Immediate delivery is indicated

380. All of the following are TRUE of HELLP syndrome EXCEPT

(A) the majority of women complain of right upper quadrant or epigastric pain with nausea and vomiting

(B) platelet count is < 100,000/mL

(C) urinalysis is positive for protein

(D) 10 percent calcium gluconate should be administered

(E) hypertension is key to the diagnosis

381. All of the following are TRUE of premature rupture of membranes (PROM) EXCEPT

(A) the finding of a "ferning" pattern is diagnostic of amniotic fluid

(B) nitrazine paper changes to dark blue

(C) the pH of amniotic fluid is 4.5 to 6.0

(D) 90 percent of term patients with PROM will go into labor within 24 h

(E) infections can precipitate PROM

382. All of the following are TRUE of infections during pregnancy EXCEPT

(A) 40 percent of *Cytomegalovirus* infections are transmitted to the fetus

(B) to be effective, *Varicella zoster* immune globulin should be given to seronegative women within 24 h of chicken pox exposure

(C) erythema infectiosum exposure can cause SAB

(D) infection with rubella in the first trimester is associated with congenital rubella syndrome

(E) fetuses exposed to maternal toxoplasmosis have a 10 percent chance of contracting congenital toxoplasmosis

383. All of following are TRUE of asthma in pregnancy EXCEPT

(A) asthma worsens in about one-third of cases

(B) oral steroids should not be prescribed

(C) β-agonists are the mainstay of therapy

(D) chest radiographs should be ordered for the same indications as for nonpregnant patients

(E) pulmonary function tests are not significantly changed during pregnancy

384. All of the following statements are TRUE of endometritis EXCEPT

(A) the incidence is greater in patients who have had a cesarean section than in those who have had a spontaneous vaginal delivery

(B) many infections are polymicrobial

(C) when patients present with endometritis 48 h to 6 weeks after delivery, chlamydia and mycoplasma should be considered as primary etiologies

(D) the speculum examination always reveals a purulent discharge

(E) the clinical diagnosis is based on the symptoms of fever, malaise, lower abdominal pain, and foul-smelling lochia

385. All of the following are TRUE of trauma in pregnancy EXCEPT

(A) rapid deceleration may cause uterine rupture

(B) pelvic fractures preclude a woman from having a vaginal delivery

(C) life-threatening hemorrhage is most often localized to the retroperitoneum

(D) splenic rupture, kidney injury, and liver laceration are the most common intraabdominal injuries

(E) the Kleihauer-Betke assay is recommended

386. To make the diagnosis of toxic shock syndrome, all of the following must be present EXCEPT

(A) hypotension

(B) temperature greater than 38.9°F

(C) rash with subsequent desquamation

(D) negative serologic test for streptococcal infection

(E) involvement of three of the following organ systems: gastrointestinal, musculoskeletal, renal, mucosal, hepatic, hematologic, or central nervous system

387. All of the following are indications for maternal transport to a tertiary perinatal center EXCEPT

(A) placental bleeding

(B) premature labor with cervical dilation to 6 cm

(C) blood pressure of 160/110 mm Hg and proteinuria

(D) premature rupture of membranes

(E) term labor in a insulin-dependent diabetic

388. When a gravid female presents in cardiac arrest, all of the following statements are TRUE EXCEPT

(A) the "human wedge" is useful in bystander CPR

(B) ideally, a Cardiff wedge should be placed under the patient's left hip and flank

(C) manual displacement of the uterus off the inferior vena cava helps increase venous return

(D) pregnant women are in an edematous state that can make intubation difficult

(E) the use of a femoral line to deliver medications should be discouraged

389. Any pregnant woman beyond 20 weeks of gestation who presents to the ED and appears to be actively contracting may need an emergent delivery. All of the following are TRUE of emergency delivery EXCEPT

(A) inability to detect fetal heart tones does not rule out a viable pregnancy

(B) amniotomy may result in prolapse of the umbilical cord

(C) once the mother feels an urge to push, she should be encouraged to proceed

(D) if the physician delivering the baby notices a "turtle sign," an assistant should apply suprapubic pressure

(E) once the head is delivered, it is imperative to check for a nuchal cord (present in 25 percent of deliveries)

390. Laparoscopy is being used more frequently to aid in the diagnosis of pelvic disease and to perform gynecologic surgeries. When a patient presents to the ED after one of these procedures, all of the following are TRUE EXCEPT

(A) free air under the diaphragm is a normal finding 1 week after surgery

(B) pelvic infections are uncommon after this procedure

(C) a traumatic bowel injury is less problematic than a thermal injury

(D) infection is an infrequent complication

(E) patients with increasing abdominal pain after the procedure have perforated bowel until proven otherwise

391. Which of the following statements is TRUE concerning genital herpes?

(A) HSV-1 accounts for up to 50 percent of the cases of genital herpes

(B) Systemic acyclovir decreases the frequency of recurrences

(C) Systemic symptoms are common with the initial presentation of genital herpes

(D) Tzanck smears are positive in the majority of cases

(E) Cultures of fluid obtained from herpes vesicles are positive only a third of the time

OBSTETRIC AND GYNECOLOGIC EMERGENCIES

ANSWERS

368. **The answer is C.** *(Chapter 101)* The etiologies of SAB can be divided into two categories: fetal and maternal. Fetal chromosomal abnormalities are the major cause of SAB. Maternal factors include uterine anomalies, incompetent cervix, progestin deficiency, and chronic medical problems such as diabetes mellitus and thyroid disease. Although the majority of spontaneous abortions occur before the 8th or 9th week of gestation, they can occur up to the 20th week. The incidence of SAB rises with increased maternal and paternal age and with parity. Pain associated with abortion usually follows the commencement of vaginal bleeding and is typically midline and crampy. This is in contrast to ectopic pregnancy or ruptured cyst in which pain is typically acute, severe, and unilateral.

369–370. **The answers are D and B, respectively.** *(Chapters 98, 100)* Because of the life-threatening potential of ectopic pregnancy, it is critical to determine whether a woman with pelvic pain is pregnant. A qualitative test for the β subunit of human chorionic gonadotropin (βhCG) can be performed immediately at the bedside and thus is the first test indicated for any female patient of child-bearing age who is complaining of abdominal pain.

Ectopic pregnancy must be considered in every woman of child-bearing age who comes to the ED complaining of pain, even if she denies pregnancy. Ovarian torsion is uncommon, but when it occurs it causes unilateral pelvic pain. Endometriosis should be considered in any woman of reproductive age complaining of one or a combination of the following signs and symptoms: acute adnexal pain, premenstrual pelvic pain, worsening dysmenorrhea, and dyspareunia. Appendicitis is always in the differential of right lower quadrant pain. The key to the diagnosis of Mittelschmerz or "middle pain" is the fact that it occurs in mid-cycle, thus making it unlikely in this patient. A history of similar pain with each menstrual cycle may be elicited.

371. **The answer is C.** *(Chapter 101)* The possibility of ectopic pregnancy must be considered in every patient who presents with abnormal uterine bleeding or pelvic pain. A focused bedside ultrasound is consistent with ectopic pregnancy if there is no identifiable gestational sac or intrauterine pregnancy visualized. Less commonly, an adnexal mass may be present, but the mass does not always represent an ectopic pregnancy. Rhesus (Rh) status should be assessed. Rh-negative women with antepartum bleeding must receive RhoGAM to prevent antibody formation that would endanger future pregnancies. Serial βhCG levels may be indicated in hemodynamically stable patients and should double in 48 h in a normal pregnancy. Urinalysis should be performed on patients with threatened abortion to rule out infection as a precipitant.

372. **The answer is A.** *(Chapter 100)* With the advent of bedside ultrasound, the use of culdocentesis has decreased. However, this simple test still has a role in the pregnant patient with signs and symptoms of ectopic pregnancy when ultrasound is not available. A needle is inserted into the cul de sac just inferior to the cervix. A culdocentesis is positive if non-clotting blood is obtained and negative if clear fluid is aspirated. Failure to aspirate blood is nondiagnostic and may represent technical problems. Culdocentesis is positive in the majority of patients with ectopic pregnancies, ruptured and unruptured (85 and 65 percent, respectively). A positive test is not specific for ectopic pregnancy but occurs with any process that produces blood in the pelvis.

373. The answer is E. *(Chapter 105)*   PID occurs in women from all socioeconomic backgrounds. Risk factors for the development of PID include a history of gonococcal infection, sexual promiscuity, adolescence, and IUD use. Instrumentation of the uterus and tubes may predispose patients to the development of endometritis and salpingitis.

374. The answer is A. *(Chapter 105)*   The Centers for Disease Control and Prevention publishes guidelines delineating several appropriate treatments for PID. The presence of penicillinase-producing gonorrhea dictates a careful choice of antibiotics. If ceftriaxone is used to treat outpatient PID, the dose is 250 mg intramuscularly as opposed to the dose of 125 mg intramuscularly for simple cervicitis.

375. The answer is E. *(Chapter 104)*   The most common causes of vulvovaginitis include (1) infections with *Gardnerella, Candida albicans, Trichomonas,* and herpes simplex; (2) contact vulvovaginitis; (3) foreign bodies; and (4) atrophic vaginitis. Bacterial vaginosis is the most common form, followed by candidiasis. Whereas 80 percent of patients with *Trichomonas vaginalis* have diffuse erythema of the vaginal vault, only 2 percent present with a "strawberry cervix" (secondary to diffuse punctate hemorrhages). Normal acidic vaginal secretions help to limit infection. In older women, because of scant nerve endings in the vagina, symptoms of vulvovaginitis do not present until advanced disease is present. Young children may present with vaginal itching and irritation secondary to pinworms.

376. The answer is A. *(Chapter 99)*   All organ systems are affected by the physiologic changes of pregnancy. Although tidal volume is increased and functional residual capacity is decreased, respiratory rate and vital capacity remain unchanged. The other changes listed are all seen with normal pregnancy.

377. The answer is D. *(Chapters 99, 102)*   Erythromycin base is safe to use in pregnancy, but erythromycin estolate should not be used because of drug-related hepatotoxicity. Other antibiotics considered safe in pregnancy include cephalosporins, nitrofurantoin, penicillin, and azithromycin. Heparin and insulin are large molecules that do not cross the placenta and are therefore safe in pregnancy.

378. The answer is B. *(Chapters 99, 102)*   The most recent evidence suggests that 10 rad is the threshold for human teratogenesis and that the fetus is most vulnerable at 8 to 15 weeks of gestation. The position of the American College of Radiology is that there is no single test that results in radiation doses that threaten the well-being of the developing embryo or fetus. Radiation exposure is as follows: two-view chest radiograph with abdominal shielding, 0.00005 rad; head CT, ≤ 0.1 rad; lumbrosacral spine series, 0.168 to 0.359 rad; IVP, 0.686 to 1.398 rad; and abdominal CT, 5.0 rad.

379. The answer is D. *(Chapter 101)*   Etiologies of third-trimester abdominal pain include placental abruption, labor contractions, hypertension with hemolysis, elevated liver enzyme and low platelet (HELLP) syndrome, appendicitis, and rarely placenta previa from uterine irritation. Classically, placental abruption presents with vaginal bleeding; however, when the separation is central, bleeding is concealed. Ultrasound does not detect all abruptions. A speculum examination is safe and appropriate in the management of this patient. Digital examinations are contraindicated when the diagnosis of placenta previa is being considered. Immediate delivery is indicated if the patient is eclamptic or the fetus is in danger for another reason. CBC, electrolytes, BUN, creatinine, LFTs, and a urinalysis may help detect an infection, HELLP syndrome, or hemorrhage.

380. The answer is D. *(Chapter 101)*   Preeclampsia (pregnancy-induced hypertension) occurs in about 7 percent of all pregnancies. It can present with a wide variety of symptoms. The classic triad is hypertension, proteinuria, and edema. The HELLP (hemolysis, elevated liver enzymes, and low platelets) syndrome represents an unusual presentation of this disease. Magnesium sulfate is indicated for seizure prophylaxis in patients with severe preeclampsia. Calcium gluconate is the antidote for magnesium toxicity. Obstetrical management is based on the degree of preeclampsia and the gestational age of the fetus; if term or near term, delivery is indicated.

381. The answer is C. *(Chapter 103)*   Premature rupture of membranes is defined as the rupture of membranes before the onset of labor. The cause of PROM is not well understood, but there is strong evidence that inflammation from infections affecting the membranes is a precipitant. The diagnosis of PROM is made by a combination of history and physical examination. Speculum examination should be performed to look for vaginal fluid pooling in the posterior fornix. Normal vaginal fluid pH is 4.5 to 6.0; amniotic fluid has a pH of 7.1 to 7.3. Nitrazine paper turns dark blue in the presence of amniotic fluid. If vaginal fluid is placed on a slide and allowed to dry, a "ferning" pattern is diagnostic for amniotic fluid.

382. The answer is B. *(Chapter 150)*   The TORCH infections can cause perinatal morbidity and mortality: T, toxoplasmosis; O, "other" such as human parvovirus (B19), hepatitis B infection, and syphilis; R, rubella; C, chicken pox or varicella infection; and H, herpes simplex. All have serious effects on fetuses. Patients exposed to varicella or hepatitis B who do not have adequate protective titers need immune globulin. For varicella, the immune globulin should be administered within 96 h of exposure.

383. The answer is B. *(Chapter 102)*   Inhaled β agonists are the cornerstone of therapy. Steroids should be added in moderate and severe exacerbations, either inhaled or orally. Concomitant respiratory infections should always be considered and a chest radiograph ordered if management would be changed based on the results. Adequate oxygenation of the mother is the key to a healthy fetus.

384. The answer is D. *(Chapter 101)*   Patients with postpartum endometritis complain of lower abdominal pain, fever, and foul-smelling discharge. The speculum examination often shows a purulent discharge but only scant discharge may be present, especially in patients with group A β-hemolytic streptococci. Cervical cultures should be obtained in all patients. Although many infections are polymicrobial, within the first 48 h postpartum, group A and B *Streptococcus*, *Staphylococcus*, and *Clostridium* should be considered as primary etiologies. Infections that present later are more commonly caused by chylamdia and mycoplasma.

385. The answer is B. *(Chapter 246)*   Pelvic deformity may interfere with the normal passage of the fetus through the pelvic inlet during labor and delivery, but cesarean section is only necessary 5 to 10 percent of the time after pelvic fracture. The Kleihauer–Betke test of maternal blood is used to detect fetal cells in the maternal circulation. Although it is difficult to perform and often unavailable in emergency situations, it should be ordered to detect the rare large fetal transfusions that require specific fetal blood therapy.

386. The answer is D. *(Chapter 138)*   Fever, hypotension, multiorgan involvement, and rash must be present to make the diagnosis of toxic shock syndrome. In addition, negative serologies for measles, leptospirosis, mononucleosis, and Rocky Mountain spotted fever are required. Negative serologic studies for streptococcal infection play no part in the diagnosis. In fact, streptococcal infections have been implicated as an etiology of the syndrome.

387. The answer is B. *(Chapter 101)*   The transferring physician must abide by federal regulations outlined in the Emergency Medical Treatment and Active Labor Act when arranging a transfer. The most common indications for maternal transport to a tertiary perinatal facility (higher level of care) are premature rupture of membranes and preterm labor. Other reasons to initiate transport include preeclampsia, placental bleeding, and diabetes mellitus. If the patient is in active labor (having contractions and dilated to 6 cm or more), any transport is contraindicated and the physician attending the patient should prepare for immediate delivery.

388.   **The answer is B.**   *(Chapter 12)*   Several physiologic changes of pregnancy must be considered during cardiopulmonary resuscitation (CPR). Mucosal engorgement and increased friability make the pregnant patient's airway more likely to bleed and swell during intubation. The enlarged uterus compresses the inferior vena cava when the woman is supine during CPR. The gravid uterus should be displaced off the inferior vena cava to the right by using the "human wedge," Cardiff wedge, a roll, or manual displacement. Infradiaphragmatic vessels are suboptimal for medication administration secondary to poor venous return.

389.   **The answer is C.**   *(Chapter 103)*   In the setting of emergency delivery, bimanual pelvic examination should be performed unless placenta previa is suspected. The cervix should be checked for dilation, effacement, and presenting part. If the mother pushes before the cervix is 100 percent effaced, a serious laceration may occur. Amniotomy is not appropriate in the ED because it may result in prolapse of the cord if the baby's head is not engaged. Nuchal cords and shoulder dystocia are problems that may arise during delivery. The "turtle sign" (fetal head pulled tight into the perineum) indicates shoulder dystocia. After a generous episiotomy is performed and the bladder is emptied, suprapubic pressure should be applied by an assistant to aid delivery of the shoulders.

390.   **The answer is A.**   *(Chapter 108)*   Major complications associated with laparoscopy are (1) thermal injuries to the bowel; (2) bleeding; (3) rarely, ureteral, bladder, and large bowel injury; and (4) infections or abscess formation. Traumatic injury to the bowel is generally less worrisome than thermal injury from the instruments used during the procedure. Typically when bowel trauma occurs, it is the result of a small-diameter needle and is recognized when the needle is withdrawn. Peritonitis rarely develops after this complication. Perforated viscus must be ruled out in patients with persistent or increasing abdominal pain. Air insufflated during the procedure should be absorbed within 3 days.

391.   **The answer is C.**   *(Chapter 104)*   Genital herpes is a sexually transmitted disease caused by a DNA virus specific to humans. There are two antigenic types of herpes simplex virus (HSV), denoted HSV-1 and HSV-2. The overwhelming majority of genital infections are caused by HSV-2. In the past HSV-1 was thought to cause only oral infections, but it is now known to be responsible for up to 30 percent of the genital infections. The initial presentation of herpes occurs 1 to 45 days after exposure and is usually accompanied by constitutional symptoms such as fever, malaise, and headache. Some people have asymptomatic infections, defined as culture-positive viral shedding in the absence of symptoms or lesions. Tzanck smears identify multinucleated giant cells in up to 50 percent of cases. Cultures are positive 85 to 95 percent of the time. Acyclovir provides partial control of the signs and symptoms and accelerates healing of the lesions. This antiviral medication does not affect the frequency or severity of recurrences.

ORTHOPEDIC EMERGENCIES

QUESTIONS

DIRECTIONS: Each question below contains five suggested responses. Choose the **one best** response to each question.

392. All of the following statements regarding bone remodeling are TRUE EXCEPT

(A) young children have a greater capacity for remodeling than adults
(B) remodeling is related to the degree of angulation
(C) angulation near the end of a long bone will remodel more satisfactorily than angulation near the midshaft
(D) angulation in the natural plane of the joint motion will remodel more successfully than angulation outside the plane of joint motion
(E) injuries involving the epiphyseal plate are more likely to remodel successfully

393. Which of the following statements about lunate fractures is FALSE?

(A) The most common mechanism is a fall on an outstretched hand
(B) Lunate fractures are the third most common type of carpal fracture
(C) The lunate occupies two thirds of the radial articular surface
(D) X-rays reliably demonstrate the fracture
(E) This fracture may be associated with avascular necrosis of the lunate

394. A 25-year-old female presents with right elbow pain after a fall while doing gymnastics. The elbow is deformed and flexed at 45 degrees. Plain radiographs show an elbow dislocation, with both radius and ulna displaced posteriorly. Which of the following neurovascular structures is most likely to be injured?

(A) Axillary nerve
(B) Radial nerve
(C) Ulnar nerve
(D) Radial artery
(E) Brachial plexus

395. A 2-year-old male is brought to the ED by his parents for refusing to use his right arm. He was well until 30 min before, when his cousin tried to lift him up a curb by that arm. He now holds the elbow slightly flexed and pronated and will not use the injured arm. Which is the MOST appropriate initial approach?

(A) Obtain emergent orthopedic consultation
(B) Order plain radiographs of the elbow
(C) Attempt to reduce the elbow by pronation and extension
(D) Attempt to reduce the elbow by supination and flexion
(E) Prepare to reduce the elbow under conscious sedation

396. All of the following statements about Volkmann's ischemic contracture are TRUE EXCEPT

(A) Volkmann's ischemic contracture is a complication of supracondylar fracture
(B) signs include refusal to open the hand in children, pain with passive extension of fingers, and forearm tenderness
(C) local edema causes decreased venous outflow and arterial inflow, resulting in local tissue ischemia
(D) muscle and nerve necrosis may occur, leading to permanent disability
(E) absence of radial pulse is diagnostic

397. A 27-year-old male presents with left wrist pain after falling on an outstretched hand. He has an obvious deformity of the wrist but is neurovascularly intact. X-ray shows a transverse distal radius fracture with dorsal angulation. On the lateral view, the ulna is displaced dorsally. Which of the following terms describes this fracture?

(A) Galeazzi's fracture
(B) Monteggia's fracture
(C) Colles' fracture
(D) Smith's fracture
(E) Barton's fracture

398. Which of the following statements about sternoclavicular dislocations is FALSE?

(A) The medial clavicular epiphysis is the last epiphysis of the body to close (at age 22–25 years)
(B) CT is the imaging modality of choice
(C) Anterior dislocations are more common than posterior dislocations
(D) Closed reduction is frequently successful
(E) Posterior dislocations are associated with injuries to thoracic structures

399. Which of the following is TRUE regarding scapular fractures?

(A) Most are treated with open reduction and internal fixation
(B) Approximately 50 percent are associated with intrathoracic injuries
(C) They frequently result in long-term disability
(D) They account for approximately 8 percent of all fractures
(E) The mechanism of injury is from direct blow, trauma to the shoulder, or fall on an outstretched arm

400. A 26-year-old soccer player presents after a direct blow to the shoulder. On examination, she has tenderness over the acromioclavicular joint, but no step-off or deformity. X-rays show no fracture, subluxation, or dislocation. Which of the following is the most appropriate management?

(A) Arrange immediate orthopedic follow-up for possible operative repair
(B) Place the shoulder in a figure-of-eight brace, with orthopedic follow-up in 1 to 2 weeks
(C) Place the shoulder in a simple sling, with instructions for early range of motion
(D) Place the shoulder in a shoulder immobilizer for 2 to 3 weeks
(E) Tell the patient that immobilization is not necessary but that she should apply ice and use analgesics as needed for pain control

401. Which of the following statements about anterior shoulder dislocations is FALSE?

(A) Nerve injury occurs in 10 to 25 percent of acute dislocations
(B) Most neural injuries involve the axillary nerve
(C) Successful reduction occurs in 70 to 90 percent of cases, regardless of technique
(D) Associated rotator cuff injuries occur in 80 percent of patients older than 60 years
(E) Vascular injuries are rare but, when they occur, tend to involve the brachial artery

402. Which of the following mechanisms is most likely to result in an anterior glenohumeral dislocation?

(A) Abduction, extension, and external rotation
(B) Forceful internal rotation and adduction
(C) Electric shock
(D) Seizure
(E) Direct force to the anterior shoulder

403. All of the following statements about fractures of the proximal humerus are TRUE EXCEPT

(A) any fracture involving the surgical neck may result in compromised blood supply to the articular segment
(B) fracture of the lesser tuberosity suggests a potential posterior shoulder dislocation
(C) significant displacement of a greater tuberosity fragment implies a possible rotator cuff tear
(D) markedly angulated surgical neck fractures are at risk for neurovascular damage
(E) emergent orthopedic consultation is recommended for multipart fractures

404. Which type of pelvic fracture is MOST often associated with severe hemorrhage?

(A) Anterioposterior compression
(B) Vertical shear
(C) Lateral compression
(D) Crush injuries
(E) Combination injuries

405. Which of the following statements about management of hemorrhage in pelvic fractures is FALSE?

(A) Patients with double breaks in the ring require blood products more often than those with single breaks
(B) Aggressive fluid and blood replacement is a mainstay of therapy
(C) An external fixator may be useful to reduce bleeding in some pelvic fractures
(D) Angiography and embolization can be done to control small bleeding sites
(E) Laparotomy provides definitive therapy

406. Which of the following hip fractures is MOST likely to disrupt perfusion of the femoral head?

(A) Subcapital fracture
(B) Intertrochanteric fracture
(C) Subtrochanteric fracture
(D) Pubic ramus fracture
(E) Avulsion of the greater trochanter

407. Which of the following statements regarding hip dislocations is FALSE?

(A) The risk of avascular necrosis increases if reduction is delayed
(B) Traumatic hip dislocations in children are rare
(C) Reduction should be done as soon as possible and always within 6 h
(D) In patients with anterior dislocations, the extremity is shortened and internally rotated
(E) Posterior dislocations are more common than anterior dislocations

408. A 13-year-old male is brought in by his parents for right hip stiffness and groin discomfort after activity. He feels well otherwise and denies fevers or chills. On examination he is ambulatory with a slight limp and mild discomfort with internal rotation. Which of the following is the MOST likely diagnosis?

(A) Congenital hip dislocation
(B) Septic arthritis
(C) Transient synovitis
(D) Legg-Calvé-Perthes disease
(E) Slipped capital femoral epiphysis

409. Which of the following injuries is MOST likely to be associated with disruption of the cruciate ligaments?

(A) Patellar fracture
(B) Femoral condyle fracture
(C) Avulsion of the tibial tuberosity
(D) Tibial plateau fracture
(E) Tibial spine fracture

410. The anterior drawer sign, Lachman's test, and the pivot shift are used to measure stability of which knee structure?

(A) Medial collateral ligament
(B) Lateral collateral ligament
(C) Anterior cruciate ligament
(D) Posterior cruciate ligament
(E) Medial meniscus

411. A 35-year-old male presents after a significant hyperextension injury to the right knee while playing soccer. On examination the knee is severely unstable in both anteroposterior and lateral directions. A palpable hematoma is present in the popliteal fossa. Plain films demonstrate no bony abnormality. Which of the following tests must be performed emergently?

(A) Magnetic resonance imaging of the knee
(B) Arteriography
(C) Bone scan
(D) CT of the knee
(E) Electromyography

412. What is the MOST common site for a compartment syndrome?

(A) Anterior compartment of the lower leg
(B) Peroneal compartment of the lower leg
(C) Deep posterior compartment of the lower leg
(D) Volar compartment of the forearm
(E) Dorsal compartment of the forearm

413. Which of the following is the most common ligament injured during ankle sprain?

(A) Anterior talofibular ligament
(B) Posterior talofibular ligament
(C) Calcaneofibular ligament
(D) Deltoid ligament
(E) Anterior tibiofibular ligament

414. A 35-year-old female presents with posterior ankle pain, which occurred suddenly while playing volleyball. Thompson's test is positive. What is the MOST likely diagnosis?

(A) Posterior talofibular ligament injury
(B) Achilles tenosynovitis
(C) Achilles tendon rupture
(D) Posterior talotibial dislocation
(E) Calcaneal fracture

415. A 45-year-old male presents with foot pain after an automobile accident. The examination shows tenderness, swelling, and ecchymosis over the midfoot. X-ray shows fracture of the base of the second metatarsal and lateral displacement of the second, third, fourth, and fifth metatarsals. What is the optimal management of this patient?

(A) Posterior splint, with orthopedic follow-up as needed
(B) Urgent orthopedic consultation for possible open reduction and internal fixation
(C) Splint the patient in equinus and follow up with orthopedics in 2 to 3 days
(D) Cast the foot and follow up with orthopedics in 2 to 3 days
(E) Hard-sole shoe, weight bearing as tolerated, follow-up in orthopedics as needed

ORTHOPEDIC EMERGENCIES

ANSWERS

392. The answer is E. *(Chapter 259)* Injury to the epiphyseal plate is a poor prognostic indicator. Specific predictors of satisfactory remodeling include youth, proximity of the fracture to the end of the bone, and angulation in the plane of natural joint motion.

393. The answer is D. *(Chapter 262)* Diagnosis of lunate fractures can be difficult because wrist x-rays may or may not show the abnormality. Missed diagnosis or improper management may result in avascular necrosis of the lunate (Kienbock's disease). The most common mechanism is a fall on an outstretched hand.

394. The answer is C. *(Chapter 261)* Neurovascular complications occur in 8 to 21 percent of patients with elbow dislocations, the most frequent injury being the ulnar nerve. Vascular complications occur in 5 to 13 percent, with the brachial artery being most commonly injured. The axillary nerve is at risk after anterior shoulder dislocation. Supracondylar humeral fractures are associated with radial nerve and artery injuries.

395. The answer is D. *(Chapter 261)* Subluxation of the radial head (nursemaid's elbow) is common among children 1 to 4 years old. It occurs with sudden traction on the hand, with the elbow extended and the forearm pronated. During forceful traction, fibers of the annular ligament become trapped between the radial head and the capitellum. To reduce the subluxation, the examiner's thumb should be placed over the patient's radial head, with the other hand on the patient's wrist. The forearm is then supinated, and the elbow is flexed. Reduction is successful when a palpable "click" is felt. Orthopedic consultation is not necessary if the history and physical are consistent with the diagnosis and reduction is successful. Plain radiographs are not diagnostic. Systemic sedation is not typically required to reduce nursemaid's elbow.

396. The answer is E. *(Chapter 261)* Volkmann's ischemic contracture is the most serious complication of supracondylar fracture. Local edema compromises tissue perfusion, which, if unrelieved, leads to tissue necrosis and permanent disability. Diagnosis is based on signs and symptoms such as refusal to open the hand, pain with passive extension of the fingers, and forearm tenderness. Lack of a radial pulse without these signs does not necessarily indicate ischemia but may represent disruption of vascular structures.

397. The answer is A. *(Chapter 262)* Galeazzi's fracture, sometimes called *reverse Monteggia's fracture*, describes a fracture of the distal third of the radial shaft with associated distal radioulnar joint dislocation. The distal radioulnar joint injury can be subtle, with the anteroposterior radiograph showing only slightly increased distal radioulnar joint space. On the lateral view, the ulna is displaced dorsally. Monteggia's fracture–dislocation is a fracture of the proximal third of the ulna associated with radial head dislocation. Colles' fracture refers to a distal radius fracture with dorsal angulation. Fractures of the distal radius with volar angulation are Smith's fractures (or *reverse Colles'*). Barton's fracture is a fracture of the dorsal or volar rim of the distal radius, in which the carpal bones are displaced in the direction of the fracture.

398.   The answer is D. *(Chapter 263)*   In reducing sternoclavicular dislocations, closed reduction is usually attempted first, but operative intervention is often required. The medial clavicular epiphysis is the last to appear (age 18 years) and the last to close (age 22–25 years). As a result, physeal injuries may be misdiagnosed as a dislocation. Routine radiographs may not be diagnostic, and computed tomography (CT) is the imaging procedure of choice. Anterior dislocations are more common than posterior dislocations. Posterior dislocations may impinge on thoracic structures, causing pneumothorax, and compression or laceration of the great vessels, trachea, or esophagus.

399.   The answer is E. *(Chapter 263)*   Most scapular fractures are treated nonsurgically, with a sling for immobilization. Such fractures require high energy, and more than 80 percent are associated with thoracic and shoulder girdle injuries. Long-term disability is typically the result of associated injuries, not of the fracture itself. Scapular injuries are rare, accounting for fewer than 1 percent of fractures. The mechanism is most commonly a direct blow to the scapula, trauma to the shoulder, or fall on an outstretched arm.

400.   The answer is C. *(Chapter 263)*   The patient has a type I acromioclavicular joint injury. Although various straps and braces have been used to reduce the dislocation, none have proved successful. A simple sling is most convenient and effective. Patients should be instructed to rest, apply ice, use analgesics, and begin early range-of-motion exercises to prevent a frozen shoulder. Mild acromioclavicular joint injuries do not require operative repair.

401.   The answer is E. *(Chapter 263)*   Although vascular injuries are rare, they tend to occur in elderly patients and involve the axillary artery. Signs of axillary artery injury include absent radial pulse, axillary hematoma, ecchymosis of the lateral chest wall, and an axillary bruit. Neural injuries occur in 10 to 25 percent of acute dislocations, most often secondary to traction neuropraxia. Axillary nerve sensation must be assessed before and after reduction because it is the most commonly injured nerve. The injury is typically transient and tends to resolve spontaneously. Successful reduction occurs in 70 to 90 percent of cases, regardless of reduction technique. Rotator cuff injury is a frequent complication in patients older than 60 years.

402.   The answer is A. *(Chapter 263)*   Shoulder dislocation is the most common major joint dislocation. Approximately 98 percent of glenohumeral dislocations are anterior. Abduction, extension, and external rotation comprise the classic mechanism. The other listed possibilities are likely to cause a posterior dislocation.

403.   The answer is A. *(Chapter 263)*   Any fracture involving the anatomic neck or the articular surface may result in compromise of the blood supply to the articular segment. Ischemic necrosis of the articular segment may ultimately require insertion of a humeral head prosthesis for these relatively rare fractures.

404.   The answer is B. *(Chapter 265)*   Hemorrhage is a major cause of death in patients with pelvic fractures. Of those with vertical shear injuries, approximately 75 percent suffer severe hemorrhage. Retroperitoneal bleeding is an inevitable complication, and up to 4 L of blood can accumulate in this space. Other complications of vertical shear injuries include bladder rupture (15 percent) and urethral injuries (25 percent).

405.   The answer is E. *(Chapter 265)*   Patients with double breaks in the ring require blood products more often than those with single breaks. Patients with significant injuries require aggressive volume resuscitation with fluid and blood replacement. An external fixator device can help control hemorrhage. In patients who are exsanguinating, angiography permits embolization of smaller vessels. Laparotomy can release a tamponade and precipitate uncontrolled hemorrhage.

406. The answer is A. *(Chapter 265)* Displaced subcapital fractures of the femoral head and neck can compromise the femoral neck vessels through shearing or compression from intracapsular hemarthrosis. The blood supply through the ligamentum teres may not be adequate to supply the entire femoral head. Avascular necrosis occurs in 15 percent of nondisplaced fractures and in 90 percent of completely displaced fractures. Fractures below the capsule (intertrochanteric and subtrochanteric) rarely disrupt important vessels. Pubic ramus fractures do not involve the femoral head.

407. The answer is D. *(Chapter 265)* Patients with posterior dislocations present with the extremity shortened and internally rotated. Those with anterior dislocations present with the extremity shortened and externally rotated. Posterior dislocations account for 80 to 90 percent of hip dislocations. Prompt reduction is important to avoid avascular necrosis. General anesthesia may be required.

408. The answer is E. *(Chapter 132)* Slipped capital femoral epiphysis occurs primarily in obese male children aged 10 to 16 years. Symptom onset is insidious. Patients often complain of hip stiffness, mild limp, and groin discomfort after activity. Initial radiographs may be normal initially but subsequently may show a posterior slip of the epiphyseal plate. The patient should be made non–weight bearing, and orthopedic consultation should be obtained.

409. The answer is E. *(Chapter 266)* Isolated injuries of the tibial spine are uncommon and usually result in damage to the cruciate ligaments. The injury is caused by an anterior–posterior force directed against the flexed proximal tibia. This may cause incomplete or complete avulsion of the tibial spine, with or without displacement. If the fracture is nondisplaced, it is treated by immobilization in full extension. Displaced fractures may require open reduction and internal fixation.

410. The answer is C. *(Chapter 266)* All three tests measure stability of the anterior cruciate ligament. The anterior drawer sign has been used for a long time, but it is not very sensitive. The test is performed with the hip flexed at 45 degrees and the knee flexed at 90 degrees. The examiner forwardly displaces the tibia from the femur. A displacement of greater than 6 mm relative to the opposite knee is considered positive. The Lachman's test is similar but is more sensitive. The test is done with 20 degrees of flexion at the knee, with the knee on a pillow. The femur is stabilized, and an anterior force is applied against the tibia. A displacement of more than 5 mm or a soft, mushy endpoint suggests an injury to the anterior cruciate ligament. In the pivot shift test, valgus stress and internal rotation is applied, and then the examiner slowly begins to flex the knee. A visible, audible, or palpable reduction may occur when the anterior subluxation is reduced.

411. The answer is B. *(Chapter 266)* The patient's history is suggestive of a knee dislocation, which may have spontaneously reduced in the field. Knee dislocations should be suspected in patients with gross instability in multiple directions. Frequently they reduce spontaneously. A high index of suspicion is important because these injuries are often associated with popliteal artery injuries (50 percent incidence) and peroneal nerve injuries. If knee dislocation is suspected, an arteriogram must be performed emergently.

412. The answer is A. *(Chapter 267)* The anterior compartment of the leg is the most common site of compartment syndrome. A tibial fracture is the usual etiology. Other causes include trauma without associated fracture, electrical injury, infectious disease (e.g., myositis), hyperthermia, hypothermia, toxins, snake bite, polymyositis, arterial embolism, seizures, and prolonged immobility that may occur after stroke or drug overdose. A high index of suspicion is important because irreversible muscle damage can occur in 4 to 6 h. Symptoms include pain with passive range of motion, paresthesias, and tense or rock-hard compartments. Poor capillary refill and pulselessness are late findings. The treatment of compartment syndrome is emergency fasciotomy.

413. **The answer is A.** *(Chapter 268)* More than 90 percent of all ankle sprains involve the lateral ligaments. Of lateral ligament injuries, 90 percent involve the anterior talofibular ligament, with 65 percent of these sprains being isolated and 25 percent with concomitant injury to the calcaneofibular ligament. If both the anterior talofibular ligament and the calcaneofibular ligament are disrupted, the anterior drawer sign will be positive.

414. **The answer is C.** *(Chapter 268)* Achilles tendon rupture is often missed by the physician on initial examination, and it may be misdiagnosed as an ankle sprain. Tendon rupture tends to occur with forceful dorsiflexion of the ankle. There is edema of the distal calf and a palpable defect in the tendon 2 to 6 cm proximal to the calcaneus. Thompson's test is positive when the foot fails to plantar flex with calf compression or squeezing. It is diagnostic of Achilles tendon rupture.

415. **The answer is B.** *(Chapter 269)* The patient has a fracture–dislocation of the tarsal–metatarsal joint, known as Lisfranc's joint. A fracture at the base of the second metatarsal is almost pathognomonic of a disrupted joint. Treatment is difficult and may require open reduction and internal fixation. It is important to obtain orthopedic consultation as early as possible.

PEDIATRIC EMERGENCIES

QUESTIONS

DIRECTIONS: Each question below contains five suggested responses. Choose the **one best** response to each question.

416. All of the following suggest that a child with asthma needs to be admitted EXCEPT

(A) persistent respiratory distress after albuterol and glucocorticoid treatments
(B) a peak flow of < 60 percent predicted in a cooperative child
(C) persistent vomiting of medications
(D) underlying bronchopulmonary dysplasia, congenital heart disease, or cystic fibrosis
(E) Sao$_2$ < 95 percent on room air upon arrival

417. A 4-month-old infant presents with a rectal temperature of 38.7°C, a respiration rate (RR) of 60, a heart rate (HR) of 160, and an SpO$_2$ on room air of 92 percent. He is smiling, drooling, and taking his bottle well, despite prominent intercostal retractions. On auscultation, he has diffuse coarse breath sounds with sibilant wheezes at both bases. All other household members have colds. There is no family history of atopy or asthma; no one smokes. ED therapy for this child could include all the following EXCEPT

(A) supplemental O$_2$ (by blow-by or nasal cannula as tolerated by the child)
(B) a trial of nebulized albuterol
(C) a trial of nebulized racemic epinephrine
(D) a dose of glucocorticoids
(E) admission

418. An 18-month-old male is brought to the ED for evaluation of a brief episode of tonic–clonic extremity movements immediately after a spanking in the grocery store. The child reportedly screamed, became limp and pale, fell to the ground, and exhibited the unusual movements. The episode lasted about 1 min and occurred about 30 min before. The toddler is now interactive, appears healthy, and has normal vital signs. What is the MOST likely diagnosis?

(A) Breath-holding spell
(B) Head trauma
(C) Toxic ingestion
(D) Prolonged QT syndrome
(E) Idiopathic (afebrile) seizure of childhood

419. One day after discharge from the normal newborn nursery, a jaundiced infant exhibits fleeting bicycling movements of the limbs, sucking of the lips, and occasional apneic episodes with color change. You interpret these as possible neonatal seizures. Work-up and treatment should include all of the following EXCEPT

(A) evaluation for inborn errors of metabolism (including urine for reducing substances, organic amino acids, serum for lactate, pyruvate, and ammonia)
(B) correction of electrolyte, calcium, magnesium, glucose, and acid–base imbalances
(C) sepsis work-up
(D) administration of diazepam as a first-line drug to control seizures
(E) loading with phenobarbital

420. Which one of the following is the LEAST consistent with a diagnosis of intussusception?

(A) Intermittent colicky abdominal pain, interspersed with symptom-free periods
(B) Grossly normal appearing stool
(C) Normal plain films of the abdomen
(D) Previously healthy 9-year-old child
(E) Altered, lethargic appearance

421. A previously healthy 9-month-old child presents with a soft, nontender abdomen and a history of vomiting at home. Which of the following strongly suggests a non-surgical etiology for the emesis?

(A) No bile present in the emesis
(B) Negative blood in stool by guaiac
(C) Normal KUB and left lateral decubitus film
(D) Soft, nontender belly without masses
(E) None of the above

422. Which of the following is the LEAST consistent with a clinical diagnosis of acute appendicitis?

(A) Normal temperature
(B) Normal white blood cell (WBC) count
(C) Presence of hunger
(D) Vomiting preceding the onset of abdominal pain
(E) Recent gastroenteritis

423. Which of the following groups of pediatric patients are at increased risk for hypoglycemia?

(A) Patients with glycogen storage disease type I
(B) Children younger than 18 months, after a period of fasting
(C) Children who have ingested alcohol but have no clinical signs of intoxication
(D) Children with an abdominal mass
(E) All of the above

424. All of the following are typical of a failure-to-thrive (FTT) baby EXCEPT

(A) alopecia over a flattened occiput
(B) inappropriate wide-eyed, affectionate reaction to strangers
(C) increased muscle tone and scissoring
(D) a relatively larger deviation from the weight curve than predicted by length or head circumference
(E) poor hygiene

425. An 8-year-old female is brought to the ED because of longstanding vague abdominal complaints, with new onset of dysuria. An extensive medical and social history and physical examination (including inspection of the genitourinary area) are unremarkable. The maternal grandmother, who is the patient's guardian, suspects that the child may have been a victim of sexual abuse. Which of the following statements is TRUE?

(A) Because the genitourinary examination is normal, sexual abuse is unlikely
(B) A pelvic examination is necessary to rule out abuse and sexually transmitted diseases (STDs)
(C) Vaginal secretions should be sent for rapid antigens to detect STDs
(D) Syphilis and HIV serologies should be sent
(E) Social service should be called and child protective services (CPS) involved even if the general physical and genitourinary examinations are normal

426. A 3-year-old preschool male presents with a 3-day history of high fever accompanied by sore throat, mild abdominal pain, headache, and vague pain "all over." Examination shows a diffuse erythematous rash, especially in the perianal area. He complains of itching in areas where the rash is peeling. You also note red oral mucosa, prominent papillae consistent with strawberry tongue, and cervical adenopathy. Appropriate actions at this point could include all the following EXCEPT

(A) performing a culture of the throat to rule out group A β-hemolytic strep (GABHS)
(B) treating for presumptive GABHS with oral or intramuscular penicillin
(C) giving intravenous gamma globulin
(D) delaying treatment until you have the results of a complete blood count (CBC) with differential, ESR, and LFTs
(E) administering oral diphenhydramine

427. A 16-month-old child presents with seven watery, nonmucoid, nonbloody stools beginning that day. The mother is not sure when he had his last void because the diaper is always wet with stool. The mother inserted a trimethobenzamide (Tigan) rectal suppository 1 h before. The child seems thirsty but has occasional clear emesis when he takes fluids. Vital signs are remarkable for a rectal temperature of 38.0°C, RR of 30, and pulse of 160, all taken while the child is screaming in triage. He appears vigorous but has a dry mouth and no tears. Appropriate ED management for this child would include all of the following EXCEPT

(A) oral rehydration solution, 5 cc by mouth at a time, every 5 min

(B) intravenous rehydration with 20 to 40 cc/kg LR or NS

(C) oral rehydration at home with clear liquids, followed by the BRATT diet in 24 h

(D) regular milk within the first 24 h

(E) discontinue and discourage use of antiemetic/antimotility agents

428. Which one of the following children with diarrhea requires antibiotics?

(A) A 3-month-old infant whose rectal swab from three nights before grew *Salmonella*

(B) A 10-year-old patient with stool culture positive for *Salmonella* whose bowel movements have decreased in frequency and volume

(C) A 4-year-old patient with sickle cell trait whose stool grew *Salmonella*

(D) A 12-month-old with mild dehydration whose rectal swab from a previous ED evaluation grew *Salmonella*

(E) A 5-year-old patient with moderate bloody diarrhea that began after completing a course of amoxicillin for otitis media

429. An 8-month-old nontoxic infant is brought to the ED with a new rash. Physical examination shows numerous 0.5- to 1.0-cm bullae and red, round, denuded lesions of similar size scattered all over but primarily in the diaper area. Because the child has spent the weekend at the father's house, where many people smoke, the mother is concerned that these may represent cigarette burns. What is the MOST appropriate action?

(A) Apply neomycin ointment to the lesions and call social services

(B) Administer topical mupirocin and local wound care

(C) Give oral cephalexin and local wound cleaning

(D) Admit for intravenous cephalosporin therapy

(E) Perform a Tzanck smear, invoke isolation precautions, and begin acyclovir

430. A 14-month-old irritable but nontoxic toddler presents with several days of upper respiratory infection (URI) symptoms and a rectal temperature of 40.0°C. On examination you do not find a specific source for the fever but note a few urticarial and nonblanching tiny petechiae on the baby's lower abdomen. Which of the following is the MOST appropriate action?

(A) CBC, blood and urine cultures, oral antibiotics, and close outpatient follow-up

(B) CBC, blood and urine cultures, home *without* medications, and follow-up every 24 h pending culture results

(C) Immediate respiratory isolation; CBC; blood, urine, and cerebrospinal fluid (CSF) cultures; intravenous antibiotics; admission

(D) Diphenhydramine for the urticaria, home with follow-up in 24 h or sooner if worse

(E) immediate respiratory isolation; CBC, blood and urine cultures; intravenous antibiotics; admission

431. An 11-month-old patient with no primary care physician is called back to the ED for reevaluation because blood that was drawn the day before as part of a work-up of fever is positive for *N. meningitidis*. The clinical impression at discharge was otitis media, and the patient was treated with amoxicillin and acetaminophen. The patient is now afebrile and playful. What is the MOST appropriate action?

(A) Repeat blood culture, intravenous ceftriaxone, admit

(B) Repeat blood culture, perform lumbar puncture and CSF culture, start intravenous ceftriaxone, admit

(C) Repeat blood culture, intramuscular ceftriaxone, home with follow-up in 24 h

(D) Repeat blood culture, continue oral amoxicillin, follow up in 24 h or sooner if worse

(E) Home after thorough history and physical examination, with reassurance to the parents

432. A 2-week-old vaginally delivered infant with an unremarkable perinatal course presents with a rectal temperature of 38.0°C and reluctance to feed for 1 day. There is no history of URI symptoms, vomiting, diarrhea, or rash. The baby's siblings (aged 13 months and 3 years) have colds, but no one else at home is ill. The infant's only medication is acetaminophen, administered by the mother 3 h before arrival at the ED. What is the MOST appropriate course of action?

(A) Home after blood culture
(B) Home after blood culture, CBC with differential, catheterized urine and urine culture
(C) Admit after blood, catheterized urine, CSF cultures, CBC, urinalysis, and intravenous ampicillin and gentamicin
(D) Admit after blood, urine, and CSF cultures for intravenous ampicillin and ceftriaxone
(E) Home with close follow-up on no medications

433. A 3-week-old infant with a 2-day duration of whitish eye drainage presents to the ED. The child had a normal spontaneous vaginal delivery. The mother reports mild URI symptoms for the past 3 days, but the older siblings (13 months and 3 years) also have colds. The child is eating and acting normally. Which of the following is MOST appropriate?

(A) Fluorescein staining of the cornea; if no dendritic changes, Gram stain and culture of the eye drainage for gonorrhea; if the Gram stain is negative for gram-negative diplococci, obtain a culture of nasopharyngeal aspirate for chlamydia; prescribe oral antibiotics
(B) Fluorescein staining of the cornea; if no dendritic changes, Gram stain for gonorrhea, culture eye drainage for chlamydia and gonorrhea; prescribe topical eye drops
(C) Topical antibiotic eye drops
(D) Treat with hot packs and lacrimal duct massage for presumptive lacrimal duct stenosis
(E) Fluorescein staining of the cornea; if no dendritic changes, topical antibiotic eye drops

434. An unimmunized 5-month-old infant presents with an indurated, red-violet quarter-sized area on the cheek and a fever of 39.5°C of 1 day's duration. He is irritable but consolable and has a supple neck. What is the MOST appropriate action?

(A) Admit after blood cultures, catheterized urine, wound aspirate, lumbar puncture, CBC, and intravenous ceftriaxone
(B) Admit after blood cultures, catheterized urine, wound aspirate, and intravenous ceftriaxone
(C) Home with close follow-up after wound-edge aspirate cultures, intramuscular ceftriaxone
(D) Home with close follow-up after blood cultures and oral amoxicillin
(E) Home with close follow-up after blood cultures and oral amoxicillin-clavulanic acid

435. Risk factors for SIDS include all of the following EXCEPT

(A) sleeping in the supine position
(B) being born to a mother with a substance-abuse problem during pregnancy
(C) prematurity or low birth weight
(D) having a sibling with SIDS
(E) history of a previous apneic episode of life-threatening proportions (ALTE)

436. A 2-week-old infant presents with congestion, mild wheezing, and a history of a "feeling warm." Except for wheezing and mildly increased respiratory effort, the baby has normal vital signs and a normal examination. All the following historical elements would place this child at increased risk for apnea EXCEPT

(A) sluggish feeding and progressive increase in constipation
(B) frequent paroxysms of cough, often followed by emesis, but no color change
(C) 1-week duration of symptoms
(D) 2-day duration of symptoms
(E) premature birth

437. Which of the following is TRUE regarding treatment of a child with diabetic ketoacidosis (DKA)?

(A) Volume replacement is the mainstay of therapy and should be generous and rapid
(B) An initial bolus of 0.1 U/kg insulin must be given before beginning an insulin infusion
(C) The insulin infusion should be discontinued once the patient's glucose has fallen below 200 to 250 mg/dL
(D) Cerebral edema may occur 6 to 8 h into therapy, after apparent clinical improvement
(E) Potassium supplementation is not needed in the child with DKA who is still acidotic, provided the serum potassium is normal

438. A 3-year-old female with hemoglobin sickle cell (HbSS) disease presents with a fever of 38.5°C after several days of URI symptoms, lower leg pain, and abdominal pain in the usual locations of her pain crises. She has scleral icterus and a spleen tip palpable on abdominal examination. The mother is concerned that the patient looks pale. RR is 18, HR is 110, blood pressure is 100/62, and O_2 saturation is at 90 percent. She takes penicillin and folic acid daily. Work-up and treatment should include all of the following EXCEPT

(A) normal saline infusion at twice maintenance levels
(B) CBC with differential, reticulocyte count, blood and urine cultures, CXR, blood for type and screen
(C) presumptive treatment with parenteral antibiotics, active against encapsulated organisms
(D) opioids in adequate doses, at frequent intervals to control the pain
(E) O_2 for hypoxia

439. When evaluating for possible otitis media, which of the following is of the LEAST diagnostic value?

(A) History of a new onset of ear pulling starting several days after URI
(B) Presence of the light reflex
(C) Translucency of the tympanic membrane (TM)
(D) Mobility in response to pneumatoscopy
(E) Fluid level behind the TM

440. During initial evaluation of a 1-month-old distressed infant with URI symptoms, a heart murmur is detected. Which of the following would be LEAST helpful in providing evidence for congenital heart disease?

(A) CXR
(B) Baseline CBC, blood gas, and blood chemistries
(C) Finding of a rounded liver edge 2 cm below the right costal margin
(D) Detecting a holosystolic murmur with radiation to the back
(E) EKG

441. A 1-week-old cyanotic infant presents in shock. History is significant for feeding difficulties and worsening URI symptoms over the past 2 days. The baby is limp, minimally responsive to noxious stimuli, and has an O_2 saturation of 72 percent on room air (with little change after oxygen administration). RR is 60, HR is 200, blood pressure is undetectable, and rectal temperature is 38.0°C. Chest auscultation shows rales but no murmur. What is the BEST course of action?

(A) Oxygen, prostaglandin E_1 titrated to effect, and consultation with a tertiary pediatric institution for possible transfer
(B) Morphine, oxygen, and phenylephrine; place the infant in the knee-to-chest position
(C) A septic work-up and antibiotics; defer lumbar puncture until the baby is stabilized
(D) A and C
(E) B and C

442. What is the MOST common cause of preload disorders in children?

(A) Distributive shock
(B) Hypovolemic shock from vomiting and diarrhea
(C) Congestive heart failure
(D) Severe anemia
(E) Hypoxemia

443. An otherwise healthy 7-week-old baby presents with a rectal temperature of 40.0°C. Thorough physical examination does not show a source for the fever. Which of the following tests is MOST likely to show a source of infection?

(A) Culture of a catheterized urine specimen
(B) Peripheral blood culture
(C) CBC and differential
(D) Culture of the CSF
(E) CXR

444. A nontoxic, playful, 18-month-old toddler is febrile to 40.5°C but has no focus for fever on examination. A 24-h follow-up visit is arranged. Which of the following would be INAPPROPRIATE management?

(A) Blood and urine cultures; intramuscular ceftriaxone
(B) Blood and urine cultures, intramuscular ceftriaxone only if WBC > 15,000
(C) Intramuscular ceftriaxone, no cultures
(D) Blood and urine cultures, no antibiotics
(E) B, C, and D are all inappropriate

445. Which of the following represents INAPPROPRIATE management of fever in children?

(A) Unwrapping the bundled child and retaking the temperature after 15 min

(B) Documenting the temperature accurately by using a tympanic thermometer, especially in infants

(C) Ibuprofen orally in a maximum dose of 40 mg/kg/day divided between 6 and 8 h

(D) Slow cooling by sponging with tepid water

(E) Administration of ibuprofen and acetaminophen simultaneously

446. A 3-month-old male presents with a fever of 39.5°C for several days, occasional vomiting with a few loose watery stools, mild URI symptoms, and a decreased appetite. He is irritable but consolable and appears nontoxic. Which of the following tests would be MOST likely to show the source of this child's fever?

(A) CBC with differential

(B) Blood culture

(C) Urine culture

(D) CSF culture

(E) Chest x-ray

447. Which of the following methods is MOST appropriate for collecting a urine specimen for culture?

(A) Bag specimen in a circumcised infant boy

(B) Suprapubic tap in an infant girl with labial fusion

(C) Catheterization in a circumcised, toilet-trained 3-year-old boy

(D) Catheterization in an uncircumcised, toilet-trained 5-year-old boy

(E) Clean catch in an uncircumcised, toilet-trained 5-year-old boy

448. All of the following statements regarding hyponatremic dehydration in children are TRUE EXCEPT

(A) serum sodium is less than 130 mEq/L

(B) sodium deficit exceeds water deficit

(C) osmolar load is less in the intracellular fluid (ICF) than in the extracellular fluid (ECF) compartment

(D) water shifts from the ECF compartment into the ICF compartment during equilibration

(E) possible sequelae include decreased circulatory volume, cerebral edema, seizures, and coma

449. All of the following statements regarding a child with hypernatremic dehydration are TRUE EXCEPT

(A) there is at least a 10 percent fluid deficit

(B) the skin may appear dry or doughy

(C) muscle tone is increased

(D) the sensorium fluctuates between lethargy and hyperirritability

(E) rapid rehydration is indicated

450. All of the following statements regarding isotonic dehydration in children are TRUE EXCEPT

(A) it is the most common type of dehydration

(B) serum sodium remains within the normal range of 130 to 150 mEq/L

(C) sodium and water deficits are proportionate

(D) calculated fluid deficit should be replaced at a uniform rate over 24 h

(E) initial fluid boluses should be subtracted from the calculated fluid deficit

451. A 1-year-old baby presents with signs of severe dehydration and shock during a severe bout of gastroenteritis. Which of the following is the MOST appropriate fluid therapy?

(A) Isotonic crystalloid bolus of 20 mL/kg

(B) Isotonic crystalloid infusion at 20 mL/kg/h

(C) D_5W 0.45 NS bolus of 20 mL/kg

(D) D_5W 0.45 NS infusion at 20 mL/kg/h

(E) D_5W 0.25 NS infusion at 20 mL/kg/h

452. You are writing admitting orders for a 25-kg toddler who requires observation after a motor vehicle accident. The trauma team requests that you keep her NPO for the first day. What are the 24-h intravenous maintenance fluid requirements for this child?

(A) 1200 mL

(B) 1300 mL

(C) 1400 mL

(D) 1500 mL

(E) 1600 mL

453. A 1-year-old boy presents to the ED with gastroenteritis that is unresponsive to oral rehydration attempts. After physical examination, your assessment is that this 10-kg child has 5 percent dehydration. Which of the following represents the total 24-h fluid requirement?

(A) 1100 mL

(B) 1200 mL

(C) 1300 mL

(D) 1400 mL

(E) 1500 mL

454. All of the following statements are TRUE about moderate dehydration in an infant EXCEPT

(A) the skin has decreased turgor
(B) mucous membranes are dry
(C) tears are diminished
(D) the child is irritable
(E) oliguria, tachycardia, and profound shock are present

455. All of the following statements about hemorrhagic shock and encephalopathy syndrome are TRUE EXCEPT

(A) the etiology is unknown
(B) the prodrome is usually a mild, nonspecific illness
(C) profuse, watery diarrhea progresses to bloody diarrhea
(D) hypoperfusion, seizures, metabolic acidosis, and DIC occur
(E) laboratory abnormalities are limited to acid–base and hematologic dysfunction

456. A 10-year-old female presents to the ED with left upper extremity pain and swelling after a fall onto an outstretched arm 2 h before. She has a tense forearm, moderate swelling at the elbow, and tenderness to palpation of the distal humerus. Passive extension of the fingers elicits pain, and she complains of tingling in the hand. Radial and ulnar pulses are present. What are the MOST appropriate immediate actions?

(A) Splint the arm in flexion and send the patient to x-ray
(B) Splint the arm in flexion, consult orthopedics, and send the patient for x-ray
(C) Splint the arm in flexion, start an intravenous line, obtain immediate x-ray, consult orthopedics, and prepare to reduce the fracture
(D) Splint the arm in extension and send the patient for x-ray
(E) Splint the arm in extension, start an intravenous line, obtain immediate x-ray, consult orthopedics, and prepare to reduce the fracture

457. Regarding supracondylar fractures, which of the following radiographic finding is LEAST likely?

(A) Subtle or nonvisible fracture line
(B) Posterior fat pad sign
(C) Loss of angulation of the anterior capitellum
(D) Imaginary anterior humeral line bisects the anterior capitellum
(E) Imaginary anterior humeral line bisects the posterior two-thirds of the capitellum

458. A 14-year-old male presents with acute onset of inability to walk and severe pain in the left groin, thigh, and knee. He is afebrile and appears nontoxic but is obviously distressed. Examination shows an externally rotated thigh and apparent limb shortening. What is the MOST likely diagnosis?

(A) Legg-Calvé-Perthes disease (coxa plana)
(B) Slipped capital femoral epiphysis (SCFE)
(C) Septic arthritis of the hip
(D) Toxic tenosynovitis of the hip
(E) Osgood-Schlatter's disease

459. Aspirin therapy is used in all of the following conditions EXCEPT

(A) Kawasaki syndrome
(B) polyarticular juvenile rheumatoid arthritis
(C) acute rheumatic fever
(D) Henoch-Schönlein purpura
(E) Kohler disease

460. A 2-year-old male presents to the ED with a 5-day history of a high fever, malaise, and irritability. Vital signs are a HR of 130, blood pressure of 84/44, RR of 24, and temperature of 40°C. Examination shows an alert, uncomfortable-appearing boy, with bilateral non-purulent conjunctivitis, no nuchal rigidity, a strawberry tongue, bilateral enlarged cervical nodes, palmar and plantar erythema, and a polymorphous rash over the trunk. Chest x-ray is normal, as are a lumbar puncture and urinalysis. Blood cultures are sent, and empiric antibiotics are started. Which of the following is the MOST appropriate treatment?

(A) Admit and start aspirin
(B) Admit and start glucocorticoids
(C) Admit and start IVIG
(D) Start aspirin and discharge with next-day follow-up
(E) Start glucocorticoids and aspirin and discharge with next-day follow-up

PEDIATRIC EMERGENCIES

ANSWERS

416. The answer is E. *(Chapter 120)* Misdiagnosis and undertreatment of pediatric asthma occur frequently. The prevalence, severity of disease, and death rate from asthma in pediatric patients has increased significantly during the past 20 years. History of intubation, two or more hospitalizations or three or more ED visits for asthma in the past year, and glucocorticoid dependence or increased use of β agonists are all associated with a higher risk of death. A peak flow of < 60 percent predicted in a patient old enough to cooperate and demonstrate good effort is an objective measure that indicates the child will probably relapse at home if not admitted. Underlying chronic pulmonary or cardiac conditions portend a more complicated course for asthma exacerbations, particularly when associated with some viruses (e.g., respiratory syncytial virus, or RSV). Initial room air oxygen saturation by itself is not a reliable indicator of need for admission.

417. The answer is D. *(Chapter 120)* Despite extensive study, glucocorticoids have not been shown to improve the course of illness in bronchiolitis. However, both nebulized racemic epinephrine and nebulized β_2 agonists are beneficial treatments. Oxygen supplementation is often helpful in decreasing respiratory rate, accessory muscle use, and the general degree of respiratory distress, even when the SpO_2 is within acceptable range on presentation. Fever in bronchiolitic children is a common finding and is frequently associated with otitis media.

418. The answer is A. *(Chapter 121)* A "breath-holding spell" typically occurs after an abrupt trauma (fall, spanking) or a verbal reprimand. It is typified by a sudden cry, followed by prolonged inhalation or exhalation (resulting in no air exchange), and a Valsalva maneuver with vagotonic effects (bradycardia). A brief tonic seizure, not considered to be epileptic, occurs. Head trauma in this child would be an unlikely cause of seizure because the child is neurologically normal. Toxic ingestion is always a consideration in this age of greater mobility, curiosity, and dexterity. However, some aberration in mental status or vital signs would be expected with ingestion severe enough to cause a seizure. Congenital heart disease can produce paroxysmal events at all ages. Pulmonary hypertension, tetralogy of Fallot, acquired cardiomyopathies, and prolonged QT syndrome should be considered. Idiopathic seizures account for up to 47 percent of afebrile seizures in children.

419. The answer is D. *(Chapter 121)* Multifocal, fragmentary seizures are common in newborns. Autonomic seizures can also occur and manifest as variable changes in respiration, temperature, and color. Hypoxia, sepsis, hypoglycemia, and hereditary or acquired metabolic disorders are the most common causes. In the absence of an obvious etiology, newborns should be treated with vitamin B_6, glucose, calcium, and magnesium as indicated. In infants younger than 7 days, phenobarbital is the antiseizure drug of first choice. Phenytoin (or fosphenytoin) is the drug of second choice. Diazepam should be used with caution because of its propensity for respiratory depression and potential to worsen hyperbilirubinemia.

420. The answer is D. *(Chapter 123)* Intermittent colicky pain, occurring about every 20 min, is the typical history for intussusception. Because the child looks and acts completely normal between pain episodes, the diagnosis is often overlooked. The stool commonly appears grossly normal until ischemia progresses and "currant jelly" stools develop. Although a mass effect in the right upper quadrant on x-ray or palpation is suggestive of the diagnosis, up to one-third of plain films are normal. The usual age range for presentation is between 3 months and 6 years. Intussusception should be considered in the differential diagnosis of any child with unexplained altered level of consciousness because up to 10 percent of children present with apathy and lethargy alone.

421. **The answer is E.** *(Chapter 123)* Vomiting is a common problem in childhood, with variable etiology. It can occur with both obstructive and nonobstructive conditions. Although a surgical condition may eventually lead to bilious emesis, at onset vomitus may be simple regurgitation of frothy, nonbilious stomach contents. Bleeding from the gastrointestinal tract may be caused by minor (fissure, milk allergy) or major (intestinal obstruction, gangrenous bowel) problems. Plain films have a low sensitivity for intussusception (normal in up to 30 percent of cases). Masses are infrequently detected during the abdominal examination in children who are later found to have intussusception, malrotation, or even pyloric stenosis. Thus, physical examination alone is not reliable to rule out a surgical condition. Observation may be the best course of action for stable children with an unclear etiology for emesis.

422. **The answer is D.** *(Chapter 123)* The classic progression of symptoms of appendicitis occurs more commonly in older children and adults. Children younger than 2 years often present when the appendix is already perforated because the preceding symptoms are too nonspecific to call attention to the pathology. Lack of anorexia or fever and normal WBC counts are common findings in pediatric patients. Gastroenteritis is often associated with appendicitis, possibly on the basis of an acutely, but secondarily, inflamed appendix. Vomiting more commonly presents *after* the onset of abdominal pain.

423. **The answer is E.** *(Chapter 125)* Nonketotic hypoglycemia is more of a physiologic alteration than true pathology; it usually presents in children younger than 18 months who have had a long fast and do not have adequate gluconeogenic precursors available to keep the blood sugar elevated and the stress hormones in check. It is most often seen on holidays and weekends, when parents sleep late and unintentionally extend the time the child has gone without eating. A child with an abdominal mass may have an enlarged liver, the result of the accumulation of abnormal products of metabolism, such as those seen in glycogen storage disease, fatty acid oxidation, or other metabolic abnormalities. Ethanol ingestion is far more likely to cause hypoglycemia in children than in adults, not only because of the higher glucose utilization in children but also because of the relatively greater effect of ethanol on gluconeogenesis. This is true even when the ethanol levels are too low to cause clinical intoxication.

424. **The answer is B.** *(Chapter 289)* Although FTT babies are usually brought to the ED for evaluation of other conditions, there are many clues that these babies are victims of nonnurturing environments. Poor physical hygiene may be obvious, but other signs may be subtle. These may include occipital flattening and alopecia, a result of the baby remaining unattended in a supine position all day. However, because the American Academy of Pediatrics officially recommends supine positioning in infancy to prevent sudden infant death syndrome (SIDS), more normally nurtured babies have been manifesting this sign. Although these infants may appear to act as if starved for affection, more commonly such babies are apathetic to, and withdrawn from, their environment, appearing to prefer self-stimulatory activities (sucking, self-regurgitation). The lower extremities of FTT infants often exhibit markedly increased tone and scissoring. The weight curve of the neglected but physically normal baby markedly deviates from the curve of the normal baby.

425. **The answer is E.** *(Chapter 289)* The absence of physical signs does not rule out sexual abuse. A speculum pelvic examination is not generally indicated in prepubertal

children, except under anesthesia in the case of severe unexplained vaginal bleeding or for vaginal foreign-body removal. Inspection of the introital area and cultures obtained from the vagina are usually sufficient. Syphilis and HIV serologies are more indicative of baseline status and should only be collected if there is an associated STD, a suspicion of these in the assailant, *and* counseling for the patient to explain the ramifications of positive results of such tests. Currently rapid antigen tests for STDs are not considered reliable in children. All suspected abuse must be reported to CPS.

426. The answer is C. *(Chapter 131)* This child's picture suggests a streptococcal scarlet fever variant. Perianal rash is a prominent feature. If the family is reliable, treatment can be based on results of culture and laboratory tests. If follow-up is a concern, presumptive treatment for GABHS without culture is the more prudent course of action. Treatment is thought to prevent the rare, nonsuppurative sequelae of rheumatic fever and possibly glomerulonephritis. If the patient's presentation were more consistent with Kawasaki's disease (e.g., a more prolonged course of fever), intravenous gamma globulin would be indicated to prevent future development of coronary artery aneurysms. Diphenhydramine provides symptomatic relief from the itchy rashes of both strep and Kawasaki's disease, especially in the peeling phase.

427. The answer is C. *(Chapter 122)* The presence of two of the four physical signs predictive of dehydration (ill appearance, capillary refill > 3 s, dry mucous membranes, and absent tears) suggest this baby to be moderately (≈ 5 percent) dry. Mild dehydration is also shown by tachycardia and relative tachypnea. A trial of oral rehydration solutions consisting of the appropriate osmolality (≈ 300 mOsm/L) and a 2:1 ratio of glucose to Na^+ (millimoles), given in small volumes as frequently as every 5 min is appropriate but very labor intensive. This would be impractical in most ED settings. Intravenous rehydration with normal saline (NS) or LR in volumes of 20 to 40 cc/kg in the ED can be followed by discharge to home with a combination of oral rehydration solution (maximum of 150 cc/kg/day) and regular diet. Commonly recommended soft drinks and the BRATT diet are high in carbohydrates and osmolality and low in nutritive value and should not be used. Antiemetics and antimotility agents should be avoided in children.

428. The answer is A. *(Chapter 122)* Because infants younger than 6 months are at risk for bacteremia, they need antibiotic therapy when stool cultures are positive for *Salmonella*. Lumbar puncture and parenteral antibiotics are advocated by some sources. Patients with hemoglobinopathies are also at risk for the suppurative complications of *Salmonella* infections. Sickle cell trait, however, does not portend increased vulnerability. Neither the 10-year-old nor the 12-month-old child with culture-proven *Salmonella* gastroenteritis needs antibiotic treatment if the symptoms are mild and the child appears nontoxic. The child who develops bloody diarrhea while on antibiotics likely has colitis caused by *Clostridium difficile*; this usually resolves with discontinuation of the antibiotics and possibly the addition of cholestyramine anion-exchange resin to absorb the *C. difficile* toxin.

429. The answer is C. *(Chapter 131)* This child most likely has staphylococcal impetigo. The pathogen produces an epidermolytic toxin that gives rise to different-sized bullous lesions. These are flaccid and thin walled and rupture easily, leaving a moist denuded base that can be mistaken for a cigarette burn. The lesions of bullous impetigo are most often found on the extremities but can be found anywhere. Except in extreme cases, routine hygiene, wound cleaning, and oral antistaphylococcal antibiotics are all that is necessary for treatment. Neomycin ointment is not effective topically. Although mupirocin is effective topically, it is expensive and its use should be restricted to infections covering a limited area.

430. The answer is C. *(Chapter 110)* The presence of petechiae in a febrile child, particularly if the petechiae cannot be attributed as secondary to pressure (e.g., in an extremity, distal to where a tourniquet has been placed), suggests *Neisseria meningitidis* or *Haemophilus influenzae* bacteremia and meningitis. In *N. meningitidis*, the rash may start out urticarial and maculopapular but usually progresses to petechiae or purpura. Children should be placed in respiratory isolation. They need a complete sepsis work-up (to include blood and CSF cultures) followed by prompt administration of broad-spectrum antibiotics and admission. Because of the potential for rapid deterioration in patients with *N. meningitidis* or *H. influenzae* bacteremia, all the other less aggressive choices are inappropriate. Cultures eventually positive for either of these organisms usually require prophylaxis for family members and health-care workers who have had close contact with the child.

431. **The answer is B.** *(Chapter 118)* Even well-appearing children require admission if their blood cultures grow either *H. influenzae* or *N. meningitidis*. Such children are at risk for bacterial sepsis and should receive a complete work-up to include CBC, repeat blood culture, catheterized urinalysis, CSF cultures, and broad-spectrum intravenous antibiotics.

432. **The answer is C.** *(Chapter 118)* Most authorities agree that a rectal temperature of 38.0°C (100.4°F) constitutes a fever during the first few months of life. Such infants may exhibit nonspecific signs and symptoms of sepsis and thus require extensive work-up (CBC with differential, blood cultures, catheterized urine, and CSF) when they present with fever. Otherwise healthy babies older than 4 weeks who present with fever and have a reliable social situation may be discharged home with close follow-up after a negative sepsis work-up. Ceftriaxone should be reserved for infants older than 1 month because it may displace bilirubin from protein-binding sites.

433. **The answer is A.** *(Chapter 117)* In the first month of life, conjunctival infection with *Herpes simplex* and *Neisseria gonorrhoeae* can cause permanent eye damage. A neonate with eye drainage must undergo fluorescein staining of the cornea to assess for dendritic changes and ulcerations, and Gram stain to rule out gram-negative diplococci. The patient in the scenario is exhibiting respiratory symptoms of onset at approximately the same time as the eye drainage. He is in the appropriate age and risk category (vaginal delivery) for chlamydial infection. Nasopharyngeal cultures or scrapings of the palpebral conjunctivae are much more sensitive than culture of the eye drainage itself for chlamydia. Oral (erythromycin), but not topical, antibiotics for 2 to 3 weeks are the most important therapy. Close follow-up is essential.

434. **The answer is A.** *(Chapter 117)* *Staphylococcus aureus*, *Streptococcus pyogenes*, and *H. influenzae*, in decreasing order of importance, are the pathogens most often associated with cellulitis in children. Fever is unusual unless *H. influenzae* is the causative organism. *Haemophilus influenzae* is an important cause for buccal cellulitis in unimmunized children. Because of the organism's invasiveness and the frequent association of unexpected meningitis, these patients need a full sepsis work-up (to include blood, urine, wound, and CSF cultures) and admission for parenteral antibiotics. Afebrile, fully immunized children can usually be treated with antibiotics and followed on an outpatient basis because they are not likely to have *H. influenzae*.

435. **The answer is A.** *(Chapter 114)* The American Academy of Pediatrics recommends that babies sleep in the supine position as protection against an apneic episode. Prematurity, previous ALTE, low birth weight, and a family history of SIDS are all risk factors.

436. **The answer is C.** *(Chapters 112, 114)* Neonates with RSV infection are at risk for central apnea during the first 3 or 4 days of illness. When RSV testing is available in the ED, it can help identify patients who may require admission. Children who have been symptomatic for longer than 4 days tend to do well (unless the work of breathing is such that they tire to the point of apnea). Pertussis in this as yet unimmunized child is a real risk. Although paroxysmal hacking cough is characteristic, infants may have apnea and no "whoop." Botulism may first manifest as constipation and then diminished gag, feeding

problems, weak cry, and decreased muscle tone before ultimately resulting in respiratory arrest. Premature infants are at higher risk for complications from RSV infection.

437. The answer is D. *(Chapter 124)*   Although volume replacement is crucial in treatment of pediatric DKA, deficit correction must proceed cautiously. Cerebral edema is unpredictable and appears late, after the patient is seemingly improved. Rapid fluid replacement and possibly speedy normalization of blood glucose may predispose to cerebral edema. The initial 0.1 U/kg bolus of insulin is no longer recommended before the insulin drip because it may exacerbate preexisting hypokalemia. Insulin infusion may be gradually decreased but should be continued until acidosis has resolved. Glucose should be added to intravenous fluids once levels have fallen to between 200 and 250 mg/dL. Correction of acidosis results in intracellular potassium shifts; osmotic diuresis further promotes potassium loss. Hence, potassium replacement is usually required early in therapy.

438. The answer is A. *(Chapter 133)*   In children with HbSS disease, infection is the most common cause of death; acute splenic sequestration is the second most common cause. Despite penicillin prophylaxis, this febrile child is at risk for infectious complications from encapsulated organisms. Furthermore, a palpable spleen tip is suggestive of sequestration crisis, extremity pain suggests vasoocclusive crisis, and a viral cause of the URI symptoms may have precipitated an aplastic crisis. Prompt administration of antibiotics and a moderate fluid bolus of one-half NS at 1.5 times maintenance are indicated. A chest x-ray to look for pneumonia or early acute chest syndrome should be obtained. The child requires supplemental oxygen to correct hypoxia (up to an O_2 saturation of 95 percent). Oximetry probes should be placed on the ear lobes or nasal bridge because the extremities in vasoocclusive crisis may not provide accurate readings.

439. The answer is B. *(Chapter 116)*   The light reflex can often be visualized in an abnormal ear. Gauging decreased translucency of the TM and evaluating for the presence of a fluid level behind the TM requires experience, but these are good indicators of infection when detected. Mobility in response to pneumatoscopy is also quite sensitive in practiced hands. New-onset ear pulling after URI is frequently associated with otitis media.

440. The answer is B. *(Chapter 115)*   Although blood work is rarely helpful in the acute management of such an infant, improved saturation in response to oxygen may suggest a pulmonary rather than a cardiac problem. Chest x-ray is helpful to assess the size and shape of the heart. Hepatomegaly usually develops late and may be manifested solely by the subtle rounding of the previously sharp liver edge. Although murmurs may occur in up to 30 percent of normal children, these are generally brief, systolic, and without radiation. "Physiologic" murmurs can be loud, but they are not holosystolic. An electrocardiogram (EKG) is useful for the evaluation of cardiac conduction and, indirectly, the heart's chamber size and electrical axis.

441. The answer is D. *(Chapter 115)*   The diagnosis of decompensated congenital heart disease is often difficult in very young infants. Borderline cardiac reserves are suggested by exercise intolerance, which, in this age group, most reproducibly manifest as difficulty in feeding, diaphoresis, increased time to take a bottle, and staccato cough-interrupted feeds. Babies often have been evaluated several times for "URI" symptoms before decompensation occurs. Shunt-dependent lesions start to decompensate when the ductus arteriosus begins to close, at around the second week of life. Prostaglandin E_1 infusions are successful in reopening the ductus arteriosus in a majority of such hemodynamically unstable patients. Although oxygen should always be administered, phenylephrine and the knee-to-chest position (for a presumptive "tet spell") would not be appropriate. Sepsis should always be considered in a baby with unexplained shock, but lumbar puncture should be deferred until the child is stabilized.

442. **The answer is B.** *(Chapter 115)* Preload is the amount of blood that the heart receives to distribute to the body. In addition to heart rate, afterload, and cardiac contractility, preload determines cardiac output. In children, the most common cause of decreased preload is hypovolemia, usually from vomiting and diarrhea. Distributive shock secondary to sepsis, neurogenic spinal shock, or anaphylaxis is a less common cause of preload reduction. Acute anemia may also be associated with decreased preload. Congestive heart failure is a frequent complication in children with congenital heart disease. Increased preload results in elevation of left atrial pressure leading to pulmonary edema and decreased oxygenation. Hypoxemia is a *result* of preload disturbance rather than a primary cause.

443. **The answer is A.** *(Chapter 110)* Urinary tract infections (UTIs) are the most common bacterial infection in this age group. UTIs may not produce any symptoms other than fever, and the urinalysis may be misleadingly normal. A culture of an appropriately collected urine sample (catheterized specimen or suprapubic tap) should be sent. Serious bacterial infections, including bacteremia and meningitis, have an incidence of up to 4 percent in these young infants. Aseptic meningitis may have a slightly higher incidence. Although a CBC may be suggestive of bacteremia (WBC count outside the range of 5000 to 15,000, with more than 7500 bands), it is neither sensitive nor specific. If respiratory signs or symptoms were present, a chest x-ray would be of higher yield.

444. **The answer is E.** *(Chapter 110)* Expectant antibiotic use in febrile children is controversial. Early antibiotic administration diminishes the incidence of bacteremia, and parenteral antibiotics may reduce the incidence of meningitis in bacteremic children. Current recommendations suggest that well-appearing children between 3 and 36 months of age, with no focus of infection and fever higher than 40.0°C, should probably receive antibiotics after cultures are drawn, irrespective of WBC count. A broad-spectrum, third-generation, long-acting cephalosporin is administered parenterally once daily for 48 h until the cultures are negative. In this age group, blood and urine cultures should always be performed, but clinical appearance can guide the need for laryngopharyngeal (LP) and CSF cultures. Children who appear ill on presentation or for whom close follow-up cannot be definitively arranged should be admitted to the hospital for parenteral antibiotics.

445. **The answer is B.** *(Chapter 110)* The aim of reducing fever is to make the child more comfortable and reduce the risk of febrile seizures. Simple unbundling of a warmly dressed baby often results in a decrease in temperature of several degrees after a short period of equilibration. The child should be dressed with similar level of warmth-giving apparel as others in the same ambient temperature. TM thermometers are notoriously unreliable, often underestimating the true degree of fever. Because the extent of a workup is sometimes determined solely by the degree of fever in a young, otherwise well-appearing infant, the temperature must be accurately documented, preferably with a rectal thermometer. Ibuprofen is given in the lower dose range of 5 mg/kg for fever temperatures below 39°C (102.2°F) and in the higher dose range of 10 mg/kg for temperatures above 39°C. The combination of antiinflammatory medications (aspirin or ibuprofen) with acetaminophen results in a more sustained antipyretic effect than either is capable of producing alone.

446. **The answer is C.** *(Chapter 136)* In young febrile infants, the rate of UTI is between 7 and 17 percent. Uncircumcised boys have an approximately three times greater incidence of UTI than girls. The rate of positive blood cultures in febrile infants is about 3 to 5 percent; CSF cultures and chest x-ray are positive much less frequently. The CBC with differential is only a qualitative screening test and is not helpful in determining the cause of fever.

447. **The answer is E.** *(Chapter 136)* In general, any child who is toilet trained and has the appropriate supervision can provide a suitable clean catch urine sample for culture. By 4 years of age, the foreskin can be completely retracted in more than 90 percent of uncircumcised boys. Labial fusion is common in infant girls, especially after a bout of diaper dermatitis. The labia can usually be easily separated by water-soluble surgical lubricant, at which point catheterization can be performed without difficulty. Suprapubic aspiration would only be necessary if labial separation were unsuccessful. Bagged specimens are never appropriate, even in circumcised boys.

448. **The answer is C.** *(Chapter 128)* Hyponatremic dehydration creates a state in which the osmolar load in the ECF compartment is lower than that in the ICF compartment. This occurs when fluid losses have been replaced with hypotonic, low-sodium solutions. The subsequent movement of water from the ECF into the ICF decreases the circulatory volume and causes cerebral edema and central nervous system dysfunction. Seizures and coma can occur when the serum sodium is less than 120 mEq/L or when the sodium level falls rapidly.

449. **The answer is E.** *(Chapter 128)* Signs of hypernatremic dehydration include dry rubbery skin, increased muscle tone, and altered level of consciousness. A hypernatremic child should be rehydrated slowly to avoid a rapid reexpansion of intracellular volume that could lead to cerebral edema. A good guide is to replace the fluid deficit over 48 to 72 h. Serum sodium should not be lowered more than 10 to 15 mEq/L over 24 h.

450. **The answer is D.** *(Chapter 128)* Calculated fluid deficit is replaced over 24 h, but half of the fluid should be administered over the first 8 h and the other half over the next 16 h. A child with mild (5 percent) dehydration has lost 5 percent of body weight in kilograms. This converts to a fluid deficit of 50 mL/kg. With moderate dehydration, the deficit increases to 100 mL/kg. Initial boluses are subtracted from the calculated fluid deficit. After calculating the proportionate rates to replace the deficit, the patient's maintenance fluid schedule must be added. Appropriate rehydration fluids include D_5 0.2 NS or D_5 0.45 NS. Once urine output is established, 40 mEq/L of potassium should be added to the intravenous solution to correct the deficit.

451. **The answer is A.** *(Chapter 128)* Regardless of the type of dehydration, if shock is present, immediate volume replacement is needed. Initially, a 20 mL/kg bolus of isotonic crystalloid (0.9 percent normal saline or lactated Ringer's solution) over 5 to 20 min is indicated. If shock persists on reassessment of the patient's heart rate, skin color, pulses, mental status, and urine output, another 20 mL/kg bolus should be administered. Any baby with change in mental status needs a bedside glucose check.

452. **The answer is E.** *(Chapter 128)* Maintenance fluid requirements are 100 mL/kg for ≤ 10 kg, 1000 mL + 50 mL/kg for 11 to 20 kg, and 1500 + 20 mL/kg for each kilogram over 20. This 25-kg patient requires 1500 mL + 20 mL/kg × 5 kg, or 1600 mL.

453. **The answer is E.** *(Chapter 128)* Maintenance requirements can be calculated by using the formula in answer 452, for a total of 1000 mL for 24 h. A state of 5 percent dehydration represents a fluid deficit of 50 mL/kg or 500 mL in this 10-kg child. Therefore, the total requirement is 1000 mL + 500 mL, or 1500 mL.

454. **The answer is E.** *(Chapter 128)* Children with moderate dehydration manifest compensated shock. Oliguria is present, but the blood pressure is normal. The sensorium ranges from restlessness to irritability. Children with severe dehydration may be hyperirritable or lethargic.

455. **The answer is E.** *(Chapter 126)* Hemorrhagic shock and encephalopathy syndrome occurs from unknown etiology in previously healthy infants after a prodrome of nonspecific illness. Profuse, watery diarrhea becomes bloody and then seizures occur. Laboratory examinations show evidence of multiorgan dysfunction. Renal, hepatic, pancreatic, and myocardial abnormalities are present.

456. **The answer is E.** *(Chapter 132)* This child has clinical evidence of a supracondylar fracture with neurovascular compromise. While preparations are made for immediate reduction, the arm should be splinted in extension to help decrease further movement and soft tissue injury. Intravenous access is needed for titration of analgesic and sedative agents. Radiographs and orthopedic consultation should be obtained expeditiously. The emergency physician should proceed with the reduction if the consultant is not immediately available. If neurovascular integrity is not restored by the reduction or if compartment syndrome is suspected, emergent forearm decompression may be necessary to prevent permanent disability.

457. **The answer is E.** *(Chapter 132)* Supracondylar fractures are the most common type of pediatric elbow fractures. In an intact upper arm, the capitellum angulates anteriorly, and an imaginary anterior humeral line would bisect the posterior two-thirds. If a supracondylar fracture were present, an anterior humeral line would bisect the anterior part of the capitellum. A posterior fat pad, if present, is always abnormal and indicates an elbow effusion. Although the fracture line itself may be subtle, the combination of bisection of the anterior capitellum and a posterior fat pad is highly suggestive of supracondylar fracture.

458. **The answer is B.** *(Chapter 132)* With SCFE, the femoral head subluxes on the femoral neck, with different degrees of displacement. If untreated, avascular necrosis ensues. SCFE risks are multifactorial and include puberty, obesity, trauma, a male-to-female predominance of 8:3, a genetic predisposition, and endocrinologic conditions. The peak incidence is between 12 and 15 years in males and between 10 and 13 years in females. SCFE is more common in blacks than in whites. Patients with SCFE are generally admitted and made non–weight bearing. Definitive orthopedic treatment consists of open reduction and fixation. Legg-Calvé-Perthes disease is characterized by avascular necrosis of the femoral head and a subsequent subchondral stress fracture. A patient with tenosynovitis of the hip may not appear toxic, but a patient with septic arthritis often will. A widened joint space is seen in radiographs of patients with Legg-Calvé-Perthes disease, tenosynovitis, and septic arthritis of the hip. Osgood-Schlatter disease is an inflammatory reaction to trauma to the tibial tuberosity.

459. **The answer is E.** *(Chapter 132)* Kohler disease, an avascular necrosis of the tarsal navicular bone that affects boys four times more frequently than girls, is not treated with aspirin. The etiology is repetitive compressive stress of the tarsal navicular, the last bone to ossify in childhood. Treatment consists of crutches for the first 3 weeks with a short-leg walking cast. Kawasaki syndrome is a systemic vasculitis affecting small and medium-sized arteries. Primary therapy consists of intravenous immunoglobulin (IVIG), with aspirin as an important adjunctive treatment. Polyarticular juvenile rheumatoid arthritis results from an inflammatory response to unknown antigens. Acute rheumatic fever is a systemic, multiorgan inflammatory disease triggered by an antecedent β-hemolytic streptococcal infection. Henoch-Schönlein purpura is a common, small-vessel vasculitis mediated by immune complexes and alternate complement pathways. A polymigratory periarticulitis occurs in most affected children and is treated with aspirin.

460. **The answer is C.** *(Chapter 132)* This patient meets all the major and minor criteria for Kawasaki syndrome. The most ominous complication is coronary aneurysm. In the United States, Kawasaki syndrome affects 3000 to 5000 children per year and is 15 times more common in boys. Treatment with IVIG is key. Adjunctive aspirin therapy is used in anti-inflammatory doses for the first 14 days and then at lower doses for its antiplatelet adhesion effect during the time that children are at risk of coronary thrombosis.

PULMONARY EMERGENCIES

QUESTIONS

DIRECTIONS: Each question below contains five suggested responses. Choose the **one best** response to each question.

461. Which of the following is the MOST common effect of pregnancy on an asthma patient?

(A) An improvement in respiratory function
(B) An exacerbation of asthma symptoms
(C) A decrease in asthma symptoms
(D) A worsening in overall respiratory function
(E) An increase in maternal complications and perinatal mortality

462. Which one of the following pulmonary function tests is the MOST useful at the bedside?

(A) Peak expiratory flow rate (PEFR)
(B) Forced expiratory volume in 1 s (FEV_1)
(C) Forced vital capacity (FVC)
(D) Total lung capacity
(E) Arterial blood gas

463. Which one of the following indicates severe asthma?

(A) Pulsus paradoxus $<$ 20 mm Hg
(B) Pulsus paradoxus $<$ 10 mm Hg
(C) Pulsus paradoxus $>$ 20 mm Hg
(D) Pulsus paradoxus $>$ 10 mm Hg
(E) Pulsus paradoxus $<$ 30 mm Hg

464. All of the following increase the likelihood of the need for hospital admission in an asthma patient EXCEPT

(A) multiple previous admissions
(B) a second ED visit within the preceding 3 days
(C) medication regimen includes systemic steroids at the time of ED presentation
(D) third-trimester pregnancy
(E) history of previous intubation due to asthma

465. All of the following may have a role in the acute management of severe asthma EXCEPT

(A) magnesium
(B) salmeterol
(C) halothane
(D) helium
(E) ketamine

466. β_2-adrenergic medications include all of the following EXCEPT

(A) isoproterenol
(B) metaproterenol sulfate
(C) salmeterol
(D) terbutaline
(E) carbuterol

467. All of the following statements are TRUE regarding aerosolized anticholinergic medications for asthma management EXCEPT

(A) the effect is additive when they are used in combination with β-adrenergic agonists
(B) they affect large central airways
(C) they can cause clinically significant adverse mucous plugging and systemic toxicity
(D) results of studies comparing them with β-adrenergic agonists are conflicting
(E) they may reduce symptoms in patients with chronic obstructive pulmonary disease (COPD)

468. Symptoms heralding respiratory arrest during an asthma exacerbation include all of the following EXCEPT

(A) lethargy
(B) severe respiratory alkalosis and the use of accessory muscles of respiration
(C) a normal pCO_2 on arterial blood gas
(D) a silent chest on auscultation
(E) agitation

469. Strategies for the management of uncomplicated COPD include all of the following EXCEPT

(A) broad-spectrum antibiotics
(B) cromolyn sodium
(C) glucocorticoid therapy
(D) anticholinergics
(E) β-adrenergic agonists

470. Which one of the following is considered the hallmark of COPD?

(A) Exertional dyspnea
(B) Chronic dry cough
(C) Chronic cough productive of yellow sputum accompanied by global diminution of breath sounds
(D) Increased anteroposterior diameter
(E) Pursed-lip exhalation

471. On chest x-ray, an increased anteroposterior diameter, flattened diaphragms, increased parenchymal lucency, and an attenuation of pulmonary vasculature are MOST consistent with which one of the following?

(A) Chronic bronchitic disease
(B) Bronchiectasis
(C) Dominant bronchitic disease in COPD
(D) Emphysema
(E) Pneumonia

472. Which statement about antibiotic therapy is TRUE for COPD patients?

(A) Broad-spectrum antibiotic therapy is indicated to treat tracheobronchitis only when it is mucopurulent
(B) In mild to moderate cases of bronchitis, antibiotic therapy should be started selectively only after sputum culture and sensitivities are available
(C) In mild to moderate cases of bronchitis, broad-spectrum antibiotics can be started before the availability of results of sputum culture and sensitivities
(D) Antibiotic therapy is reserved for the treatment of coexistent pneumonia
(E) Antibiotics are reserved to treat pneumonia and severe cases of bronchitis

473. Which of the following treatments is safe for a patient who is a lung transplant candidate?

(A) Withhold broad-spectrum multiple-drug antibiotic regimens unless fever is higher than 40°C
(B) Intubation
(C) Nonsteroidal antiinflammatory therapy
(D) Glucocorticoids
(E) Blood transfusion

474. A 24-year-old unhelmeted motorcycle rider is declared brain dead 2 days after hitting a truck at freeway speeds. Per his prior expressed wishes, his family wants him to be considered for organ donation. During your night shift, the ICU nurse calls you because he is concerned that the patient's blood pressure is falling. For this patient to be considered an organ donor, all of the following are TRUE EXCEPT

(A) he should receive CMV-negative blood transfusions to maintain a hematocrit of at least 30 percent
(B) central venous pressure must be sustained at > 10 cm H_2O
(C) pO_2 must be > 80 mm Hg, pCO_2 must be 35 to 45 mm Hg, and pH must remain between 7.30 and 7.45
(D) the patient must have a negative chest x-ray
(E) HLA matching must be performed

475. All the following are major side effects of immunosuppressant drugs used in lung transplant patients EXCEPT

(A) hypokalemia
(B) hypertension
(C) bilirubinemia
(D) gastric dysmotility
(E) neurotoxicity

476. Initial ED tests for a patient status post lung transplant could include all of the following EXCEPT

(A) chest x-ray
(B) arterial blood gas
(C) cyclosporine level
(D) azathioprine level
(E) complete blood count (CBC) with differential

477. Which one of the following can cause pancreatitis?

(A) Azathioprine
(B) Prednisone
(C) Cyclosporine
(D) Tacrolimus
(E) All of the above

478. Clinical features consistent with acute rejection in a lung transplant patient include all of the following EXCEPT

(A) bilateral interstitial infiltrates
(B) cough, chest tightness, and fatigue
(C) a rise in temperature of 0.5°C over baseline
(D) a normal chest x-ray
(E) FEV_1 drop of at least 25 percent below baseline over 48 h

479. Cyclosporine levels are affected by all the following EXCEPT

(A) type of laboratory assay
(B) use of nonsteroidal antiinflammatory drugs
(C) length of time since the transplant was performed
(D) use of macrolides and antiepileptics
(E) use of calcium channel blockers

480. Which one of the following has the highest sensitivity for pulmonary embolism?

(A) A high-probability ventilation-perfusion radionuclear scan
(B) A medium-probability ventilation-perfusion radionuclear scan
(C) A low-probability ventilation-perfusion radionuclear scan
(D) Transesophageal echocardiography (TEE)
(E) Dynamic (spiral) computed tomography (CT)

481. Which one of the following $\dot{V}/\dot{Q}$ findings (coupled with the clinical description) is LEAST suggestive of pulmonary embolism?

(A) Multiple matched defects between ventilation and perfusion scans with a low clinical index of suspicion
(B) One moderately sized mismatched defect between ventilation and perfusion scans with a low clinical index of suspicion
(C) Bilateral mismatched defects between ventilation and perfusion scans with a moderate clinical index of suspicion
(D) A low-probability scan with a high clinical index of suspicion
(E) An intermediate-probability scan with a low clinical index of suspicion

482. All of the following statements are TRUE regarding dynamic CT of the chest EXCEPT

(A) a negative study does not rule out pulmonary embolism (PE)
(B) it can detect pneumonia and acute aortic dissection
(C) its specificity is lower than that of a high-probability $\dot{V}/\dot{Q}$ scan
(D) it is most reliable for pulmonary emboli that extend up to the subsegmental level of the pulmonary vessels
(E) it requires the injection of contrast material

483. Which of the following is NOT characteristic of pneumococcal pneumonia?

(A) Acute onset, tachycardia, and tachypnea
(B) Recurrent rigors
(C) Pleuritic chest pain
(D) Thick, rusty sputum
(E) Malaise, flank or back pain, and vomiting

484. Which of the following chest x-ray findings is LEAST consistent with pneumococcal pneumonia?

(A) Single, lobar consolidation
(B) Pleural effusion
(C) Patchy, multilobar involvement
(D) Pneumothorax
(E) Bulging fissure

485. Which of the following is NOT characteristic of *Klebsiella* pneumonia?

(A) Most frequently occurs in alcoholics and patients with diabetes and COPD
(B) Empyema and abscess formation are common complications
(C) Pleuritic chest pain is a common symptom
(D) Sputum is often brown and proteinaceous
(E) Patients usually respond to outpatient antibiotics

486. Which of the following is TRUE regarding *Legionella* pneumonia?

(A) Accounts for less than 2 percent of bacterial pneumonias
(B) Has a higher incidence in the winter and spring
(C) Mode of transmission is through person-to-person contact
(D) Usually resolves without sequelae, even if not treated with antimicrobials
(E) The organism is a gram-negative rod

487. Which of the following is NOT a clinical characteristic of *Legionella* pneumonia?

(A) Toxic appearance
(B) Lack of GI symptoms
(C) Pleuritic chest pain and hemoptysis
(D) Relative bradycardia
(E) Mental status changes

488. Which of the following organisms is associated with multilobar involvement, large pleural effusions, a rapidly progressive course, and a high mortality?

(A) Group A streptococcal pneumonia
(B) Staphylococcal pneumonia
(C) *Haemophilus influenza* pneumonia
(D) *Mycoplasma* pneumonia
(E) Pneumococcal pneumonia

489. Which of the following patient groups is LEAST likely to require admission for pneumonia?

(A) Pregnant patients
(B) Immunocompromised or debilitated patients
(C) Patients toxic in appearance
(D) Patients unable to care for themselves at home
(E) Patients with mild hypoxia on blood gas analysis

490. Which of the following regarding viral pneumonia is FALSE?

(A) Hantavirus has a high associated mortality
(B) Influenza vaccine is generally ineffective in preventing influenza pneumonia
(C) Viral pneumonias often occur as epidemics, but sporadic cases may be seen
(D) Complications include bacterial superinfection, respiratory failure, and bronchiolitis obliterans-organizing pneumonia (BOOP)
(E) Supportive care is the mainstay of treatment

491. Complications of *Mycoplasma* pneumonia infection include all of the following EXCEPT

(A) Guillain-Barré syndrome
(B) aseptic meningitis and encephalitis
(C) hemolytic anemia
(D) pericarditis and myocarditis
(E) septic arthritis

492. What is the MOST common chest x-ray finding seen in patients with *Mycoplasma* pneumonia?

(A) Acute interstitial, patchy infiltrates
(B) Lung abscess
(C) Large pleural effusions
(D) Mediastinal lymphadenopathy
(E) Cavitary lesions

493. Treatment for atypical pneumonia includes all of the following EXCEPT

(A) erythromycin
(B) azithromycin
(C) tetracycline
(D) penicillin and/or cephalosporins
(E) bronchodilators, expectorants, and cough suppressants

494. Which of the following is NOT a chlamydial organism that can cause pneumonia?

(A) *C. trachomatis*
(B) *C. psittaci*
(C) The TWAR agent
(D) Mycoides
(E) All of the above are chlamydial agents that cause pnuemonia

495. Which of the following immunocompromised patients are NOT at increased risk for contracting fungal pneumonia?

(A) Patients with acquired immunodeficiency syndrome (AIDS)
(B) Organ transplant patients
(C) Patients on chronic steroids
(D) Cancer patients
(E) Patients with sickle cell disease or splenectomy

496. Which of the following laboratory values is LEAST consistent with *Pneumocystis carinii* pneumonia (PCP) infection?

(A) Elevated WBC count
(B) Low CD4 count
(C) Elevated LDH and ESR
(D) Marked hypoxia on arterial blood gas
(E) Increased A-a gradient on arterial blood gas

497. Which of the following BEST characterizes the typical chest x-ray findings seen in PCP infection?

(A) Normal chest x-ray
(B) Diffuse bilateral interstitial infiltrates
(C) Hilar lymphadenopathy
(D) Pneumothorax
(E) Pleural effusions

498. What is the method of choice for diagnosing PCP?

(A) Gallium scan
(B) Cytologic sputum analysis
(C) Fiberoptic bronchoscopy
(D) Direct fluorescence of sputum with monoclonal antibodies
(E) Fungal culture

499. What is the drug of choice for the endemic fungal pneumonias (histoplasmosis, Blastomycosis, and coccidioidomycosis)?

(A) Amikacin
(B) Amphotericin B
(C) Rifampin
(D) Pentamidine
(E) Fluoroquinolones

500. The severity of pulmonary injury from aspiration is based on all of the following factors EXCEPT

(A) the presence of bacterial contamination
(B) the pH of the aspirate
(C) the volume of the aspirate
(D) the presence of particulate matter
(E) the position of the patient at the time of aspiration

501. Which of the following are complications of aspiration pneumonia?

(A) Lung abscess
(B) Pulmonary fibrosis
(C) Hemoptysis
(D) Empyema
(E) All of the above

502. Which of the following chest x-ray findings favors lung abscess over empyema?

(A) An air–fluid level at the site of a previous pleural effusion
(B) A cavity with an air–fluid level that tapers at the pleural border
(C) An air–fluid level that crosses a fissure
(D) An air–fluid level that extends to the lateral chest wall
(E) None of the above

503. Which of the following is beneficial if pulmonary aspiration has occurred?

(A) Irrigation of the tracheobronchial tree with neutral or alkaline saline
(B) Steroids
(C) Prophylactic antibiotics
(D) Bronchoscopy
(E) All of the above

504. What is the drug of choice for treatment of uncomplicated lung abscess?

(A) Clindamycin
(B) Ceftriaxone
(C) Gentamicin
(D) Erythromycin
(E) Tetracycline

505. Which of the following groups has a high prevalence of tuberculosis?

(A) Elderly and nursing home patients
(B) Immigrants
(C) HIV-infected patients
(D) Alcoholics and illicit drug users
(E) All of the above

506. Which of the following BEST describes the classic chest x-ray findings in primary tuberculosis?

(A) Parenchymal infiltrates in any area of the lung with unilateral lymphadenopathy
(B) Infiltrate or nodule with calcification
(C) Infiltrates of the upper lobe or superior segment of the lower lobes
(D) Cavitary lesions
(E) Pleural effusion

507. Which of the following is an appropriate initial treatment for pulmonary tuberculosis?

(A) INH
(B) INH plus rifampin
(C) INH, rifampin, and ethambutol
(D) INH, rifampin, ethambutol, and pyrazinamide
(E) INH, rifampin, ethambutol, and streptomycin

508. Risk factors for spontaneous pneumothorax include all of the following EXCEPT

(A) smoking
(B) Marfan's syndrome
(C) female sex
(D) sarcoidosis
(E) COPD

509. Which of the following is the BEST view to request when assessing for the presence of pneumothorax on chest x-ray?

(A) Supine anteroposterior
(B) Upright posteroanterior (PA)
(C) Inspiratory PA
(D) Lateral decubitus with the patient lying on the unaffected side
(E) Expiratory PA

510. What is the BEST position in which to place a patient with massive hemoptysis?

(A) Affected side up
(B) Affected side down
(C) Trendelenburg
(D) Reverse Trendelenburg
(E) None of the above

511. Hypercapnia can result from all of the following EXCEPT

(A) rapid, shallow breathing
(B) increased CO_2 production
(C) small tidal volume
(D) underventilation of the lung
(E) reduced respiratory drive

512. Which of the following is NOT a cause of peripheral cyanosis?

(A) Congestive heart failure
(B) Peripheral vascular disease
(C) Cold exposure
(D) Intracardiac shunting
(E) Arterial or venous obstruction

PULMONARY
EMERGENCIES

ANSWERS

461. **The answer is E.** *(Chapter 64)* The effect of pregnancy on asthma is unpredictable. Respiratory status and asthmatic symptoms can worsen, improve, or remain unchanged. However, maternal complications are slightly increased, and perinatal mortality nearly doubles. Premature births are also more common in asthma patients.

462. **The answer is A.** *(Chapter 64)* Of the listed tests, PEFR is the most helpful at the bedside in an ED. Both PEFR and FEV_1 are useful in assessing the severity of an asthma attack and the adequacy of the response to treatment. However, FEV_1 is difficult to perform at the bedside in an acutely ill patient, and FVC is poorly tolerated because of the need to forcefully exhale the entire vital capacity. Arterial blood gas measurement has limited use, particularly with the advent of pulse oximetry and the emergence of noninvasive $ETCO_2$ monitors. The decision to intubate an asthma patient should be based on clinical grounds, not on blood gas results.

463. **The answer is C.** *(Chapter 64)* A pulsus paradoxus is an accentuation of the decrease in systolic blood pressure that normally occurs during inspiration. A drop in blood pressure of greater than 20 mm Hg (i.e., pulsus paradoxus > 20 mm Hg) indicates excessive negative intrathoracic pressure and correlates with severe asthma. In this situation, left ventricular afterload and venous return to the right heart are increased, thereby causing a transient reduction in cardiac output and systolic blood pressure.

464. **The answer is D.** *(Chapter 64)* All of the listed factors except third-trimester pregnancy increase the likelihood that a patient will require hospitalization. Although oral steroid therapy on ED discharge is common, it is unclear whether it results in a reduction in relapse rate and subsequent need for admission. Systemic steroid dependence at the time of ED presentation increases the likelihood of admission and of death from asthma. Pregnancy increases the risk of maternal complications and perinatal mortality but is not considered a risk factor for hospital admission.

465. **The answer is B.** *(Chapter 64)* Magnesium, halothane, helium (heliox), and ketamine have been advocated for the acute management of severe asthma. They have no role in mild to moderate cases. Salmeterol xinafoate is a β_2-adrenoreceptor agonist with a greater affinity than albuterol. It is used for maintenance therapy in a twice-a-day dosing and should not be used more frequently. Therefore, it has no role in the acute management of asthma.

466. **The answer is A.** *(Chapter 64)* β-adrenergic agonists are the treatment of choice for acute asthma. Isoproterenol is a nonselective β-adrenergic agonist with a short duration of action. The other listed agents have β_2 selectivity. They are the preferred drugs because they have less β_1-specific side effects such as tachycardia.

467. **The answer is C.** *(Chapter 64)* Anticholinergic medications affect large central airways by blocking vasoconstriction induced by vagal innervation (cholinergic mediated).

They can cause adverse reactions such as dry mouth, thirst, irritability, confusion, tachycardia, ileus, blurry vision, and increased intraocular pressure. Fortunately, the advent of an aerosolized form (ipratropium) has minimized these systemic effects and the associated concerns about mucous plugging. Although results of studies comparing anticholinergic medications with β-adrenergic agonists are conflicting, the combination of the two agents has an additive benefit.

468.   The answer is B.   *(Chapter 64)*   Lethargy, exhaustion, agitation, confusion, and the appearance of paradoxical respiration herald respiratory arrest. A silent chest with little wheezing on auscultation, acidosis, and a "normal" or elevated pCO_2 are all worrisome signs and may indicate imminent respiratory failure. Respiratory alkalosis and the use of accessory muscles of respiration are consistent with a severe attack but do not necessarily indicate fatigue and impending ventilatory arrest.

469.   The answer is B.   *(Chapter 65)*   All the listed items except cromolyn sodium are appropriate treatments for COPD. Other therapies include oxygen, mobilization of secretions, adequate respiratory vaccinations, and the treatment of complications. Cromolyn sodium is used prophylactically in asthma patients to prevent mast cell degranulation. It has no role in the treatment of acute asthma attacks.

470.   The answer is A.   *(Chapter 65)*   All the listed clinical features can manifest in COPD. However, exertional dyspnea is considered the hallmark of the disease. COPD should be considered in the differential diagnosis of every patient who presents with a new complaint of dyspnea on exertion.

471.   The answer is D.   *(Chapter 65)*   Disease that is predominantly emphysematous is associated with the described radiographic changes. Chest x-ray findings in COPD differ depending on the predominant clinical features. Dominant chronic bronchitic disease is often associated with subtle findings or a normal chest x-ray.

472.   The answer is C.   *(Chapter 65)*   In mild to moderate cases of bronchitis, broad-spectrum antibiotics can be started before the availability of results of sputum culture and sensitivities. Antibiotics are indicated for mucopurulent or severe tracheobronchitis and cases of coexisting pneumonia. Smokers with bronchitis may also benefit from antibiotics. The trend for treatment of bronchitis in nonsmokers is toward the use of bronchodilators and away from the use of antibiotics. With the emerging threat of antibiotic-resistant bacteria, antibiotic treatment should be reserved for those patients in whom it would be expected to improve clinical outcome.

473.   The answer is C.   *(Chapter 66)*   Nonsteroidal antiinflammatory agents interfere with immunosuppressant drug levels and must be avoided in lung transplant recipients but not in transplant candidates. Pretransplant blood transfusions can lead to antibody formation and increase the risk of acute rejection. Before transfusion, blood must be screened for *Cytomegalovirus* (CMV) to avoid infecting the transplant candidate. Intubation can lead to respiratory muscle deconditioning and nosocomial infections. Noninvasive positive-pressure mask ventilation can help avoid intubation until a suitable organ is available. Broad-spectrum multiple-drug antibiotic regimens are used to prevent the development of pan-resistant chronic infections and should not be withheld based on the degree of fever. Glucocorticoids in large doses can worsen airway healing after a transplant and are contraindicated.

474.   The answer is E.   *(Chapter 66)*   Current time constraints preclude HLA matching between donor and recipient before transplant. Fluids, vasopressors, and CMV-negative blood transfusions should be administered to maintain a blood pressure that is adequate to perfuse the potentially transplantable organs. Accepting transplant centers usually require a negative chest radiograph.

475. The answer is A. *(Chapter 66)* Cyclosporine can cause hyperkalemia and gastric dysmotility. Hyperbilirubinemia, jaundice, and cholestasis have been reported with cyclosporine and azathioprine. However, none of the immunosuppressants used in lung transplant recipients cause hypokalemia. Hypertension is a side effect of cyclosporine and prednisone. Both cyclosporine and tacrolimus can cause neurotoxicity.

476. The answer is D. *(Chapter 66)* Initial ED tests typically include all those listed except for an azathioprine level. Unlike cyclosporine, such a level is not typically measured. Chest x-ray and arterial blood gases are useful in assessing the patient for the most frequent complications: rejection and infection. A CBC can rule out deleterious effects of immnosuppressant drugs on cell counts.

477. The answer is A. *(Chapter 66)* Immunosuppressant drugs have multiple gastrointestinal (GI) side effects. Azathioprine (Immuran) can cause pancreatitis. Cyclosporine and azathioprine can result in gastric atony and cholestasis. Prednisone can cause gastritis and is also implicated in peptic ulcer disease.

478. The answer is E. *(Chapter 66)* Acute rejection is common in lung transplant patients. It should be suspected when the temperature rises 0.5°C over baseline and when FEV_1 decreases by 10 percent or more from baseline over 48 h. Bilateral interstitial infiltrates and a normal chest x-ray are possible (a "radiologically silent" rejection). Cough, chest tightness, and fatigue are frequent presenting symptoms.

479. The answer is B. *(Chapter 66)* Antiinflammatory nonsteroidal drugs should be avoided in lung transplant patients because they react synergistically with cyclosporine and can exacerbate renal insufficiency. They do not, however, affect cyclosporine blood levels. Cyclosporine levels are dependent on the method used by the laboratory and the length of time since the transplant was performed. Toxic levels can result from drugs that inhibit hepatic P450 enzymes such as macrolides, calcium channel blockers, ketoconazole, and cimetidine. Drugs that induce hepatic enzymes such as phenytoin, barbiturates, and rifampin could precipitate rejection.

480. The answer is E. *(Chapter 67)* The sensitivity of spiral CT for pulmonary embolism has been reported at 86 to 91 percent. It exceeds that of $\dot{V}/\dot{Q}$ scans and TEE. Its specificity is nearly as good as that of a high-probability $\dot{V}/\dot{Q}$ scan. High- and medium-probability $\dot{V}/\dot{Q}$ scans have a higher specificity than low-probability scans. Their sensitivity however, is significantly lower than that of dynamic CT.

481. The answer is A. *(Chapter 67)* Results of $\dot{V}/\dot{Q}$ scanning must be used in conjunction with pretest probability (clinical suspicion) to assess the likelihood of pulmonary embolism. A mismatched defect between ventilation and perfusion scans is most consistent with a pulmonary embolism, and the scan would be read as moderate or high probability. Bilateral mismatched defects between ventilation and perfusion scans suggest a high probability of recurrent pulmonary emboli. Many pulmonary diseases can cause ventilation and perfusion abnormalities. These include COPD, pneumonia, and chronic fibrosis. The $\dot{V}/\dot{Q}$ scan is "low probability" when matched, but no unmatched, defects are present. There is only about a 4 percent incidence of pulmonary embolism if a low-probability $\dot{V}/\dot{Q}$ scan is coupled with a low clinical suspicion.

482. The answer is C. *(Chapter 67)* The specificity of dynamic CT for PE is high (78–95 percent) and comparable to that of a high-probability $\dot{V}/\dot{Q}$ scan (88 percent). Because $\dot{V}/\dot{Q}$ scans are read as "high probability" less than 20 percent of the time, the overall specificity of dynamic CT for PE is higher than that for $\dot{V}/\dot{Q}$. The sensitivity of dynamic CT for PE is greater than or equal to 90 percent and is most reliable for emboli that extend to the segmental divisions of the pulmonary vessels. Spiral CT has an advantage over $\dot{V}/\dot{Q}$ scan in that it can also detect pneumonia, aortic dissection, tumors, and effusions.

However, a negative spiral CT does not rule out PE. Magnetic resonance imaging can detect pulmonary emboli with a sensitivity of about 70 percent and a specificity similar to that of spiral CT.

483. The answer is B. *(Chapter 59)* Pneumococcal pneumonia is the most common community-acquired pneumonia, with peak incidence in the winter and spring. It is characterized by acute onset, with associated symptoms that include fever, tachycardia, tachypnea, pleuritic chest pain, malaise, back or flank pain, and vomiting. Cough is a common symptom and usually productive of rusty, thick sputum. A single rigor lasting minutes is common, but recurrent rigors suggest another diagnosis.

484. The answer is D. *(Chapter 59)* Pneumococcal pneumonia typically presents with single lobe involvement, most often the right middle, right lower, and the left lower lobes. Occasionally, patchy involvement can occur, particularly in the elderly and in infants. Pleural effusions occur in about 10 percent of cases, and the effusion is generally small. As in *Klebsiella* pneumonia, a bulging fissure can be seen. A pneumothorax is uncommon and suggests another diagnosis, such as *Staphylococcus aureus* or *Pneumocystis carinii* pneumonia. However, chest x-ray findings must be considered in the context of clinical presentation. Blood cultures are now thought to be more useful in identifying the causative organism of pneumonia than either chest x-ray or sputum Gram stain.

485. The answer is E. *(Chapter 59)* *Klebsiella* pneumonia is most commonly found in alcoholics and patients with diabetes and COPD. It is usually a lobar (right upper lobe), necrotizing pneumonia, often with empyema and abscess formation. Patients are generally toxic on presentation, with rigors, shortness of breath, cyanosis, and pleuritic chest pain. Sputum is often thick and currant-jelly like and can result in airway compromise. Admission is recommended for treatment with intravenous aminoglycosides and cephalosporins.

486. The answer is E. *(Chapter 59)* *Legionella* is a gram-negative rod accounting for up to 6 percent of all bacterial pneumonias. It occurs sporadically, with peak incidence in the summer and fall. Transmission is usually airborne through heat-exchange units, air conditioners, respiratory therapy devices, whirlpools, and cooling devices. Individuals at risk are males with a history of alcoholism, diabetics, patients with COPD, smokers, postsurgical patients, immunocompromised hosts, and people who work near construction or excavation sites. Mortality approaches 75 percent without early treatment.

487. The answer is B. *(Chapter 59)* Patients with *Legionella* pneumonia appear toxic. Fever, chills, malaise, and headache are common clinical features. More than half of patients exhibit GI symptoms, including nausea, vomiting, and diarrhea. Pleuritic chest pain is common, and a relative bradycardia may also be seen. Patients often present with mental status changes ranging from confusion to coma.

488. The answer is A. *(Chapter 59)* Group A streptococcal pneumonia is rapidly progressive and has a high mortality rate. Clinically, patients appear toxic with sudden onset of fevers and chills, a productive cough, and pleuritic chest pain. Pulmonary examination ranges from fine crackles to focal consolidation. Chest x-ray often shows multilobar involvement, with large pleural effusions. Sputum is usually bloody and purulent. Treatment includes intravenous fluids and antibiotics. Penicillin is the antimicrobial treatment of choice. A high index of suspicion must be maintained to diagnose this rare cause of pneumonitis.

489. The answer is E. *(Chapter 59)* Patients requiring admission include those at the extremes of age, immunocompromised or debilitated patients, and those who are unable to care for themselves. Anyone toxic on presentation, with a significantly elevated respiratory rate, moderate to severe hypoxemia (pO_2 60–70 mm Hg), or evidence of cardiovascular instability should also be admitted. Pneumonia and pregnancy carries an increased risk of mortality to both the mother and the fetus, especially if the woman is infected with varicella pnuemonia.

490. **The answer is B.** *(Chapter 59)* Viral pneumonia is common and clinically manifests as anything from self-limited disease to a life-threatening condition. Epidemics are common, but sporadic cases may occur. Complications include superinfection with bacteria, respiratory failure, and BOOP. Hantavirus, which is primarily seen in the southwestern United States, can be associated with hemorrhagic fever and confers a mortality of up to 70 percent. Management of viral pneumonia consists of supportive care, with bed rest, fluids, analgesics, and expectorants. The influenza vaccine is usually effective against influenza A and B viruses. It is recommended for patients with cystic fibrosis, COPD, the elderly, and health-care workers.

491. **The answer is E.** *(Chapter 59)* Most patients with mycoplasma pneumonia have a self-limited course. However, pulmonary complications include hypoxemia, respiratory distress syndrome, pneumothorax, pleural effusion, and lung abscess. Extrapulmonary manifestations include aseptic meningitis and encephalitis, Guillain-Barré syndrome, hemolytic anemia complicated by renal failure, and disseminated intravascular coagulation. Cardiac manifestations include pericarditis and myocarditis, congestive heart failure, and dysrhythmias. Septic arthritis is not a common complication of mycoplasma infection.

492. **The answer is A.** *(Chapter 59)* Mycoplasma pneumonia is characterized by patchy densities to dense consolidation involving an entire lobe of the lung. An acute interstitial pattern (similar in appearance to adult respiratory distress syndrome) can also be seen and lead to significant functional impairment. Cavitary lesions, lung abscesses, large pleural effusions, mediastinal lymphadenopathy, and atelectasis are also seen but less commonly. Their presence suggests bacterial infection or another diagnosis.

493. **The answer is D.** *(Chapter 59)* Erythromycin is the drug of choice for atypical pneumonias, including *Mycoplasma* and chlamydial infection. Newer-generation macrolides, doxycycline, and tetracycline are also effective. Because these organisms lack a cell wall, penicillin and cephalosporins are ineffective. Treatment with bronchodilators, expectorants, and cough suppressants provides symptomatic relief.

494. **The answer is D.** *(Chapter 59)* The three groups of chlamydial organisms that cause pneumonia are *C. trachomatis*, *C. psittaci*, and the TWAR agent. Infected patients experience a prodrome of upper respiratory infection, followed by chest pain and cough with mucoid sputum production. Pulmonary examination can range from fine crackles to focal consolidation. Treatment consists of either a macrolide or tetracycline. Mycoides is not a chlamydial organism.

495. **The answer is E.** *(Chapter 59)* Patients with T-cell defects (lymphoma, AIDS, steroid-dependent patients, cancer and chemotherapy patients, and organ transplant patients on immunosuppressive drugs) and granulocyte defects (neutropenia, leukemia, steroid dependence, and cancer patients undergoing chemotherapy) are prone to bacterial and fungal infections. Patients with sickle cell anemia or status post splenectomy are also prone to bacterial illness (particularly with encapsulated organisms) but not to fungal pneumonias.

496. **The answer is A.** *(Chapter 59)* Although leukopenia, anemia, or thrombocytopenia secondary to drug therapy may be present, the total WBC count is typically normal in patients with PCP. CD4 counts are almost invariably reduced; most PCP infections occur in patients with CD4 counts less than 200. Elevated LDH and ESR are common but are relatively nonspecific findings. Severe hypoxemia is a frequent complication. A pO_2 of less than 70 portends a worse prognosis. The A-a gradient is also increased, and this increase can be accentuated through mild exercise.

497. **The answer is B.** *(Chapter 59)*   The chest radiograph is abnormal in up to 90 percent of patients with significant PCP infection. The classic chest x-ray pattern is diffuse bilateral interstitial infiltrates in the "bat wing" distribution. PCP can also present as asymmetrical infiltrates, with a cavitary or cystic appearance. Unilateral or bilateral pneumothoraces, bronchopleural fistulas, hilar lymphadenopathy, and pleural effusions can also be seen but are less common. A normal chest x-ray, as seen in 10 to 20 percent of cases, does not rule out PCP.

498. **The answer is C.** *(Chapter 139)*   Fiberoptic bronchoscopy is the method of choice for diagnosing PCP. The combination of transbronchial biopsy, bronchial washings, and bronchoalveolar lavage has a diagnostic yield of nearly 100 percent. Gallium scans have a sensitivity of 90 to 98 percent but a low specificity. Cytologic sputum yields are inconsistent, with a negative predictive value of only about 50 percent. Direct flourescent antibodies have a sensitivity of nearly 90 percent.

499. **The answer is B.** *(Chapter 66)*   Amphotericin B is the drug of choice for the endemic fungal pneumonias. Ketoconazole is also effective. Amikacin is used for the treatment of *Mycobacterium avium* complex, rifampin for tuberculosis, and pentamidine for PCP pneumonia. Fluoroquinolones are not effective in this setting.

500. **The answer is E.** *(Chapter 60)*   Clinical outcome after pulmonary aspiration depends on the pH and volume of the aspirate. A pH of less than 2.5 and a large volume cause more severe injury. The presence of particulate matter can result in persistent inflammatory changes and hemorrhagic pneumonitis and form a chronic granulomatous reaction. Bacterial contamination is another complicating factor, particularly if *Pseudomonas*, *Proteus*, *Escherichia coli*, or anaerobes are involved. The position of the patient at the time of aspiration does not affect the severity of injury.

501. **The answer is E.** *(Chapter 60)*   Acutely, respiratory failure is the most serious complication of aspiration pneumonia. Chronic sequelae include lung abscess, pulmonary fibrosis, and empyema. Mortality is high, ranging from 40 to 70 percent when the aspirate pH is low. Grossly contaminated aspirate, as seen with aspiration in the setting of bowel obstruction, carries a mortality approaching 100 percent.

502. **The answer is E.** *(Chapter 60)*   All of the listed findings favor empyema over lung abscess. The chest x-ray of a patient with lung abscess demonstrates a cavity, usually with an air–fluid level. The most common sites for aspiration-induced abscesses are the posterior segment of the right upper lobe and the superior segments of the right and left lower lobes. Lung abscess secondary to parenchymal disease, carcinoma, opportunistic infection, or septicemia can occur anywhere in the lung.

503. **The answer is D.** *(Chapter 60)*   Bronchoscopy is indicated for removing large particles and clearing the airway after aspiration. The tracheobronchial tree should not be irrigated because this can push the aspirate deeper into the lungs and result in increased mortality. Steroids and prophylactic antibiotics have no value and should not be administered.

504. **The answer is A.** *(Chapter 60)*   The drug of choice for an uncomplicated lung abscess is clindamycin, 600 mg IVPB, every 6 h until the patient has been afebrile for 5 days. Patients should be continued on oral clindamycin for 6 to 8 weeks thereafter. Penicillin, metronidazole, and cefoxitin are reasonable alternatives. Bronchoscopy evaluates for tumor or foreign body and is useful to obtain material for culture.

505. **The answer is E.** *(Chapter 61)*   All of the listed patient groups have a high prevalence of tuberculosis. Other high-risk groups include residents and staff of homeless shelters and prisons. Tuberculosis is the leading cause of death from a single infectious agent. Rates of infection are increasing, mostly from multi–drug-resistant strains.

506. The answer is A. *(Chapter 61)* The chest x-ray for patients with primary tuberculosis classically shows parenchymal infiltrates with unilateral lymphadenopathy. Calcification, when present, is a late finding. Reactivation tuberculosis infections usually involve the upper lobes or the superior segment of the lower lobes. Other findings can include a miliary pattern, pleural effusion (usually unilateral), atelectasis, and pulmonary fibrosis. Because tuberculosis can present as any abnormality on chest x-ray, comparison should be made with previous films, if available.

507. The answer is D. *(Chapter 61)* With the increased incidence of multi–drug-resistant tuberculosis, the CDC currently recommends four-drug therapy until susceptibility tests are available. Beginning therapy should include isoniazid, rifampin, pyrazinamide and either ethambutol or streptomycin for 2 months. Patients should be treated for at least 6 months (9 months if HIV infection coexists).

508. The answer is C. *(Chapter 62)* Patients who are smokers, male, between the ages of 20 and 40 years, and have a higher height-to-weight ratio are at increased risk for developing spontaneous pneumothoraces. In addition, Valsalva maneuvers (such as can occur with smoking marijuana or cocaine), underlying pulmonary disease (such as COPD and sarcoidosis), and Marfan's and Ehler-Danlos syndromes are risk factors.

509. The answer is E. *(Chapter 62)* The size of the hemithorax decreases with expiration, which makes a pneumothorax more likely to be visible on an expiratory film or a lateral decubitus film with the patient lying on the affected side. Comparing inspiratory and expiratory views can help to distinguish a pneumothorax from skin folds and other artifacts.

510. The answer is B. *(Chapter 63)* The optimal positioning for patients with massive hemoptysis is with the bleeding lung down. This minimizes contamination of blood from the affected to the unaffected lung and helps prevent compromise of oxygenation and ventilation. Tracheal intubation is indicated if there is respiratory failure or the patient is unable to clear blood from the airway.

511. The answer is B. *(Chapter 58)* Hypercapnia results from alveolar hypoventilation and is arbitrarily defined as a pCO_2 of greater than 45 mm Hg. It can result from a variety of causes, including rapid shallow breathing, underventilation, small tidal volumes, and a blunted respiratory drive. An increase in the anatomical dead space can also lead to a decrease in alveolar ventilation. With severe hypercapnia, seizures, coma, and cardiovascular collapse can occur. In contrast to acute hypercapnia, chronic hypercapnia can be well tolerated, even with a pCO_2 greater than 80 mm Hg.

512. The answer is D. *(Chapter 58)* Cyanosis, a bluish discoloration of the skin, results from an increased amount of reduced hemoglobin, usually > 5 g in 100 mL capillary blood. Central cyanosis can be seen in conditions that are characterized by unsaturated arterial blood or abnormal hemoglobin. Peripheral cyanosis is secondary to the slowing of blood to an area or an abnormally great extraction of oxygen from normally saturated arterial blood. All of the listed conditions except intracardiac shunting may lead to peripheral cyanosis.

RENAL AND UROLOGIC EMERGENCIES

QUESTIONS

DIRECTIONS: Each question below contains five suggested responses. Choose the **one best** response to each question.

513. A 60-year-old male with history of benign prostatic hypertrophy presents complaining of nausea and vomiting. Laboratory values include serum Na of 145 mmol/L, blood urea nitrogen (BUN) of 45 mg/dL, creatinine of 2.0 mg/dL, urine Na of 10, and urine creatinine of 80. Which of the following is the MOST likely diagnosis?

    (A) Prerenal failure
    (B) Acute tubular necrosis (ATN)
    (C) Glomerulonephritis
    (D) Postrenal failure
    (E) Pyelonephritis

514. All of the following can cause acute renal failure (ARF) EXCEPT

    (A) rhabdomyolysis
    (B) nonsteroidal antiinflammatory drugs (NSAIDS)
    (C) ethylene glycol
    (D) penicillin
    (E) iron

515. Which of the following patients with pyelonephritis can be safely treated as an outpatient?

    (A) A 75-year-old diabetic female
    (B) A 20-year-old 20-week pregnant female with mild abdominal cramping
    (C) A 30-year-old female with persistent vomiting and fever
    (D) A 33-year-old male with renal calculi
    (E) None of the above can be safely treated as outpatients

516. Which of the following is NOT an appropriate treatment for priapism?

    (A) Terbutaline 0.25 mg administered subcutaneously in the deltoid
    (B) Aspiration of corporeal blood
    (C) Ice-water enema
    (D) Neo-Synephrine instillation into the corpora cavernosa
    (E) Exchange transfusion

517. A 19-year-old male complains of acute onset of scrotal pain. Which of the following procedures is LEAST indicated?

    (A) Treat with cefixime and azithromycin and discharge home
    (B) Radionulide scan of the testes
    (C) Attempt manual detorsion
    (D) Urinalysis
    (E) Doppler ultrasound

518. Renal transplant patients should receive all of the following measures to prevent infection EXCEPT

    (A) measles, mumps, rubella (MMR) vaccine
    (B) nystatin
    (C) pneumococcal vaccine
    (D) hepatitis B vaccine
    (E) prophylaxis for dental procedures

519. A chronic renal dialysis patient is brought to the ED in cardiac arrest. The MOST likely cause is

    (A) pericardial effusion
    (B) hyperkalemia
    (C) hypocalcemia
    (D) malignant hypertension
    (E) postdialysis hypotension

520. Patients with renal stones should be admitted in all of the following cases EXCEPT

(A) associated urinary tract infection
(B) single kidney with obstruction
(C) uncontrolled pain
(D) stone > 6 mm
(E) all of the above

521. A 22-year-old previously healthy male complains of dysuria. Genital examination is normal. Urinalysis shows 5 to 10 white blood cells per high power field. Which of the following antibiotic regimens is MOST appropriate?

(A) Ciprofloxacin, 500 mg orally twice a day for 2 weeks
(B) Trimethoprim-sulfamethoxazole, two tablets orally twice a day for 3 days
(C) Azithromycin, 1 g orally once, and ofloxacin, 400 mg orally once
(D) Cephfalexin, 500 mg orally for 7 days
(E) Ciprofloxacin, 500 mg orally once

522. Which of the following is NOT a common cause of hematuria?

(A) Urinary tract infection (UTI)
(B) Rapidly progressing glomerulonephritis
(C) Renal stone
(D) Cancer
(E) HIV nephropathy

523. Which of the following structures needs to be repaired in a fractured penis?

(A) Tunica albuginea
(B) Corpus spongiosum
(C) Corpora cavernosum
(D) Buck's fascia
(E) Urethra

524. All of the following substances cause urinary retention EXCEPT

(A) methamphetamines
(B) ephedrine
(C) cogentin
(D) β-blockers
(E) tricyclic antidepressants

525. All of the following are causes of postrenal failure EXCEPT

(A) bladder tumor
(B) phimosis
(C) neurogenic bladder
(D) urethral prolapse
(E) retroperitoneal fibrosis

526. Which of the following is the MOST appropriate treatment for a patient with chronic renal failure and a clotted hemodialysis shunt?

(A) Irrigate with heparinized saline
(B) Angiogram to delineate the lesion
(C) Consult a vascular surgeon
(D) Give systemic urokinase 100,000 U
(E) Initiate broad spectrum antibiotics

527. What percentage of urological stones are radiopaque?

(A) 15
(B) 30
(C) 50
(D) 75
(E) 90

528. What is the MOST common causative organism for uncomplicated UTI?

(A) *Chlamydia trachomatis*
(B) *Klebsiella*
(C) *Proteus* species
(D) *Escherichia coli*
(E) *Staphylococcus saprophyticus*

529. All of the following are risk factors for UTI EXCEPT

(A) sexual intercourse
(B) uterine prolapse
(C) use of diaphragm and spermacide
(D) irregular menses
(E) lack of estrogen in postmenopausal women

530. Which of the following statements regarding infection in patients with continuous ambulatory peritoneal dialysis (CAPD) is TRUE?

(A) Gram-negative bacteria are responsible for most cases of CAPD peritonitis
(B) Confirmed peritonitis in a CAPD patient requires admission for parenteral antibiotics
(C) Cell count in cases of peritonitis is at least 250 leukocytes
(D) Infection is the most frequent complication of CAPD
(E) The peritoneal catheter should be changed at the first sign of peritonitis

RENAL AND UROLOGIC EMERGENCIES

ANSWERS

513. The answer is A. *(Chapter 88)* Fractional excretion of sodium [FENa(%)] is used in determining the cause of renal failure. FENa(%) = (urine sodium/serum sodium)/(urine creatinine/serum creatinine) × 100. The following table illustrates the laboratory findings in the different types of renal failure. Pyelonephritis should not cause renal failure.

	Prerenal	Intrinsic renal	Postrenal
FENa(%)	< 1	> 2	> 2
Urine Na	< 20	> 40	> 40
Serum BUN:Cr	> 20:1	10:1	< 10:1
Urine:serum Cr ratio	> 40:1	< 20:1	< 20:1

514. The answer is E. *(Chapter 88)* Myoglobinuria from rhabdomyolysis can cause acute tubular necrosis. NSAIDs cause preferential reduction in renal blood flow, leading to renal failure from hypoperfusion. Ethylene glycol can cause intraparenchymal obstruction in the kidneys, leading to ARF. Penicillin is a cause of allergic interstitial nephritis. Iron does not usually have renal toxicity.

515. The answer is E. *(Chapter 90)* Young, otherwise healthy, women with uncomplicated acute pyelonephritis may be treated as outpatients. Patients with comorbid diseases, immunosupression, most pregnant women, and patients with unremitting fever or inability to tolerate oral fluids or medications should be admitted. Other risk factors for worse prognosis include old age, diabetes, renal calculi, urinary obstruction, recent hospitalization or instrumentation, and sickle cell anemia. These groups of patients should also be treated as inpatients with parenteral antibiotics.

516. The answer is C. *(Chapter 91)* Priapism is a painful, pathologic erection secondary to engorgement of the corpora cavernosa but not the glans or corpus spongiosum. There are multiple etiologies for priapism including sickle cell anemia, medications, spinal cord injury, leukemic infiltration, and idiopathic. Neither sedation nor ice-water enema is effective in reducing the erection. Shunt surgery is necessary in some cases.

517. The answer is A. *(Chapter 91)* Testicular torsion is a urologic emergency. It can be difficult to distinguish clinically from torsion of the appendix testis or epididymitis. Urologic consultation for operative exploration should be obtained immediately when testicular torsion is suspected. Radionuclide scans and Doppler ultrasound studies can help confirm the diagnosis, but these are time consuming in a condition for which even a short delay could mean loss of the testicle. Manual detorsion can be attempted in the ED while awaiting surgical consultation.

518. The answer is A. *(Chapter 96)* Renal transplant patients are treated with immunosuppressive agents to prevent graft rejection. Important measures to prevent infection in these patients include pneumococcal vaccine, hepatitis B vaccine, trimethoprim-sulfa prophylaxis for *Pneumocystis carinii* pneumonia, and nystatin to prevent oral candida. MMR vaccine is an attenuated live vaccine and is potentially virulent in immunosuppressed patients. *Cytomegalovirus* is the most common infectious agent in transplant patients and may be suppressed with gancylcovir.

519.   **The answer is B.** *(Chapter 89)*   Although all of these choices can lead to cardiac arrest in chronic dialysis patients, hyperkalemia is the most common cause. Treatment should start with intravenous calcium gluconate and then continue with dextrose and insulin and with sodium bicarbonate. Other electrolyte disturbances seen in uremic patients include hypokalemia, hypocalcemia, and hypermagnesemia.

520.   **The answer is E.** *(Chapter 92)*   Renal colic patients with any of these features should be hospitalized for management and urologic consultation. Patients with renal insufficiency, severe underlying disease, or evidence of complete obstruction should be considered for admission and discussed with a urologist. Uncomplicated patients whose pain can be controlled with oral medications may be discharged home with a urine strainer and close follow-up with a urologist.

521.   **The answer is C.** *(Chapter 90)*   Men younger than 35 to 40 years with urinary tract signs and symptoms should be evaluated and treated presumptively for sexually transmitted urethritis. Cultures for *Chlamydia* and gonorrhea should be sent and empiric treatment for both administered. Appropriate treatment includes coverage of *Chlamydia* with doxycycline, 100 mg orally for 1 week, or a single dose of 1 g azithromycin. Gonorrhea can be treated with a single dose of ceftriaxone 250 mg intramuscularly, a single dose of cefixime 400 mg orally, ofloxacin 400 mg orally, or ciprofloxacin 500 mg orally. Ciprofloxacin, 500 mg twice a day for 2 weeks, is appropriate treatment for pyelonephritis, and trimethoprim-sulfamethoxazole will treat uncomplicated urinary tract infection in young women. The patient should be advised to have his sexual partners checked and to use condoms.

522.   **The answer is E.** *(Chapter 93)*   HIV nephropathy causes protein wasting in the urine. All the other choices are included in the broad differential diagnosis for hematuria. Trauma, instrumentation, bladder stones, and sickle cell anemia may also result in hematuria. The patient's age, history, and urinalysis results help to determine etiology. For example, bacteria and white blood cells are seen with infection. Red cell casts are found in rapidly progressive glomerulonephritis (usually associated with acute renal failure). Cancer is more likely in older smokers presenting with painless hematuria.

523.   **The answer is A.** *(Chapter 91)*   Tear of the penile tunica albuginea, the thick fascial layer around the corpora cavernosa, can occur during sexual intercourse or other sexual activity. The urethra is rarely injured, but a retrograde urethrogram may be necessary for full evaluation. The tunica albuginea should be surgically repaired. Buck's fascia is a thin layer of fascia encasing both the corpora cavernosa and the corpus spongiosum.

524.   **The answer is D.** *(Chapter 91)*   Urinary retention is frequently caused or exacerbated by pharmaceutical agents. Some of the most commonly implicated medications include antihistamines, anticholinergics, and antispasmodic agents. Sympathomimetics may cause urinary retention through their α-adrenergic stimulation. β-blockers can cause erectile dysfunction but do not contribute to urinary retention.

525.   **The answer is D.** *(Chapter 88)*   Postrenal failure can be caused by obstruction anywhere along the urinary tract, from the kidney and the ureters (usually bilateral involvement) to the bladder and the urethra. Bladder neck obstruction may result from neurogenic bladder or medications. Prostatic hypertrophy and functional bladder neck obstruction are the most common causes of postrenal failure. Urethral prolapse should not cause urinary obstruction.

526. The answer is C. *(Chapter 89)* Clotting and infection are the most frequent complications of vascular access shunts. A vascular surgeon should be consulted for thrombectomy in the case of a clotted shunt. Success on shunt reopening depends on the length of time it has been clotted. Rarely, some clotted shunts may be treated with local instillation of urokinase, into the arterial and venous sides. Manipulation or irrigation of anything into the shunt may lead to embolization of the clot.

527. The answer is E. *(Chapter 92)* Most renal stones are visualized on plain x-rays or noncontrast CT scan. The majority (75 percent) of renal calculi contain calcium with either oxalate or phosphate. Struvite or magnesium–ammonium–phosphate stones account for another 10 percent and are associated with urea-splitting bacteria and staghorn calculi. Another 10 percent of stones are composed of uric acid; the remainder are caused by cystine and other uncommon minerals.

528. The answer is D. *(Chapter 90)* All of these organisms may cause uncomplicated UTIs. However, *E. coli* is by far the most common bacterium. Anaerobic bacteria do not grow in urine. Unusual organisms, such as yeast or enterococcus, are often found in complicated UTI, especially in patients with underlying renal disease, recent hospitalization, or instrumentation of the urinary tract.

529. The answer is D. *(Chapter 90)* Sexual intercourse increases the concentration of bacteria in the bladder. Women susceptible to UTI should be advised to urinate after intercourse. Some spermicides enhance vaginal colonization with *E. coli*. Uterine and bladder prolapse and neurogenic bladder cause incomplete bladder emptying and thus reduce the ability of the bladder to clear bacteria. Some patients who are nonsecretors of blood group antigens may have a genetic susceptibility to UTI. There is no relation between irregular menses and UTI.

530. The answer is D. *(Chapter 89)* Infection is the most common complication of CAPD, and the majority of cases of peritonitis are caused by *Staphylococcus* species. Peritonitis is usually defined as more than 100 leukocytes with more than 50 percent neutrophils. Therapy consists of infusion of antibiotics with the dialysate into the peritoneal cavity. Parenteral antibiotics are only indicated if the patient is bacteremic. The peritoneal catheter needs to be changed when there have been multiple episodes of peritonitis or evidence of tunnel infection or intraabdominal abscess.

TOXICOLOGIC EMERGENCIES

QUESTIONS

DIRECTIONS: Each question below contains five suggested responses. Choose the **one best** response to each question.

531. All of the following statements concerning decontamination of the poisoned patient are TRUE EXCEPT

(A) ipecac syrup continues to be a front-line tool in home management of poisoning
(B) gastric lavage is of limited utility except in selected overdoses when the airway has been adequately protected
(C) current superactivated charcoal has 1.5 times the absorptive area of older preparations
(D) cathartics may cause electrolyte derangements and dehydration
(E) whole bowel irrigation is a highly effective method for dealing with body "packers" or "stuffers" and overdoses with enteric-coated or sustained release medications

532. Which of the following toxin–antidote pairs is correct?

(A) Arsenic and British antilewisite (BAL)
(B) Lead and calcium disodium edetate or dimercaptosuccinic acid
(C) Mercury and BAL
(D) Nitrites and methylene blue
(E) All of the above

533. Which of the following is TRUE regarding tricyclic antidepressants (TCA)?

(A) TCA overdoses are the leading cause of death in intentional ingestions, with a mortality rate of 10 to 15 percent
(B) All TCAs share a general structure composed of six aromatic rings
(C) TCAs have no activity against central nervous system histamine receptors
(D) TCAs are competitive antagonists of acetylcholine at peripheral and central nicotinic receptors
(E) None of the above

534. Which of the following TCAs is capable of causing status epilepticus without QRS widening?

(A) Nortriptyline
(B) Amoxapine
(C) Maprotiline
(D) Desipramine
(E) Amitriptyline

535. A 22-year-old female presents to the ED comatose after a seizure, with a blood pressure of 80/40 and a pulse of 148. QRS duration is 280 ms. She has been depressed and began taking nortriptyline 2 weeks ago. What is the MOST appropriate initial therapeutic intervention?

(A) Intravenous access and sodium bicarbonate at a dose of 1 to 2 mEq/kg
(B) Intravenous access, gastric lavage, and diazepam to control seizures
(C) Airway control, intravenous access, and activated charcoal per nasogastric tube
(D) Airway control and mechanical ventilation, intravenous access, and sodium bicarbonate at a dose of 1 to 2 mEq/kg
(E) Physostigmine, 0.5 to 2.0 mg intravenously, diluted in 10 mL saline and given over 5 min

536. If sodium bicarbonate therapy is ineffective, which of the following antidysrhythmics may be used to treat ventricular dysrhythmias associated with TCA overdose?

(A) β-blockers
(B) Calcium channel blockers
(C) Phenytoin
(D) Lidocaine
(E) Class IA or IC antidysrhythmics

537. Which of the following statements about fluoxetine (Prozac) is FALSE?

(A) It is the most frequently prescribed antidepressant in the United States

(B) It is the most potent of the selective serotonin reuptake inhibitors (SSRIs)

(C) Seizures occur in approximately 0.2 percent of patients taking fluoxetine

(D) Fluoxetine is the most potent inhibitor of P-450 hepatic drug metabolism and may elevate TCA levels 2- to 10-fold

(E) The most common symptoms seen in fluoxetine overdose are sinus tachycardia, drowsiness, tremor, and nausea/vomiting

538. All of the following statements concerning serotonin syndrome are TRUE EXCEPT

(A) it is characterized by alterations in cognitive-behavioral ability, autonomic nervous function, and neuromuscular activity

(B) it is usually seen when monoamine oxidase inhibitors or selective serotonin reuptake inhibitors are combined with other serotonergic drugs

(C) morphine and fentanyl are contraindicated for treatment

(D) neuromuscular symptoms are greatest in the lower extremities

(E) mandatory treatment includes discontinuation of all serotonergic medications

539. Which of the following drugs can be safely used in patients taking monoamine oxidase inhibitors (MAOIs)?

(A) Codeine
(B) Dextromethorphan
(C) Ketamine
(D) Meperidine
(E) Morphine

540. Which of the following statements regarding adverse effects of neuroleptic medications is INCORRECT?

(A) Lower potency drugs such as chlorpromazine have greater anticholinergic, antiadrenergic, and antihistaminic side effects, whereas the higher potency agents such as haloperidol have mainly antidopaminergic side effects

(B) Dopamine antagonism accounts for adverse reactions, resulting in movement disorders

(C) Dystonic reactions are idiosyncratic, present early, and are seen more frequently in females

(D) Akathisia and drug-induced parkinsonism are seen early and may be treated with benztropine or amantadine

(E) Tardive dyskinesia is a late adverse effect and has no proven treatment

541. After initial stabilization of airway, breathing, and circulation in a patient with neuroleptic malignant syndrome, which of the following is the BEST initial drug therapy?

(A) Bromocriptine
(B) Dantrolene
(C) Molindone
(D) Diazepam
(E) Pancuronium

542. Which of the following statements regarding overdose of antipsychotic medications is FALSE?

(A) Seizures and dysfunction of temperature regulation may be significant findings

(B) Hypotension is due to α_1-adrenergic blockade and direct myocardial depression

(C) Tachycardia is due to anticholinergic effects, and to a reflex response to vasodilation

(D) Conduction abnormalities due to a quinidine-like action and ventricular dysrhythmias including torsades de pointes have been reported

(E) Class IA antidysrhythmics are indicated to treat neuroleptic-induced dysrhythmias

543. Which of the following factors increases the risk of lithium toxicity at standard doses?

(A) Diabetes mellitus
(B) Renal failure
(C) Advanced age
(D) Concurrent use of nonsteroidal antiinflammatory drugs (NSAIDs)
(E) All of the above

544. Which of the following statements regarding barbiturates is FALSE?

(A) Barbituric acid has no central nervous system activity

(B) In a pure barbiturate overdose, the patient's pupils will be small

(C) Barbiturates may be used to treat seizures, induce anesthesia, or manage elevated intracranial pressure

(D) A severe overdose may result in a flat-line EEG

(E) Charcoal administration and alkalinization of the urine are beneficial treatments for barbiturate overdose

545. Flumazenil is a selective antagonist of benzodiazepines. Which of the following is TRUE regarding its use in a patient with an altered level of consciousness?

(A) Flumazenil can be safely used if there is a reliable history of pure benzodiazepine overdose

(B) Benzodiazepine overdoses are usually isolated overdoses and flumazenil can be freely used with diagnostic and therapeutic benefit

(C) Administration of a trial of flumazenil has very low risk of adverse effect

(D) Few patients who overdose on benzodiazepines are physically dependent on these drugs

(E) In the ED, flumazenil is most useful for reversing effects of benzodiazepines given for diagnostic and therapeutic procedures

546. After an overdose, which of the following findings does NOT match with the listed sedative-hypnotic agent?

(A) Ethchlorvynol–prolonged coma

(B) Meprobamate–gastrointestinal concretions

(C) Methaqualone–hyperacusis and hypertonicity

(D) Chloral hydrate–vinyl-like odor on the breath

(E) Glutethimide–anticholinergic symptoms

547. Which of the following statements regarding alcohol toxicity is TRUE?

(A) Cocaethylene has 40 times higher affinity for cocaine receptors than cocaine

(B) Methanol causes a severe anion gap acidosis and is directly toxic to the optic nerve

(C) Isopropanol is strongly associated with hemorrhagic gastritis and produces a profound anion gap acidosis

(D) Ethylene glycol is commonly found in antifreeze and causes a severe nonanion gap acidosis

(E) Isopropanol is less intoxicating than ethanol

548. Which of the following drugs is the MOST efficacious for the treatment of opiate withdrawal in an intravenous drug user?

(A) Methadone
(B) Compazine
(C) Clonidine
(D) Ativan
(E) Naloxone

549. Which of the following statements regarding cocaine is TRUE?

(A) Cocaine is both a local anesthetic and a central nervous system stimulant

(B) Cocaine has a quinidine-like effect on myocardial conduction causing QRS widening and QT prolongation

(C) Cocaine inhibits presynaptic reuptake of norepinephrine, dopamine, and serotonin

(D) Overdose on cocaine predisposes to dysrhythmias, seizures, hyperthermia, and rhabdomyolysis

(E) All of the above

550. Which of the following is NOT associated with toxic doses of amphetamines?

(A) Cerebral vasculitis and choreoathetosis

(B) Cardiomyopathy and polyarteritis nodosa

(C) Urinary incontinence and dysuria

(D) Nausea, vomiting, and diarrhea

(E) Elevated thyroxine level and leukocytosis

551. Which of the following statements regarding hallucinogens is TRUE?

(A) Phencyclidine (PCP) is strongly associated with synesthesias

(B) Flashbacks are common with PCP use

(C) Patients who have ingested lysergic acid diethylamide (LSD) are prone to anxiety-induced paranoia and auditory hallucinations

(D) Complications are common with nutmeg, marijuana, mescaline, and peyote

(E) Hallucinogenic amphetamines are associated with vasculitis

552. Which of the following statements about acetaminophen poisoning is FALSE?

(A) Hepatotoxicity has traditionally been defined as an ALT or AST level > 500 IU/L

(B) The Rumack-Matthew nomogram predicts the risk of hepatotoxicity after a single overdose of acetaminophen based on blood levels obtained 4 to 24 h after ingestion

(C) The risk of death in an untreated patient whose blood level is in the "probable toxicity" zone of the nomogram is 5 to 24 percent

(D) The toxic metabolite of acetaminophen is *N*-acetyl-para-benzo-quinoneimine (NAPQI)

(E) There are four stages of acetaminophen toxicity

553. Which of the following are side effects of NSAIDs?

(A) Nausea, vomiting, and abdominal pain

(B) Headache, behavioral and cognitive problems, and aseptic meningitis

(C) Seizures

(D) Metabolic acidosis and acute renal insufficiency

(E) All of the above

554. Which of the following drugs does NOT increase the serum half-life of theophylline?

(A) Cimetidine

(B) Erythromycin

(C) Phenytoin

(D) Quinolones

(E) Allopurinol

555. Which of the following statements regarding chronic digitalis toxicity is FALSE?

(A) It is most often seen in elderly patients taking digoxin and diuretics

(B) Chronic digitalis toxicity may mimic common diseases such as influenza or gastroenteritis

(C) This toxicity may manifest as mental status changes or psychiatric symptoms

(D) Serum potassium is usually decreased or normal

(E) The serum digoxin level is markedly elevated

556. Phenytoin administration decreases the serum level of all of the following drugs EXCEPT

(A) oral anticoagulants

(B) carbamazepine

(C) methadone

(D) furosemide

(E) valproic acid

557. Which of the following is FALSE regarding toxic iron ingestions?

(A) Iron poisoning can be divided into four stages based on clinical signs and symptoms

(B) A child with nausea and vomiting, WBC > 15,000/μL, and serum glucose > 150 mg/dL is likely to have a serum iron level > 300 μg/dL

(C) A negative deferoxamine challenge test is unreliable in ruling out significant iron ingestion

(D) Deferoxamine is best administered intravenously at a rate of at least 15 mg/kg/h

(E) Total iron binding capacity (TIBC) assays are unaffected by the presence of acute iron overdose

558. Which statement about hydrocarbon toxicity is TRUE?

(A) Hydrocarbon ingestion accounts for up to 10 percent of childhood accidental ingestions in the United States and 20 percent in less developed nations

(B) Persons ingesting hydrocarbons with viscosities of < 30 Saybolt Seconds Universal (SSU) are at much lower risk of aspiration than those ingesting agents with SSU ratings of > 60

(C) Highly volatile hydrocarbons such as diesel oil have a high toxic potential when inhaled

(D) Volatile hydrocarbon inhalational solvent abuse may cause chronic encephalopathy and cerebellar ataxia

(E) All of the above

559. Which of the following statements about hydrofluoric acid exposure is FALSE?

(A) Hydrofluoric acid is a widely used industrial chemical and is formulated in solution ranging from 20 to 70 percent in strength

(B) Exposure may result in extensive burns despite minimal initial findings

(C) Subcutaneous or intramuscular calcium injection is a recommended therapy

(D) Exposure may cause life-threatening hypocalcemia and hypomagnesemia

(E) Intraarterial administration of calcium gluconate is a highly recommended therapy for extremity exposures to hydrofluoric acid

560. All of the following are signs of acetylcholinesterase inhibitor toxicity EXCEPT

(A) miosis
(B) salivation
(C) diarrhea
(D) muscle fasciculations
(E) anhydrosis

561. Which of the following plants may cause anticholinergic toxicity?

(A) *Datura stramonium*
(B) Deadly nightshade
(C) Henbane
(D) Mandrake
(E) All of the above

562. Which of the following is NOT a central nervous system finding in cyanide toxicity?

(A) Arterialization of retinal veins
(B) Headache
(C) Agitated delirium
(D) Coma
(E) Seizures

TOXICOLOGIC EMERGENCIES

ANSWERS

531. The answer is C. *(Chapter 151)* Current superactivated charcoal has three times the absorptive area of older preparations, or 3000 m²/kg. The dose is 1 mg/kg, and it may reduce absorption of ingested toxins by 50 percent. Cathartics may be dangerous, especially in pediatric patients and when given in multiple doses to poorly hydrated patients.

532. The answer is E. *(Chapter 151)* Arsenic, mercury, and gold poisoning are treated with BAL. Each milliliter of BAL in oil has 100 mg of dimercaprol in 210 mg of 21 percent benzyl benzoate and 680 mg of peanut oil. Dimercaptosuccinic acid is an oral, water-soluble preparation of BAL that can be used to treat lead poisoning.

533. The answer is E. *(Chapter 152)* TCA overdoses are the leading cause of death in intentional ingestions, with a mortality rate of 2 to 5 percent. All TCAs share a general structure composed of three aromatic rings (a central seven-member ring with two outer benzene rings) with an aminopropyl side chain connected to the central ring. TCAs are active against central nervous system histamine receptors. This results in sedation. TCAs are competitive antagonists of acetylcholine at peripheral and central muscarinic receptors.

534. The answer is B. *(Chapter 152)* TCA-induced seizures are usually single, generalized, self-limited, and brief. However, amoxapine and maprotiline can cause status epilepticus. Amoxapine seizures commonly occur without QRS widening. Seven percent of the population in the United States are "slow metabolizers" of TCAs and are prone to developing higher serum levels for a given dosage.

535. The answer is D. *(Chapter 152)* This patient is severely intoxicated due to TCA overdose. She is at high risk of further cardiopulmonary decompensation and aspiration unless immediate airway control and ventilation are initiated. After ensuring an adequate airway, intravenous access and bicarbonate therapy are the treatment priorities. Gastric lavage (if soon after the ingestion) and activated charcoal are then indicated to prevent continuing absorption of the drug. Use of physostigmine in this case may show transient improvement in level of consciousness but is contraindicated because of the risk of death.

536. The answer is D. *(Chapter 152)* Lidocaine is the second-line agent of choice in TCA overdose after sodium bicarbonate for treatment of ventricular dysrhythmias. Class IA and IC antidysrhythmics, β-blockers, calcium channel blockers, and phenytoin are contraindicated and may exacerbate TCA-related dysrhythmias. Bretylium is the third-line drug for TCA rhythm disturbances unresponsive to bicarbonate or lidocaine.

537. The answer is B. *(Chapter 153)* Paroxetine is the most potent of the SSRIs. The most serious side effect of this class of antidepressants is serotonin syndrome. Extrapyramidal symptoms, hyponatremia, hypoglycemia, and sexual dysfunction are also associated with SSRI medications.

538. The answer is C. *(Chapter 153)* Morphine and fentanyl are considered safe treatments for serotonin syndrome. The syndrome is usually seen after increasing the dose of a potent serotonin agonist or adding a second serotonergic agent (such as lithium) to a patient's regimen. Electroconvulsive therapy, cocaine, meperidine, levodopa, L-tryptophan, and other drugs may predispose patients to serotonin syndrome.

539. The answer is E. *(Chapter 154)* Drugs that are safe to use with MAOIs include aspirin, acetaminophen, ibuprofen, morphine, albuterol, epinephrine, norepinephrine, and isoproterenol. Drugs that are contraindicated if the patient is taking MAOIs include bretylium, pseudoephedrine, caffeine, levodopa, theophylline, and TCAs. MAOIs result in three basic types of drug interactions: pharmacodynamic, pharmacokinetic, and idiosyncratic. Indirect-acting sympathomimetics are the most common cause of pharmacodynamic drug interactions for the MAOI patient. The indirect-acting sympathomimetics can result in a tyramine-like hyperadrenergic state when consumed in conjunction with MAOIs. Pharmacokinetic drug interactions from MAOIs are due to inhibition of usual drug metabolism by cytochrome oxidase. Opiates and sedative-hypnotics are especially susceptible to this phenomenon.

540. The answer is C. *(Chapter 155)* Dystonic reactions are more likely to occur in males and are seen in 12 percent of patients treated with a single dose of neuroleptic. Akathisia (subjective restlessness) and acute parkinsonism are also early movement disorders associated with neuroleptic administration. Both are more likely to present in females and occur in 20 percent and 13 percent of patients, respectively. Neuroleptic malignant syndrome occurs in fewer than 3 percent of patients and is more common in males. Tardive dyskinesia is a late-appearing neurologic syndrome that occurs more commonly in females and affects 30 percent of long-term neuroleptic patients. At present, there is no effective treatment.

541. The answer is D. *(Chapter 155)* Diazepam, in large doses if necessary, is the first-line drug treatment for neuroleptic malignant syndrome (NMS). If this fails, paralytic drugs are indicated. Other drugs that may be used in the treatment of NMS include dantrolene, bromocriptine, carbidopa/levodopa, or amantadine. Presenting symptoms for NMS include hyperthermia, muscular rigidity, altered level of consciousness, and autonomic instability. Haloperidol is the most common inciting agent. Patients taking neuroleptics simultaneously with lithium, TCAs, MAOIs, or antiparkinsonian drugs are at greatest risk.

542. The answer is E. *(Chapter 155)* Seizures, tachycardia, hypotension, and atrioventricular/intraventricular dysrhythmias have all been reported in neuroleptic overdose. Hypothermia and hyperthermia can also be seen. Coma and respiratory depression are rare with isolated neuroleptic ingestion. Anticholinergic symptoms are common with overdoses of low-potency neuroleptics such as chlorpromazine and thioridazine, and extrapyramidal disorders are more likely with high-potency antipsychotics. Class IB (lidocaine or phenytoin) antidysrhythmics are indicated to treat neuroleptic-induced dysrhythmias.

543. The answer is E. *(Chapter 156)* Any factor that decreases the efficiency of the kidney to deal with chronic lithium exposure increases the risk of lithium toxicity. Pathophysiologic factors that deplete the body of water or total body sodium increase lithium toxicity. Risk factors for lithium toxicity include diabetes mellitus, hypertension, renal failure, old age, a low sodium diet, and coingestion of diuretics or NSAIDs.

544. The answer is B. *(Chapter 157)* A general rule of thumb is that 10 times the therapeutic dose of barbiturates causes severe toxicity. Overdose results in progressive central nervous system depression similar to that seen with ethanol ingestion. Hypothermia is common, skin bullae occur in 6 percent of patients, and pupils may be either constricted or dilated. Flat-line electroencephalogram (EEG) is not uncommon in severe overdose. Hence, brain death cannot be declared until the effects of the acute ingestion have resolved.

545.   The answer is E. *(Chapter 158)*   Benzodiazepine overdose is usually a mixed overdose. If the patient is prone to seizures (e.g., when TCAs are coingested), flumazenil is contraindicated. Even if the history is reliable for a pure benzodiazepine overdose, the patient may be benzodiazepine-dependent and thus at risk for intractable seizures if flumazenil is administered. Because supportive care and charcoal lead to good outcomes after most benzodiazepine overdoses, blind use of flumazenil in the ED patient with an altered level of consciousness is unwarranted.

546.   The answer is D. *(Chapter 159)*   Chloral hydrate overdose is associated with a pear-like odor of the breath. Ethchlorvynol overdose is associated with a vinyl-like odor of the breath. Glutethimide overdose may show waxing and waning sedation and can be associated with a flat-line EEG.

547.   The answer is A. *(Chapter 160)*   The combination of ethanol with cocaine produces a dangerous metabolite, cocaethylene. Risk of sudden death in coingesters is about 20 times that with cocaine alone. Toxicity from methanol and ethylene glycol results from their metabolites, formaldehyde and formic acid, not direct toxicity. Isopropanol causes hemorrhagic gastritis, and it produces an osmolal gap but not an anion gap. Both methanol and ethylene glycol cause a severe anion gap metabolic acidosis. Isospropanol is commonly used as rubbing alcohol and is approximately twice as potent as ethanol.

548.   The answer is A. *(Chapter 161)*   Methadone is an oral opiate that relieves all symptoms of opiate withdrawal except the desire to use a needle or "shoot up." Compazine, clonidine, and benzodiazepines provide partial relief of symptoms and are useful for treatment of opiate withdrawal in outpatients. Naloxone induces opiate withdrawal.

549.   The answer is E. *(Chapter 162)*   The parent compound of cocaine exists naturally in the plant *Erythroxylon coca* and is indigenous to South America. In large doses, cocaine may exert a direct negative effect on the myocardium because of its quinidine-like activity. Plasma cholinesterase converts cocaine to ecgonine methyl ester. Benzoylecgonine, the other major metabolite, is excreted in urine and assayed in most toxicology screens. It is present in the urine for 24 to 72 h after an isolated use but may persist for up to 2 weeks in chronic users.

550.   The answer is C. *(Chapter 162)*   Amphetamine intoxication causes urinary retention but not incontinence. Patients may complain of dysuria and urinary hesitancy. The other listed effects have all been reported. In addition, flushing, tachycardia, hypertension, dysrhythmias, and myocardial infarction can be caused by amphetamine ingestion. Aggressive cooling measures and even paralysis are sometimes needed to control severe hyperthermia and prevent rhabdomyolysis.

551.   The answer is E. *(Chapter 163)*   Synesthesias are common with LSD and are manifested by the "hearing of colors" and "seeing of sounds." This phenomenon is not described with PCP. Flashbacks are common with LSD but not with PCP. Patients who have ingested LSD are prone to anxiety-induced paranoia and visual, not auditory, hallucinations. Complications are rare with nutmeg, marijuana, mescaline, and peyote. Chronic use of hallucinogenic amphetamines can lead to vasculitis.

552.   The answer is A. *(Chapter 165)*   Hepatotoxicity has traditionally been defined as an alanine aminotransferase (ALT) or aspartate aminotransferase (AST) level of greater than or equal to 1000 IU/L. The Rumack-Matthew nomogram predicts the risk of hepatotoxicity after a single ingestion of acetaminophen based on a blood level obtained 4 to 24 h later. The nomogram is inaccurate if additional acetaminophen was taken in the preceding 12 to 24 h. For a patient whose level is in the "probable toxicity" zone of the nomogram who is not treated with *N*-acetylcysteine, the risk of death is 5 to 24 percent and the probability of significant hepatotoxicity is 14 to 89 percent. Significant toxicity is possible in children who consume more than 140 mg/kg or adults who take more than 7.5 g of acetaminophen acutely. When it occurs, acute liver failure typically presents 72 to 96 h after the acute ingestion, during stage III of the poisoning.

553. The answer is E. *(Chapter 166)* NSAIDs include salicylates and nonsalicylates. There are five chemical classes of nonsalicylate NSAIDs: acetic acids, propionic acids, fenamic acids, oxicams, and pyrazolones. Mefenamic acid ingestion can lead to seizures. Aseptic meningitis has been reported with NSAID use and is most often found in patients suffering from autoimmune disorders. NSAID-induced aseptic meningitis is thought to be due to drug hypersensitivity.

554. The answer is C. *(Chapter 167)* Phenytoin, rifampin, phenobarbital, and carbamazepine all decrease the half-life of theophylline. The half-life of theophylline is also reduced in children, smokers, patients with hyperthyroidism, and in those who eat charcoal-broiled foods. Drugs that increase the half-life of theophylline include erythromycin, clarithromycin, mexilitine, tocainide, and propafenone. The half-life of theophylline is also increased in patients with cirrhosis, severe obstructive airway disease, pneumonia, and congestive heart failure.

555. The answer is E. *(Chapter 168)* A high index of clinical suspicion is necessary to make the diagnosis of chronic digoxin toxicity. Chronic toxicity is usually associated with a normal or mildly elevated digoxin level. Acute, but not chronic, digoxin overdose is associated with hyperkalemia. Hypomagnesemia is a common feature of chronic overdose.

556. The answer is A. *(Chapter 172)* Phenytoin increases the serum level of oral anticoagulants, acetaminophen, and primadone. Drugs whose levels are decreased include amiodarone, disopyramide, mexilitene, and quinidine. Phenylbutazone, sulfonamides, valproic acid, high-dose salicylates, and tolbutamide increase levels of phenytoin. The mechanism for this increase in serum phenytoin level is displacement of the drug from protein binding. This increases the free fraction of phenytoin, although total drug concentration may decrease.

557. The answer is E. *(Chapter 173)* Iron poisoning can be divided into four stages based on clinical signs and symptoms. Nausea and vomiting, white blood cell (WBC) count > 15,000/μL, and serum glucose > 150 mg/dL are all highly predictive of a serum iron level > 300 μg/dL in acute iron overdose. A single negative deferoxamine challenge test should not be used to rule out significant iron ingestion in the presence of a strong history or significant signs or symptoms. TIBC assays may be falsely elevated in the setting of acute iron overdose. If the patient survives an acute ingestion, the fourth stage of toxicity may develop days to weeks later; this stage is characterized by gastric outlet or small bowel obstruction.

558. The answer is D. *(Chapter 174)* Hydrocarbon ingestion accounts for up to 10 percent of childhood accidental ingestions in the United States and between 33 and 59 percent in less developed nations. Persons ingesting hydrocarbons with viscosities of < 60 SSU are at much higher risk of aspiration than those ingesting agents with SSU ratings of > 100. Highly volatile hydrocarbons have a high toxic potential when inhaled, but diesel oil is not highly volatile.

559. The answer is C. *(Chapter 175)* Subcutaneous or intramuscular injection of calcium is useless in hydrofluoric acid exposure. The recommended methods of delivery of calcium gluconate are as a 2.5 percent gel by intradermal injection of 10 percent solution with a 30-gauge needle, or by intraarterial injection of 10 mL of 10 percent calcium gluconate diluted in 50 mL of D_5W over 4 h. Therapy is successful when the patient achieves and maintains a pain-free state. Calcium chloride should not be used because of the risk of tissue necrosis if inadvertent extravasation occurs.

560. **The answer is E.** *(Chapter 176)* Acetylcholinesterase inhibitor toxicity due to organophosphate or carbamate poisoning is characterized by diaphoresis, not by anhydrosis. Signs and symptoms of these poisonings may be classified as muscarinic, nicotinic, and central. Miosis is the most specific muscarinic finding and muscular fasciculations is the most specific finding for nicotinic receptors. The acronym *SLUDGE* (salivation, lacrimation, urination, diarrhea, gastrointestinal, emesis) describes the clinical presentation. Organophosphate binding to acetylcholinesterase becomes covalent and irreversible if not treated with pralidoxime within 24 to 36 h. Carbamate binding to acetylcholinesterase is reversible.

561. **The answer is E.** *(Chapter 177)* *Datura stramonium* is the scientific name for the plant commonly known as jimsonweed. It is a weed that is widely distributed throughout the United States, grows 3 to 6 feet high, and has large, jagged, white or purple trumpet-shaped flowers. All parts of the plant are toxic and contain atropine, hyoscyamine, and scopolamine. Mydriasis from jimsonweed may persist for up to 1 week and can result from systemic or ocular exposure ("cornpicker's" eye). The classic description of a patient with anticholinergic syndrome is: "hot as a hare, blind as a bat, dry as a bone, red as a beet, and mad as a hatter."

562. **The answer is C.** *(Chapter 182)* Agitated delirium is not a feature of acute cyanide toxicity. Cyanide results in progressive central nervous system dysfunction, with coma and death being the end result. Local effects of cyanide include oropharyngeal burns and the odor of almonds. Cardiopulmonary effects are divided into early and late stages. The early stage includes dyspnea, hypertension, tachycardia, and dysrhythmias. The late cardiopulmonary effects are bradycardia, hypotension, and cardiopulmonary arrest.

TRAUMA

QUESTIONS

DIRECTIONS: Each question below contains five suggested responses. Choose the **one best** response to each question.

563. Which one of the following statements regarding trauma epidemiology is INCORRECT?

(A) Alcohol is associated with 40 percent of motor vehicle accidents (MVAs)

(B) In the elderly, fractured hips are the most common injury sustained during a fall

(C) If involved in a motorcycle accident, you are 35 times more likely to die than if you are involved in an automobile accident

(D) Most trauma victims in the United States are transported to trauma centers for resuscitation

(E) Within the United States, trauma is the leading cause of death up to the age of 45 years

564. A 45-year-old male unrestrained driver is brought to the ED with cervical spine precautions by an EMT unit after a high-speed MVA. He has a Glasgow Coma Scale (GCS) score of 6 and no obvious signs of trauma. His shallow respirations are being inadequately assisted with a bag-valve mask. Radial pulse is thready, and the extremities are cool. Which of the following should be performed before rapid sequence intubation (RSI)?

(A) A brief neurologic examination including a check of rectal tone

(B) An immediate chin lift to clear the airway from any obstruction

(C) A full set of vital signs

(D) A lateral cervical spine x-ray

(E) Four quick tidal volume breaths with 100 percent oxygen using a bag-valve mask device

565. A 28-year-old male sustains a gunshot wound to the back, just medial to the left scapula. Field blood pressure is 98/p, pulse is 101, and respiratory rate is 38. En route to the ED, he received high-flow oxygen and 1 L normal saline. He is agitated and diaphoretic on arrival. You are unable to hear heart sounds because of ambient noise, but the neck veins appear normal. Blood pressure starts to decrease and respiratory status worsens over the next few minutes, but he is still conscious and oriented. Given that all of the following interventions are available, what is the MOST appropriate next step?

(A) Emergent bedside cardiac ultrasound

(B) Emergent thoracotomy

(C) Immediate needle decompression of the left chest

(D) Immediate blood transfusion

(E) Immediate chest x-ray

566. Which of the following statements is TRUE regarding pediatric trauma?

(A) Trauma is the leading cause of death in children younger than 1 year

(B) Because of their smaller body surface area, hypothermia is less common in children than in adults

(C) Head injury is the most frequent cause of death

(D) Initial assessment and management of an injured child differs from that of an adult

(E) Alcohol use is a factor in most trauma cases associated with MVAs

567. Which of the following statements is INCORRECT regarding the child's airway?

(A) Children are dependent on diaphragmatic excursion for breathing in order to generate adequate tidal volume

(B) In children older than 4 years, the narrowest portion of the trachea is no longer subglottic

(C) The location of the infant's larynx is more cephalad than the location of the adult's larynx

(D) Cricothyrotomy is contraindicated in small children

(E) The correct endotracheal tube size for a 4-year-old child is 5.0

568. A 6-month-old child falls and hits his head. Which of the following signs would be the MOST indicative of serious neurological injury?

(A) The parent states the child was pale and sweaty for a few minutes after the fall

(B) A single post-fall episode of emesis

(C) Lethargy immediately after the head injury

(D) Hypotension

(E) A single grand mal seizure immediately after the fall

569. Which of the following statements is INCORRECT regarding pediatric spinal cord injury?

(A) Because of a child's large head, the fulcrum of cervical motion lies at C4–5

(B) Widening of the prevertebral soft tissue of 8 mm or more anterior to C2 is abnormal

(C) In most cases, pseudosubluxation resolves if x-rays are repeated with the child in the sniffing position

(D) More than 50 percent of children with SCIWORA (spinal cord injury without radiographic abnormality) have a delayed onset of paralysis

(E) A normal spine series can be found in up to two-thirds of children with spinal cord injury

570. Which of the following is TRUE regarding geriatric patients?

(A) They fall less frequently than younger people because they are more cautious about their balance

(B) They are likely to sustain multiple orthopedic fractures after a fall

(C) They are more likely to die from an MVA than from any other traumatic injury

(D) The increased incidence in violent crimes in the United States has spared the elderly

(E) Alcohol is less likely to be associated with a fatal assault than it is for a younger person

571. Which of the following statements would be MOST CORRECT regarding evaluation of a head and neck CT of a 75-year-old male after a fall?

(A) Epidural hematomas occur more frequently in the elderly than in young adults

(B) There should be 25 to 30 percent more brain atrophy in the normal 75-year-old male than in a 30-year-old male

(C) Subdural hematomas occur less frequently in the elderly than in young adults

(D) Increased "dead space" within the skull may delay symptoms of intracranial bleeds

(E) Compared with young adults, elderly patients have an increased incidence of cervical spine injuries

572. An 83-year-old female fell while walking to the bathroom. She complains of severe pain and will not tolerate any movement of the left leg. The leg is externally rotated and shortened. Which of the following is the MOST likely location for the fracture?

(A) Intertrochanteric

(B) Transcervical

(C) Subcapital

(D) Subtrochanteric

(E) Acetabular

573. A 15-year-old male is brought to the ED after being assaulted to the head with a lead pipe. He opens his eyes briefly to deep painful stimuli, mumbles incomprehensible sounds, and withdraws to painful stimuli. What is his initial GCS?

(A) 10

(B) 9

(C) 8

(D) 7

(E) 6

574. While in the CT scanner, the patient described in question 573 develops anisocoria. Which of the following statements is INCORRECT regarding uncal herniation?

(A) Compression of cranial nerve III along the edge of the tentorium incisura causes pupillary dilation

(B) Constriction of parasympathetic fibers on the surface of cranial nerve III causes unopposed sympathetic dilation of the pupil

(C) With further compression of cranial nerve III, full oculomotor paralysis develops, causing the eye to deviate inferiorly and medially

(D) Uncal herniation can compress the corticospinal tract, leading to contralateral hemiplegia

(E) An emergency burr hole should be placed on the same side as the dilated pupil in the majority of cases

575. A 42-year-old female has a GCS of 6 after an MVA. Which of the following statements is TRUE regarding her care?

(A) If hypotension is allowed to occur, the mortality risk is more than doubled

(B) The most critical determinant of outcome in severely head-injured patients is ICP

(C) The patient should be hyperventilated to a pCO_2 of less than 25 mm Hg

(D) Hypotension in the severely brain-injured patient is usually due to the primary brain injury

(E) CT of the abdomen and head should be performed immediately in a hypotensive, severely head-injured patient

576. A 13-year-old male is involved in a water ski boat accident. Which of the following would NOT be indicative of a basilar skull fracture?

(A) Generalized bruising on the face, most notably around the eyes

(B) Bluish, dull tympanic membrane on the left side

(C) A small retroauricular ecchymosis on the left side

(D) Left-sided facial droop

(E) Medial deviation of the left eye

577. Which of the following patients does NOT require immediate neurosurgical evaluation?

(A) A 24-year-old male with a GCS score of 13 and a linear fracture of the temporal bone diagnosed by skull x-ray at an outside hospital

(B) A comatose 38-year-old female with a depressed linear skull fracture

(C) A 42-year-old male with a basilar skull fracture diagnosed by bony windows on head CT

(D) A 19-year-old female with a scalp laceration and clear discharge from the right ear after an unhelmeted fall while rollerblading

(E) A 58-year-old female with a GCS score of 4 and a negative head CT

578. A homeless, alcoholic male is brought to the ED with a mildly altered level of consciousness. Although there is no history or external signs of trauma, a head CT is obtained and it shows a large collection of blood, with slight midline shift. Which of the following statements is TRUE regarding this patient's most likely diagnosis?

(A) It is usually caused by tearing of the middle meningeal artery

(B) The patient should show signs of elevated intracranial pressure immediately after the injury

(C) Brain atrophy associated with alcoholism makes him less susceptible to this type of bleed

(D) Immediate surgery may not be necessary

(E) Morbidity and mortality are much lower than for other intracerebral bleeds

579. A 36-year-old female comes to the ED complaining of headache and nausea. She had a negative head CT 5 days earlier after a brief lapse of consciousness after an MVA. She is amnestic to the event. Which of the following statements is FALSE?

(A) The mortality rate for patients with head injury and a negative head CT approaches zero

(B) Retrograde and antegrade amnesia is common with this type of injury

(C) The patient is not at risk for significant injuries because she is 5 days out from the initial trauma and relatively asymptomatic

(D) The patient may have alterations in thinking, sleeping, or concentration abilities

(E) A new sensitivity to alcohol is normal and will probably resolve within a few weeks

580. A young female presents to the ED with a GCS score of 6 after being "t-boned" by a large pickup truck on her side of the vehicle. Initial head CT is negative for bleed. Pupils were initially normal and reactive to light but are now bilaterally dilated and sluggish. Which one of the following therapies would be LEAST beneficial for this patient?

(A) 1 L normal saline bolus

(B) Intubation and hyperventilation to keep the pCO_2 less than 25 mm Hg

(C) Mannitol 1 g/kg intravenous bolus

(D) Elevation of the head of the bed to 30 degrees

(E) Furosemide 0.3 to 0.5 mg/kg intravenously

581. Which of the following statements regarding spinal injury is TRUE?

(A) Twenty percent of patients deteriorate neurologically in the ED
(B) In a neurologically normal patient, the absence of pain or tenderness along the spine excludes spine injury
(C) Approximately 75 percent of spinal injuries occur in the cervical region
(D) Approximately 25 percent of all head-injured patients have associated spinal injuries
(E) If appropriate precautions are maintained, evaluation of the spine may be safely deferred until after intubation is performed

582. Which of the following statements is INCORRECT regarding spinal shock?

(A) Distal areflexia can persist for hours to weeks
(B) After reflexes return, the patient develops spastic paralysis
(C) Fluid resuscitation alone is generally insufficient to treat hypotension
(D) Vasomotor instability leads to hypotension and cool, moist skin
(E) Paradoxical bradycardia can coexist with hypotension

583. A 76-year-old male with severe osteoarthritis falls head first onto the cement. On ED arrival, he is confused and answers "yes" to all questions. You notice that he is not moving the upper extremities or legs. All of the following are characteristic for this type of cord syndrome EXCEPT

(A) the legs are typically weaker than the arms
(B) the hands are weaker than the proximal arm muscles
(C) prognosis is better for this syndrome than for other cord syndromes
(D) vascular compromise in the pattern of the anterior spinal artery is the cause
(E) the bladder is occasionally affected

584. Which of the following statements is INCORRECT regarding cervical spine injuries?

(A) The Jefferson fracture is due to a vertical compression injury
(B) Hangman's fracture is a bilateral fracture through the pedicles of C2
(C) A flexion teardrop fracture leaves the posterior ligaments intact
(D) A unilateral facet dislocation is diagnosed when there is anterior dislocation of 25 to 33 percent of one vertebral body on the next vertebra
(E) Bilateral interfacetal dislocation is an unstable cervical injury with total ligamentous disruption

585. A 26-year-old intoxicated male driver is involved in a high-speed MVA. Which of the following findings on cervical spine x-ray would NOT be suggestive of serious injury?

(A) An 8-mm prevertebral soft tissue swelling at C4
(B) A 4-mm anterior subluxation of C5 on C6
(C) Fanning of the cervical spinous processes
(D) A predental space of 3 mm
(E) An 18-degree change in angulation of the cervical column

586. Which of the following patients with penetrating neck trauma is MOST likely to require immediate surgical exploration?

(A) An 18-year-old asymptomatic male with a stab wound to zone II of the neck that penetrates the platysma
(B) A 12-year-old female with a BB gunshot wound to zone II of the neck who complains of a minor voice change and occasional nonproductive cough
(C) A 43-year-old female with a glass shard laceration to zone III of the neck with minimal associated bleeding
(D) A 21-year-old male with a zone I, II, and III neck laceration from a pocket knife associated with significant hemorrhage that is well controlled with a pressure dressing
(E) A 33-year-old female with a gunshot wound to zone I of the neck and anisocoria

587. Which of the following is the LEAST appropriate management of a patient with a spinal cord injury?

(A) Immobilization with a long spine board, semi-rigid cervical collar and bolstering devices

(B) Low-dose vasopressors to treat neurogenic shock

(C) Atropine to treat bradycardia

(D) Methylprednisolone 30 mg intravenous bolus and then 5.4 mg/kg/h for 23 h if administered within the first 12 h of injury

(E) Transfer to a definitive-care facility once cardiovascular stability has been achieved

588. Which of the following statements is TRUE regarding chest trauma?

(A) Thoracic injury is the cause of death in 25 percent of all trauma patients

(B) Most deaths from chest trauma occur before ED arrival

(C) Mortality is greater than 50 percent for patients who present with a blood pressure less than 80 systolic or who require intubation on arrival

(D) Twenty-five percent of blunt chest trauma patients are candidates for emergent thoracotomy

(E) Forty-five percent of penetrating chest trauma patients are candidates for emergent thoracotomy

589. A 24-year-old unrestrained male driver is involved in a high-speed MVA. GCS score is 10, and he has severe chest wall contusions and mild hemoptysis. He is intubated for respiratory distress. Within a few minutes of intubation, he suffers a cardiac arrest. Which of the following therapeutic measures would be LEAST likely to have an immediate life-saving effect?

(A) Decrease the ventilatory rate

(B) Needle decompression of the chest

(C) Pull back the endotracheal tube

(D) One liter crystalloid fluid bolus

(E) Immediate Trendelenburg position, left lateral side down

590. Which of the following patients is NOT a candidate for emergent ED thoracotomy?

(A) A 12-year-old male with a stab wound to the left axilla who loses pulses on ED arrival

(B) A 29-year-old male with a gunshot wound to the left upper quadrant, with a distending abdomen and a precipitous decrease in GCS score to 3

(C) A 42-year-old male involved in an MVA, initially alert, who arrives to the ED with pulseless electrical activity after a 6-min transport time

(D) A 36-year-old female with a stab wound to zone I of the neck who becomes altered and loses radial pulses 4 min before ED arrival

(E) An 18-year-old male who fell 12 feet from a tree, was alert in the field, but is now altered, bradycardic, hypotensive, and has a distended abdomen

591. Which of the following statements is INCORRECT regarding flail chest?

(A) The main cause of morbidity and mortality is hypoxia secondary to the patient's inability to generate adequate negative intrathoracic pressure

(B) Flail chest is characterized by paradoxical movement of the involved portion of the chest wall during respiration

(C) It may not be apparent immediately after the injury

(D) Initial therapy is aimed at immediate pain relief, generous pulmonary toilet, and fluid restriction to prevent fluid overload

(E) Prophylactic intubation decreases mortality in minimally symptomatic patients with large pulmonary contusions

592. After a moderate-speed MVA, a 32-year-old male restrained driver has a normal upright anteroposterior chest x-ray but a 2-mm pneumothorax on CT. Which of the following is the BEST indication for placement of a thoracostomy tube?

(A) One or more rib fractures

(B) Need for intubation and mechanical ventilation

(C) Pulmonary contusion

(D) Cardiac contusion

(E) $Pao_2 < 100$

593. Hamman's sign MOST likely suggests which of the following conditions?

(A) Pneumothorax
(B) Pneumomediastinum
(C) Pericarditis
(D) Pleurisy
(E) Pericardial tamponade

594. Which of the following is the LEAST reliable sign of Beck's triad in a patient with pericardial tamponade?

(A) Distended neck veins
(B) Tracheal deviation
(C) Tachycardia
(D) Hypotension
(E) Muffled heart tones

595. Which of the following statements is CORRECT regarding needle pericardiocentesis for diagnosis and treatment of penetrating cardiac injury?

(A) The false negative rate is high
(B) Most of the pericardial blood can usually be removed
(C) If successful, surgery is rarely needed
(D) Rapid aspiration of 20 mL of blood without moving the needle usually indicates successful needle placement
(E) ECG monitoring is more accurate if attached to a plastic catheter

596. Which area of the heart is MOST commonly injured in a myocardial contusion?

(A) Right ventricle
(B) Right atrium
(C) Left ventricle
(D) Left atrium
(E) Interventricular septum

597. Which of the following is the MOST common valvular injury in a patient who survives transport to the ED after blunt cardiac trauma?

(A) Papillary muscle or chordae tendineae of mitral valve
(B) Mitral valve leaflets
(C) Aortic valve
(D) Pulmonic valve
(E) Tricuspid valve

598. What is the MOST likely abnormality that would be seen on chest x-ray in a patient with traumatic rupture of the aorta after blunt injury?

(A) Superior mediastinal widening
(B) Obscuration of the aortic knob
(C) Deviation of esophagus to the left
(D) Fracture of the first or second rib
(E) Apical cap

599. Physical findings suggestive of traumatic rupture of the aorta include all of the following EXCEPT

(A) flail chest
(B) systolic murmur over the back
(C) lower extremity hypertension
(D) difference in pulse amplitudes between the upper and lower extremities
(E) hoarseness without laryngeal injury

600. Which of the following statements is TRUE regarding blunt tracheobronchial injuries?

(A) Blunt cervical tracheal injuries usually occur proximal to the tracheal cartilage
(B) Most lower tracheobronchial injuries occur 5 cm or more from the carina
(C) Common signs and symptoms include dyspnea, hemoptysis, subcutaneous emphysema, Hamman's sign, and sternal tenderness
(D) Injuries to the major bronchi are usually caused by elevated intraabdominal pressure
(E) Concurrent esophageal injuries occur in fewer than 5 percent of cases

601. Approximately how much blood is contained in an acute pericardial tamponade after penetrating cardiac injury?

(A) 10 mL
(B) 50 mL
(C) 200 mL
(D) 500 mL
(E) 1000 mL

602. In which of the following cases would a diagnostic peritoneal lavage (DPL) be the MOST useful?

(A) Blunt abdominal trauma with hypotension and free intraperitoneal fluid on ultrasound
(B) Multiple trauma with spinal cord injury and normal abdominal examination
(C) An alert patient involved in a high-speed vehicle collision with no abdominal findings
(D) Gunshot wound (GSW) to the mid-abdomen with intraabdominal bullet fragments
(E) Penetrating abdominal injury with diffuse abdominal tenderness and rebound tenderness

603. Which of the following is an indication for surgery in a patient with blunt kidney injury?

(A) Hematuria with more than 100 red blood cells (RBC)/high-power field (HPF) on an unspun urinalysis
(B) Severe flank pain unrelieved by analgesics
(C) Unexplained hypertension
(D) Flank hematoma
(E) Laceration through Gerota's fascia

604. Which of the following would NOT be considered a positive DPL in a patient with blunt abdominal trauma?

(A) > 20 mL gross blood aspirated upon catheter entry
(B) RBC count in lavage fluid 200,000 cells/μL
(C) WBC count in lavage fluid 100 cells/μL
(D) Amylase level in lavage fluid 500 U/100 mL
(E) Vegetable matter seen in lavage fluid

605. Which of the following statements regarding diaphragmatic injury after blunt abdominal trauma is MOST correct?

(A) Diaphragmatic herniation is usually apparent on initial upright chest x-ray
(B) The right side of the diaphragm is more commonly injured than the left
(C) CT and DPL are almost never helpful in diagnosis
(D) The diagnosis is usually made immediately
(E) Difficulty in passing a nasogastric tube suggests herniation of abdominal viscera into the chest

606. A 25-year-old male driver is brought to the ED by ambulance after a high-speed head-on collision. Physical examination is remarkable for a blood pressure of 70/P, heart rate of 140, abdominal tenderness, and a prominent hematoma across the mid-abdomen. Which of the following organs is MOST likely to be injured?

(A) Liver
(B) Spleen
(C) Kidney
(D) Lung
(E) Bladder

607. Which one of the following is NOT associated with penile rupture?

(A) Blood at the urethral meatus
(B) Penile pain
(C) Penile swelling
(D) Penile discoloration
(E) Priapism

608. What is the MOST commonly injured structure in the genitourinary (GU) tract?

(A) Bladder
(B) Kidney
(C) Ureter
(D) Urethra
(E) Penis

609. A young female presents to the ED with flank pain and abdominal tenderness after a high-speed MVA. Abdominal CT shows a non-enhancing kidney. Which of the following is the MOST likely diagnosis?

(A) Renal artery thrombosis
(B) Ureteral disruption
(C) Renal laceration
(D) Renal pelvis rupture
(E) Renal contusion with large subcapsular hematoma

610. All of the following statements regarding bladder injuries are TRUE EXCEPT

(A) the bony pelvis protects the bladder in adults
(B) penetrating injuries are more common than blunt injuries
(C) surgical repair is usually indicated after intraperitoneal ruptures
(D) extraperitoneal ruptures are usually treated with catheter drainage alone
(E) contusions rarely require surgical treatment

611. Which of the following is LEAST appropriate in the initial management of a patient with a pelvic fracture and ongoing hemorrhage?

(A) Placement of an external fixator device
(B) Crystalloid infusion
(C) Blood transfusion
(D) Angiography and vessel embolization
(E) Laparotomy

612. Which of the following blunt traumatic injuries would be MOST likely to result in a positive DPL?

(A) Renal pedicle injury
(B) Small bowel mesenteric tear
(C) Subcapsular splenic rupture
(D) Ureteral transection
(E) Duodenal hematoma

613. In examining a patient with blunt pelvic injury after a 20-foot fall, you find blood at the urethral meatus and a normal prostate examination. What is the MOST appropriate next step to evaluate for the cause of the urethral blood?

(A) Cystogram
(B) Intravenous pyelogram (IVP)
(C) CT with intravenous and oral contrast
(D) Foley catheter
(E) Retrograde urethrogram

614. Which of the following statements regarding wound ballistics is CORRECT?

(A) Tissue surrounding a bullet track should be excised to prevent wound necrosis
(B) Military bullets are more damaging than civilian bullets of the same size
(C) Bullets frequently tumble in flight
(D) Bullets frequently tumble in tissue
(E) Bullets of the same caliber have the same wounding potential

615. All of the following are considered passive injury countermeasures EXCEPT

(A) motorcycle helmets
(B) automobile airbags
(C) building sprinkler systems
(D) spring-loaded lawnmower shutoff switches
(E) spring-loaded circular saw blade covers

616. Which of the following statements regarding injury control is CORRECT?

(A) Educational programs are almost always valuable in changing behavior
(B) Enactment of mandatory use laws rarely affects behavior
(C) States that have repealed mandatory motorcyclist helmet laws have seen little or no increase in fatality rates
(D) Driver education has been more successful than motor vehicle engineering in reducing death rates from vehicle crashes
(E) Mandatory-use laws are difficult to enact

617. Which of the following neurological findings would MOST likely result from a nerve injury caused by a mid-shaft humerus fracture?

(A) Weakness in wrist extension
(B) Decreased sensation over the dorsum of the little finger
(C) Decreased sensation to the palmar index finger
(D) Weakness in wrist flexion
(E) Weakness in index finger abduction

618. Which of the following statements regarding scapular fractures is CORRECT?

(A) They are most common in elderly women
(B) The most common mechanism of injury is a rotational torso movement
(C) Associated injuries rarely occur
(D) Common associated injuries involve the ribs and lungs
(E) Open reduction and internal fixation is usually required

619. Which is the MOST frequently injured solid organ after penetrating trauma?

(A) Liver
(B) Spleen
(C) Pancreas
(D) Kidney
(E) Diaphragm

620. Which of the following statements regarding pancreatic injuries is CORRECT?

(A) Penetrating injuries are more common than blunt injuries
(B) The serum amylase is almost always elevated
(C) DPL is highly sensitive
(D) Complications are infrequent and of little consequence
(E) Concomitant injuries are rare

621. Which of the following urinalysis results would be an indication for IVP or abdominal CT in an adult after blunt abdominal or flank trauma?

(A) 0–5 RBC/HPF
(B) 5–10 RBC/HPF
(C) 10–20 RBC/HPF
(D) Gross hematuria
(E) Dipstick positive for blood

622. An adult patient has abdominal pain, tenderness, and a lap-belt hematoma after a vehicle crash. Which of the following is the LEAST likely to be injured?

(A) Spleen
(B) Liver
(C) Small intestine
(D) Ureter
(E) Colon

623. Which of the following knee injuries is MOST likely to be associated with vascular trauma?

(A) Tibial plateau fracture
(B) Femoral condyle fracture
(C) Anterior dislocation
(D) Posterior dislocation
(E) Lateral dislocation

624. A fracture at which of the following sites is MOST likely to be associated with a disruption of the midfoot?

(A) Base of the second metatarsal
(B) Calcaneus
(C) Base of the fifth metatarsal
(D) Navicular
(E) Cuboid

625. Regarding Achilles tendon rupture, all of the following are TRUE EXCEPT

(A) Thompson's test is usually positive
(B) a palpable tendon defect is usually present
(C) active plantar flexion excludes the diagnosis
(D) patients frequently report hearing a snap at the time of injury
(E) this injury usually occurs in middle-aged men

626. What compartment pressure indicates the need for fasciotomy in a patient with suspected compartment syndrome?

(A) 3 mm Hg
(B) 10 mm Hg
(C) 15 mm Hg
(D) 30 mm Hg
(E) 60 mm Hg

TRAUMA

ANSWERS

563. The answer is D. *(Chapter 243)* Despite the overwhelming advent of sophisticated trauma systems, the majority of trauma victims are first seen in community hospitals. This underscores the need for all emergency physicians to be well versed in trauma management. In 1988, 48,000 people were killed in MVAs. Trauma is the leading cause of death in young adults.

564. The answer is E. *(Chapter 243)* This patient clearly requires immediate intubation and ventilation. Gaining control of the airway must not be delayed to obtain x-rays, perform a neurologic examination, or even measure a full set of vital signs. A "normal" lateral cervical spine x-ray does not rule out an unstable cervical spine injury. Irrespective of x-ray findings, the same precautions (inline stabilization) must be taken during RSI. A jaw-thrust maneuver could help clear an airway obstruction, but a chin lift would be contraindicated because of a possible cervical spine injury.

565. The answer is A. *(Chapter 251)* It is unclear whether this patient has cardiac tamponade, a tension pneumothorax, or hemorrhagic shock. Cardiac tamponade is diagnosed clinically by Beck's triad (hypotension, muffled heart sounds, and elevated neck veins). However, in a hypovolemic patient, clinical assessment may be difficult. Pericardial fluid detected by bedside ultrasound confirms the diagnosis of pericardial tamponade. If present, immediate pericardiocentesis is indicated and can be lifesaving.

566. The answer is C. *(Chapter 244)* Trauma is the most common cause of death in children *older than* 1 year, with head trauma as the primary lethal injury. Infection is the first and trauma is the second leading reason for ED visits in the pediatric age group. In children younger than 1 year, suffocation is the most common cause of death due to injury. Car accidents, drowning, burns, and bicycle accidents are the most frequent reasons for accidental injury. In 25 percent of all pediatric trauma cases secondary to MVAs, alcohol is involved. Although physiologic differences must be considered; initial management of injured children is the same as that for adults. Hypothermia occurs more rapidly in children because their ratio of body surface area to mass is greater.

567. The answer is B. *(Chapter 244)* In addition to the smaller size, the pediatric airway differs from the adult airway in anatomic proportions. The subglottic area is the narrowest portion of the trachea in a child up to age 8. For this reason, uncuffed endotracheal tubes are recommended. Because children are more dependent on diaphragmatic excursion for breathing, abdominal or chest wall impedance can impede adequate oxygenation and ventilation. The infant's larynx is more cephalad than the adult's, the tongue is relatively larger, and the vocal cords are shorter and more concave. The cricoid cartilage is easily damaged, and cricothyrotomy is not recommended. A formula to approximate the endotracheal tube size required for a child up to the age of 12 years old is:

internal diameter in millimeters = (16 + patient's age in years)/4.

Another way to approximate the endotracheal tube size is to use a tube the same size as the child's nares or little finger.

568. **The answer is D.** *(Chapter 244)* Infrequently, infants become hypotensive from blood loss into either the subgaleal or epidural space after head trauma. Hypovolemia can occur because of open cranial sutures and fontanelles. Transient paleness, lethargy, diaphoresis, and emesis are common after minor head trauma and do not necessarily signify significant neurological injury. Persistence of any of these signs or symptoms, or change in mental status is concerning. Seizures may occur shortly after head injury and are usually self-limited. However, about 50 percent of patients with posttraumatic seizures have positive findings on head computed tomography (CT). Children with two or more seizures or a GCS < 8 should be strongly considered for anticonvulsant therapy.

569. **The answer is A.** *(Chapter 244)* There are a number of anatomic differences between children and adults with respect to the cervical spine. Because of the large head in children, the fulcrum of the neck becomes C2–3; as a consequence, the majority of cervical injuries occur in this area. About 40 percent of children younger than 7 years and 20 percent of children up to 16 years show anterior displacement of C2 on C3 (pseudosubluxation). In normal children without injury, 3 mm of motion of C2 on C3 is often seen with flexion and extension. Most pseudosubluxation is corrected radiographically by placing the child's head in the neutral, sniffing position. In up to two-thirds of children suffering from spinal cord injuries, a normal radiograph is found (SCIWORA). About 50 percent of children with SCIWORA have a delayed onset of symptoms. Paralysis can present up to 4 days after the initial injury.

570. **The answer is C.** *(Chapter 245)* Falls are the most common accidental injury in patients older than 75 years. Most elderly patients fall on a level surface and suffer an isolated orthopedic injury. Even though a low-height fall may result in death, MVAs are the most common mechanism of traumatic death in the elderly. In particular, elderly patients are victims of auto/pedestrian accidents more commonly than their younger counterparts. Decreased vision, hearing, and reflexes are all contributing factors. As in younger populations, alcohol is involved in the majority of fatal assaults.

571. **The answer is D.** *(Chapter 245)* As the brain ages, it undergoes atrophy and decreases in size by about 10 percent between the ages of 30 and 70 years. Atrophy causes stretching of the bridging veins, which in turn leads to an increased incidence of subdural hematomas. As the dura becomes more fibrous, it adheres to the cranium and obliterates the potential space for epidurals. Therefore, although subdural hematomas are more common in the elderly, epidural bleeds are rare. Because of the increased "dead space" in the brains of elderly patients, they often have delayed presentations of significant intracranial hemorrhages. The elderly have a decreased incidence of cervical spine injury and a different pattern of injury. There is a rise in C1–2 fractures, mostly because of the increased incidence of odontoid fractures.

572. **The answer is A.** *(Chapter 245)* Falls in the elderly are associated with high morbidity and mortality. They are the most common cause of accidental injury in patients older than 75 years and the second most common cause between the ages of 65 and 74 years. The most likely area of hip fracture is the intertrochanteric region. Pain coupled with external rotation of the leg is a classic presentation. The second most likely place for a fracture of the hip is the transcervical region.

573. **The answer is C.** *(Chapter 247)* The GCS is a standardized scoring system used to predict prognosis after head injury. The scale evaluates three aspects of the patient's responsiveness and can be used to follow changes in these parameters over time. Eye opening, best verbal response, and best motor response are each assigned a numerical value. The maximum score obtainable is 15 and the minimum score is 3. This patient opened his eyes to pain (2), withdrew to pain (4), and mumbled incoherently (2), for a total score of 8. Intubation for airway protection and to facilitate diagnostic studies should be strongly considered when the GCS score is 8 or less. A score of 8 or less persisting for 6 h or longer indicates severe neurologic injury. Children have a better prognosis than do adults at low GCS levels. The presence of drugs or alcohol may limit the usefulness of the GCS scoring system.

574. **The answer is C.** *(Chapter 247)* Uncal herniation occurs when the uncal portion of the temporal lobe is pushed through the tentorium. Because cranial nerve III lies on the edge of the tentorium, compression causes injury to the superficial parasympathetic nerves. This results in unopposed sympathetic activity and manifests as pupillary dilation on the side of the herniation. In addition, corticospinal tract fibers in the midbrain become compressed. This squeezing through the tentorium causes contralateral hemiplegia. Ipsilateral mydriasis and contralateral hemiplegia is known as *tentorial herniation syndrome.* An intracranial hematoma is most often present on the side of the pupillary dilation, and an emergent burr hole would be placed on that side. In 20 percent of cases, pupillary changes are contralateral, and motor changes are ipsilateral. This occurs when a mass or hematoma pushes the opposite side of the midbrain against the tentorial edge, resulting in a dilated pupil on the opposite side of the lesion. Hence, bilateral emergency burr holes should be placed if trephination on the first side does not improve the patient's clinical condition.

575. **The answer is A.** *(Chapter 247)* Severe head injury is defined by a GCS score lower than 8 in an adult. The most critical determinant of outcome in the head-injured patient is the cerebral perfusion pressure (CPP). The formula for CPP is [MAP (mean arterial pressure) − ICP (intracranial pressure)]. To maintain adequate brain perfusion, hypotension must be avoided. Adequate oxygenation is the other key factor. Hyperventilation to a pCO_2 of less than 25 mm Hg should be avoided because profound vasoconstriction and ischemia can result. Mortality risk is more than doubled if hypotension occurs and increases by 75 percent in severely head-injured patients who experience both hypotension and hypoxemia. Hypotension in adults is not due to the brain injury itself, except in the terminal stages when medullary failure supervenes. This patient requires assessment for internal hemorrhage, but blood pressure must be stable before considering a CT. Although they may provide less specific information, diagnostic peritoneal lavage and abdominal ultrasound have the advantage that they can be performed at the bedside.

576. **The answer is E.** *(Chapter 247)* Basilar skull fractures can occur at any point in the base of the skull, but the typical location is along the petrous portion of the temporal bone. Clinical signs of a basilar skull fracture include Battle's sign (retroauricular hematoma), raccoon eyes (retroorbital hematoma), cerebrospinal fluid leak, hemotympanum, and cranial nerve VII palsy. The cranial nerve VII palsy may appear immediately or present a few days after injury. Prognosis for recovery is better in the delayed-onset variety. Because of the force needed to cause a basilar skull fracture, a head CT is indicated to look for coexisting intracranial injuries. Palsy of cranial nerve VI has not been described with basilar skull fractures. The use of prophylactic antibiotics in the setting of basilar skull fracture is controversial and should only be initiated after consultation with the consulting neurosurgeon.

577. **The answer is C.** *(Chapter 247)* Although basilar skull fractures are indicators of significant force during the injury, they do not need immediate neurosurgical evaluation if a head CT is otherwise negative. Given the fracture over the temporal bone, under which the middle meningeal artery lies, patient A has a high likelihood of epidural hematoma. With a slightly depressed GCS, a neurosurgeon should be notified immediately. A comatose patient with a depressed linear skull fracture has a 20 times increased risk of intracranial hematoma. The patient with the rollerblade injury has a communicating, open scalp laceration and a dural tear, as shown by the otorrhea. Dural tears require early surgical repair to decrease the incidence of infection. Patient E is likely to have diffuse axonal injury requiring meticulous control of cardiovascular and neurosurgical parameters.

578. The answer is D. *(Chapter 247)* This patient likely has a subdural hematoma, a collection of blood beneath the dura and overlying the arachnoid and brain. It results from tears of bridging veins that extend from the subarachnoid space to the dural venous sinus. Patients with brain atrophy due to either aging or alcoholism are particularly susceptible to developing subdural hematomas. Acute subdurals are usually symptomatic within 24 h. Subacute subdural hematomas are symptomatic between 24 h and 2 weeks after injury, and chronic subdurals become symptomatic 2 weeks or more after the injury, when the blood clot liquefies. On CT, most acute subdurals appear hyperdense, subacute bleeds are isodense or mixed density, and chronic subdurals are hypodense. Immediate surgery may not be appropriate for chronic subdural bleeds. The morbidity and mortality of subdurals exceeds that of epidurals because of the greater severity of underlying brain injury. Epidural bleeds are associated with a tear of the middle meningeal artery.

579. The answer is C. *(Chapter 247)* This patient is suffering from postconcussive syndrome after minor head injury. Patients with minor head injury represent 80 percent of the population of patients presenting to the ED with head trauma but suffer neurological deterioration less than 2 percent of the time. Symptoms are subtle and may only be brought out by formal neuropsychological testing. Insomnia, amnesia to the event, sensitivity to alcohol, difficulty concentrating, depression, and visual changes are common. Most symptoms resolve within the first few weeks, but patients should be warned that they can persist for up to 6 months postinjury. No focal motor weakness or sensory loss has been described with this syndrome, and anyone with these signs after an accident should be further evaluated. Intracranial bleeds and posttraumatic seizures can present as late as 1 to 2 weeks after minor head trauma.

580. The answer is B. *(Chapter 247)* This multitrauma patient has a major head injury. Early intubation and maintenance of cerebral perfusion pressure are paramount. Hyperventilation to a pCO_2 of less than 25 mm Hg could cause ischemia, thereby worsening the brain injury. The ideal level of pCO_2 is between 30 and 35 mm Hg. Mannitol, and possibly furosemide, can reduce intracranial pressure but should be avoided in a hypotensive patient. Intravenous fluids should be administered as required to volume resuscitate the patient. Glucose-containing fluids can result in hyperglycemia, which has been shown to be harmful to the brain. Therefore, lactated Ringer's or normal saline solutions are recommended. Management of this critical patient should be coordinated with a neurosurgeon and a trauma surgeon.

581. The answer is E. *(Chapter 248)* Five percent of patients with spinal trauma experience onset or worsening of neurological symptoms after reaching the ED. This is usually due to either spinal cord ischemia or inadequate immobilization. As long as the spine is protected, evaluation may be deferred until the patient has been stabilized. Spinal boards are excellent transportation devices but should be removed as quickly as feasible to prevent complications such as decubitus ulcers or patient discomfort. Fifty-five percent of all spinal injuries occur in the cervical region, and only 5 percent of head-injured patients have an associated spinal injury. Lack of pain or tenderness does not preclude unstable spinal injury, particularly if the patient has a distracting injury or is under the influence of drugs or alcohol.

582. The answer is D. *(Chapter 248)* Neurogenic shock results from impairment of descending sympathetic pathways. Patients lose their vasomotor tone and sympathetic stimulation to the heart. This leads to pooling of blood and hypotension. Other potential manifestations of this autonomic nerve dysfunction include priapism, urinary retention, paralytic ileus, and loss of temperature control. The unique findings of neurogenic shock are that the skin remains warm, dry, and pink, and adequate urine output is maintained. Atropine is used to treat the paradoxical bradycardia. Hypotension is usually unresponsive to fluids alone and often requires the judicious use of vasopressors. Distal areflexia can last hours to weeks and is followed by spastic paralysis.

583. The answer is A. *(Chapter 248)* Central cord syndrome typically occurs after a hyperextension injury in an elderly patient with congenital stenosis or osteoarthritis. It is characterized by a disproportionately greater loss of motor strength in the proximal extremities than in the lower extremities. Within the upper extremities, the distal aspect is more affected than the proximal aspect. This characteristic pattern is due to disruption of the cord's vascular supply from the anterior spinal artery. Motor tracts on the innermost portion are affected first, and the distal extremities on the outer portion are affected last. The bladder is occasionally involved. Recovery progresses distally to proximally, and the prognosis is better for this syndrome than for other cord syndromes.

584. The answer is C. *(Chapter 264)* A flexion teardrop injury involves displacement of a large triangular fragment from the anterior aspect of the involved vertebral body. This results in extensive anterior and posterior ligamentous disruption. The extension teardrop fracture leaves the posterior ligaments intact. A Jefferson fracture is a burst of the ring of C1, and the hangman's fracture is a bilateral fracture through the pedicles of C2. Bilateral interfacetal dislocation shows 50 percent anterior displacement of one vertebral body on another, and unilateral facet dislocation is diagnosed when there is a 25 to 33 percent anterior dislocation. Cervical spine fractures are considered unstable when two or more columns of the spine are affected.

585. The answer is D. *(Chapter 264)* The combination of the lateral, odontoid, and anteroposterior views of the cervical spine is about 92 percent sensitive for identifying a cervical fracture. If the predental space is greater than 3 mm, there is a high likelihood of cruciform ligament disruption. Prevertebral soft tissue swelling of greater than 5 mm at C3–4 indicates a possible hematoma with associated fracture. Abrupt changes in angulation of vertebral interspaces greater than 11 degrees or anterior subluxation of greater than 3 mm is suspicious for cervical injury. Fanning of the spinous processes suggests possible posterior ligamentous injury. If three views of the cervical spine are unremarkable but clinical suspicion remains high, further studies such as flexion–extension films, CT, or magnetic resonance imaging are warranted.

586. The answer is E. *(Chapter 250)* Zone I of the neck lies below the cricoid cartilage, zone II is between the cricoid cartilage and the angle of the mandible, and zone III is above the angle of the mandible. Although the consulting surgeon might elect to take any of these patients to the operating room, the types of absolute indications for surgery are decreasing. Clear indications for operative repair include the presence of an expanding or pulsatile hematoma, hemoptysis, blood-tinged saliva, or absent pulses. Horner's syndrome (pupillary constriction, eyelid lag, and anhydrosis) indicates sympathetic ganglion injury. Because of the potential for associated carotid injury, these patients require surgical exploration. Indications for imaging (angiography, bronchoscopy, esophagoscopy, or CT) are controversial. Patients with zone I and III penetrating injuries generally undergo angiography, but CT has become a popular alternative, especially in stable patients.

587. The answer is D. *(Chapter 248)* In a patient with spinal cord injury, the primary goal is to prevent further neurologic deterioration. In North America, high-dose steroids are given to patients within 8 h of injury to reduce swelling around the cord. Hypotension and bradycardia must be reversed to prevent further cord ischemia.

588. The answer is A. *(Chapter 251)* Chest trauma carries a significant morbidity and mortality. On ED arrival, one-fifth of patients with chest trauma are hypotensive or require intubation. The majority of deaths from chest trauma occur after arrival to the ED. Mortality for unstable patients is about 20 percent as opposed to 1 percent for patients with stable vital signs on ED arrival. Fewer than 10 percent of blunt trauma patients and 15 to 30 percent of penetrating trauma patients are candidates for emergent thoracotomy.

589. **The answer is D.** *(Chapter 251)* Cardiac arrest frequently occurs in the peri-intubation period. Aggressive bagging of the intubated patient increases intrathoracic pressure, leading to a decrease in venous return. Therefore, decreasing the ventilatory rate and volume can augment cardiac output, especially in the hypovolemic patient. Tension pneumothorax is commonly precipitated by positive pressure ventilation in a patient with a visceral pleural injury. In this setting, needle decompression of the chest can reverse the cardiac arrest. Repositioning the endotracheal tube after a right mainstem intubation can also be life-saving. A patient with hemoptysis is at risk for air embolism. Trendelenburg and the left lateral decubitus position may temporarily keep the air bubbles in the venous circulation. If the arrest is secondary to hypovolemia, it is unlikely that a single liter of crystalloid will lead to return of spontaneous circulation.

590. **The answer is C.** *(Chapter 251)* The role for resuscitative thoracotomy in the ED is limited. Thoracotomy may have a role in selected patients with penetrating injury to the neck, chest, and extremities and signs of life within 5 min of arrival to the ED. A resuscitative thoracotomy is seldom of benefit for patients with cardiac arrest secondary to blunt trauma or head injury, or for those without vital signs on the scene. Blunt trauma patients with pulseless electrical activity on ED arrival have a prognosis of virtually zero and are poor candidates for resuscitative thoracotomy. It is difficult to assess the path of the weapon after blunt abdominal trauma, and emergent thoracotomy may be life-saving. Several therapeutic measures can be accomplished with ED thoracotomy: (1) evacuation of a pericardial tamponade, (2) direct control of thoracic exsanguination, (3) open cardiac massage, and (4) cross clamping of the aorta to increase blood flow to the brain and heart.

591. **The answer is A.** *(Chapter 251)* Flail chest occurs when a segment of chest wall does not have bony continuity with the rest of the rib cage, usually in the setting of multiple rib fractures. Morbidity is due to hypoxemia associated with the underlying lung injury. If there is a suspicion for a large lung contusion, prophylactic intubation (before signs of respiratory distress) can decrease mortality from 69 percent to 7 percent. The initial presentation of flail chest may be subtle due to rib splinting. The injured lung in flail chest is sensitive to under-resuscitation of shock and to fluid overload. Judicious use of fluids is required to adequately hydrate the patient without worsening the pulmonary contusion.

592. **The answer is B.** *(Chapter 251)* An "occult pneumothorax" is a small pneumothorax that is seen on CT but not on chest x-ray. Patients with occult pneumothoraces can be observed without a chest tube unless they need to be intubated. Positive pressure ventilation postintubation carries the risk of converting an occult pneumothorax into a tension pneumothorax if a thoracostomy is not performed.

593. **The answer is B.** *(Chapter 251)* With pneumomediastinum, a crunching sound known as Hamman's sign can be heard during systole secondary to mediastinal air surrounding the heart. The diagnosis of pneumomediastinum is most easily confirmed on CT but can sometimes be made with plain films. Subcutaneous emphysema in the neck is another suggestive physical finding.

594. **The answer is E.** *(Chapter 251)* Beck's triad consists of distended neck veins, hypotension, and muffled heart tones. However, even with a large tamponade (200 mL), heart sounds are usually clear. Tachycardia and tracheal deviation are not components of the triad. Beck's triad can be seen with tension pneumothorax, myocardial contusion, acute mycardial infarction, and systemic air embolism.

595. **The answer is A.** *(Chapter 251)* Pericardiocentesis is a temporizing measure until cardiac surgery is available. The false negative rate in trauma has been reported to be as high as 80 percent. Pericardial blood is difficult to remove because it has clotted. Rapid aspiration of high volumes of blood usually indicates that the needle is in the right ventricle. If it is used, the electrocardiographic (ECG) monitor is always connected to a metal needle.

596. The answer is A. *(Chapter 251)*   In both myocardial rupture and contusion, the most commonly injured part of the heart is the anterior right ventricle because of its location immediately below the sternum. Myocardial contusion can be difficult to diagnose, especially in the setting of multisystem trauma. It should be considered in any patient involved in an MVA with speeds greater than 35 miles per hour, especially if the patient's chest strikes the steering wheel.

597. The answer is C. *(Chapter 251)*   The aortic valve is the most commonly injured, followed by laceration of the papillary muscle or chordae tendineae of the mitral valve. Patients with bioprosthetic valves are more susceptible. The tricuspid valve is rarely injured. Diagnostic clues for cardiac injury include chest pain, tachycardia, dysrhythmias, heart failure, fractured sternum, widened pericardial silhouette on chest x-ray, and elevated ST segments.

598. The answer is A. *(Chapter 251)*   A high index of suspicion must be maintained to diagnose aortic rupture because at least one-third of patients have no external evidence of thoracic injury on initial examination. All the listed findings can be seen on chest x-ray after traumatic rupture of the aorta, but widening of the superior mediastinum is the most frequent abnormality. Mediastinal width is usually greater than 8.0 cm after an aortic rupture. Subadventitial and periadventitial hematomas, secondary to bleeding from small mediastinal vessels, are the primary causes of this radiologic finding.

599. The answer is C. *(Chapter 251)*   Upper, not lower, extremity hypertension has been reported in 31 to 43 percent of cases of traumatic aortic rupture. This finding was initially attributed to compression of the aorta by a periaortic hematoma. Recent evidence suggests that it may be due to aortic wall stretching and subsequent receptor stimulation. The systolic murmur is thought to occur as a result of turbulent flow across the injured area. Hoarseness and voice change are less frequent physical findings.

600. The answer is C. *(Chapter 251)*   Cervical tracheal injuries occur most frequently at the junction of the cricoid cartilage and the trachea, usually after striking the anterior neck against the dash of a car. Most lower tracheobronchial injuries occur within 2 cm of the carina. Lower tracheobronchial injuries are caused by rapid deceleration and shearing of mobile bronchi from fixed structures. Concurrent esophageal injuries occur in 25 percent of patients.

601. The answer is C. *(Chapter 251)*   In a previously normal pericardium, 200 mL of blood will create sufficient intrapericardial pressure to restrict venous filling of the heart and cause tamponade. Although it may be detected by bedside ultrasound, this amount is too small to be reliably visible on chest x-ray. Removal of as little as 5 to 10 mL of blood can be life saving by augmenting venous filling and dramatically improving stroke volume.

602. The answer is B. *(Chapter 252)*   DPL is a diagnostic option for a patient with equivocal physical findings after significant trauma. Both GSW to the mid-abdomen and fluid on ultrasound with hypotension necessitate urgent laparotomy, and DPL is not necessary Similarly, stab wounds with peritoneal irritation require laparotomy. Spinal cord injuries may make physical examination unreliable, and DPL would be one option for evaluation. Hepatic dysfunction with portal hypertension and severe coagulopathies are considered relative contraindications to DPL. With increasing availability of bedside ultrasound and rapid CT scanning, DPL is being used less frequently.

603. The answer is E. *(Chapter 254)*   Most renal injuries can be managed nonoperatively. Indications for surgery after blunt kidney injury include evidence of continued blood loss, loss of renal function, and laceration through Gerota's fascia. Hematuria is common and usually self-limited. Pain is unrelated to the necessity for surgery.

604. **The answer is C.** *(Chapter 252)* Aspiration of more than 5 mL of gross blood upon catheter entry is considered positive. In the lavage fluid, commonly accepted threshold values are RBC > 100,000/μL, white blood cell (WBC) count > 500, or amylase > 200. In addition, bile, vegetable matter, or bacteria seen on microscopic examination is considered positive. In many centers, ultrasound is replacing DPL as a less invasive, faster bedside study.

605. **The answer is E.** *(Chapter 251)* Most cases of diaphragmatic injury do not involve herniation and are difficult to diagnose. The only finding on chest x-ray may be a blurred diaphragm or an effusion, sometimes difficult to detect on a portable, supine film. Diagnosis is frequently delayed; most injuries occur on the left side. CT and DPL frequently provide evidence to suggest or confirm the presence of a ruptured diaphragm.

606. **The answer is B.** *(Chapter 252)* The spleen is the most commonly injured solid organ after blunt trauma. Clinical findings include Kehr's sign (left shoulder pain), left upper quadrant abdominal tenderness, hypotension, and tachycardia. Solid abdominal organ injury causes morbidity and mortality primarily as a result of hemorrhage. Lung injury with tension pneumothorax is another possibility in this patient, but is less likely than splenic injury.

607. **The answer is E.** *(Chapter 254)* Penile rupture is the traumatic rupture of the corpus cavernosum. It occurs during an erection but is associated with immediate detumescence. The urethra may also be torn. Management includes immediate surgical evacuation of the blood clot and repair of the torn tunica albuginea.

608. **The answer is B.** *(Chapter 254)* In one case series, 67 percent of all GU injuries were to the kidney. The bladder is the second most commonly injured structure. Kidney injuries include contusions, lacerations, ruptures, pedicle injuries, and renal pelvis ruptures.

609. **The answer is A.** *(Chapter 254)* Renal pedicle injuries include lacerations and thrombosis of the renal artery and vein. They commonly occur as a result of high-velocity deceleration forces and are frequently associated with multiple injuries. If the renal artery is occluded or divided, CT demonstrates a non-enhanced kidney with a faint capsular enhancement, known as the *rim sign*. Surgical repair should occur within 12 h to maximize the likelihood of kidney viability.

610. **The answer is B.** *(Chapter 254)* The bladder is more intraabdominal in children and is better protected within the bony pelvis in adults. Blunt injuries to the bladder are more frequent than penetrating injuries and are commonly associated with pelvic fractures. Bladder ruptures are repaired surgically if intraperitoneal and managed conservatively with bladder drainage if extraperitoneal. Contusions can usually be managed by simple observation.

611. **The answer is E.** *(Chapter 265)* Retroperitoneal bleeding can be massive and life-threatening after a pelvic fracture. Up to 4 L of blood can be held in the retroperitoneal space. Resuscitation begins with crystalloid fluid boluses, followed by blood products. The external fixator device is useful, and angiography with embolization can be life-saving in the setting of ongoing bleeding. Laparotomy is used only as a last resort because opening the abdominal cavity can relieve a tamponade and cause fatal hemorrhage.

612. **The answer is B.** *(Chapters 252, 254)* A mesenteric tear would cause sufficient bleeding to result in a positive DPL. Subcapsular splenic injuries do not bleed into the peritoneal cavity. The duodenum and kidney are in the retroperitoneum, and injuries to these structures usually do not cause the DPL to be positive.

613. The answer is E. *(Chapter 254)*   Before administering intravenous contrast, a Foley catheter should be inserted. However, blood at the meatus indicates a urethral injury, and placement of a urinary catheter can convert a partial urethral tear into a complete disruption. A retrograde urethrogram should be performed first, and, if positive, a suprapubic catheter should be inserted for bladder drainage.

614. The answer is D. *(Chapter 256)*   Clinical experience has shown that missile track excision is not necessary because wound necrosis is not a problem. Hollow and soft-point bullets used in civilian firearms often damage more tissue than military bullets. Bullets almost never tumble in the air because they spiral out of the firearm barrel, but they commonly tumble in tissue. Caliber measures the bullet's diameter. When considering wounding potential, other important characteristics are length, jacket, cartridge case, shape, construction, and composition.

615. The answer is A. *(Chapter 258)*   Active countermeasures require the conscious cooperation of the individual to be protected. Passive countermeasures exert their protective effects automatically. The motorcyclist must wear a helmet, whereas all the other measures are permanent parts of the building, automobile, or device. Passive countermeasures are usually more effective in reducing injury because they are more likely to be used.

616. The answer is E. *(Chapter 258)*   Education can be valuable but is often shown to be ineffective when evaluated critically. Mandatory-use laws (e.g., seat belt, motorcyclist helmet) are extremely effective in decreasing morbidity and mortality. States that have repealed helmet laws have seen up to a 40 percent increase in fatality rates. Vehicle engineering has resulted in a substantial decrease in death rates, whereas driver education has been largely ineffective. Mandatory-use laws are very difficult to enact (and subject to repeal), usually with the argument that they would compromise "personal freedom."

617. The answer is A. *(Chapter 259)*   The radial nerve is the one most commonly injured after a mid-shaft humerus fracture. These fractures are most often seen in active adults rather than in the elderly, in whom proximal humerus fractures are more likely. Radial nerve injuries are manifested by wrist drop (weakness on wrist extension) and decreased sensation to the dorsum of the first web space. Other complications include injuries to the brachial artery or vein and to the median or ulnar nerves.

618. The answer is D. *(Chapter 259)*   Scapular fractures occur most commonly in men age 25 to 40 years. Because the scapula is mobile, the most common mechanism of injury is a direct blow. Considerable force is required to fracture the scapula. As a result, 80 percent of such fractures are associated with injuries to the chest wall and lungs. Treatment is usually conservative, and open repair is rarely indicated.

619. The answer is A. *(Chapters 251, 252)*   The spleen is the most commonly injured organ after blunt trauma, and the liver in penetrating trauma. Small and large intestines are also frequently injured. Subcapsular hematomas, commonly seen with stab wounds, may be associated with a negative DPL.

620. The answer is A. *(Chapter 252)*   Pancreatic injury is more common with penetrating trauma. It may also occur as a result of a crushing injury that divides the pancreas over the vertebral column. Examples include steering-wheel or bicycle-handlebar injuries. Unrecognized, this injury has considerable morbidity and mortality. DPL is usually negative, and the serum amylase is usually normal.

621. The answer is D. *(Chapters 252, 253)*   Indications for radiologic evaluation have changed over the last 10 years. Whereas formerly any degree of hematuria necessitated evaluation, it is now recognized that the yield for significant urologic injury is extremely low unless the patient has gross hematuria, microscopic hematuria with shock, or a penetrating renal injury. Abdominal CT may need to be performed to assess for other injuries but is not indicated strictly on the basis of microscopic hematuria. Indications for the imaging of pediatric patients are more liberal.

622. **The answer is D.** *(Chapters 252, 254)* All of the listed structures except the ureters are commonly injured during blunt abdominal trauma. Although the ureter is occasionally injured during penetrating trauma, ureteral injuries are the rarest of all genitourinary injuries from external trauma. During blunt trauma, injury can occur at the ureteropelvic junction as a result of hyperextension of the spine, with the distal ureter fixed at the bladder.

623. **The answer is D.** *(Chapter 266)* Posterior dislocation (tibia posterior to the femur) has an approximately 50 percent likelihood of associated popliteal artery injury. In addition, the patient must be evaluated for peroneal nerve, ligamentous, and meniscal injuries. Spontaneous reduction of a posterior knee dislocation before evaluation is common. Therefore, a high index of suspicion must be maintained in any patient with a suggestive mechanism of injury and a grossly unstable joint. If not already reduced, early reduction of the dislocation is essential. Orthopedic and sometimes vascular surgery consultation are indicated.

624. **The answer is A.** *(Chapter 269)* The tarsal–metatarsal joint is referred to as Lisfranc joint. Injuries to this joint are uncommon and result from relatively severe trauma, such as motor vehicle crashes. The keystone of this joint is the second metatarsal, and a fracture at the base of the second metatarsal is almost diagnostic of a disrupted joint. A Lisfranc fracture requires prompt orthopedic consultation.

625. **The answer is C.** *(Chapter 268)* Achilles tendon rupture most commonly occurs in middle-aged men, more often on the left side, and usually during forceful dorsiflexion of the ankle. Rupture can also occur from a direct blow or secondary to a laceration. The calf squeeze test (Thompson's test) is almost always positive. Active plantar flexion may be maintained, although it is weaker than on the contralateral ankle. Definitive treatment may be conservative (with casting) or operative. Tendon rupture is commonly misdiagnosed as ankle sprain.

626. **The answer is D.** *(Chapter 270)* Compartment syndrome occurs when injured muscle within a fascial sheath swells and compresses blood vessels and nerves within the compartment. The most common sites are the four compartments in the leg: peroneal, anterior, deep and superficial posterior. Of these, the anterior compartment is the most often affected, usually secondary to a tibial fracture. Compartment syndromes can also occur in the volar and dorsal compartments of the forearm and the interosseous muscles of the hand. Compartment pressures must be measured if the diagnosis is suspected. Pressures over 30 mm Hg can cause ischemia and are an indication for emergency fasciotomy.

Notes

Notes

Notes

Notes

Notes

Notes

Notes

Notes

Notes

Notes

Notes

Notes

Notes

Notes

Notes

Notes

ISBN 0-07-135144-2

90000

9 780071 351447